OB-GYN and Genitourinary Words and Phrases

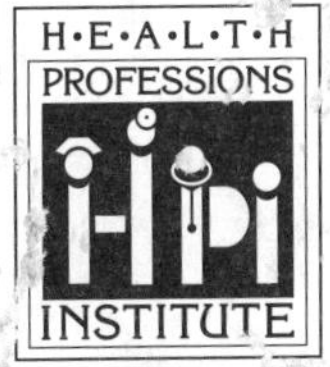

Health Professions Institute • Modesto, California • 2002

OB-GYN and Genitourinary Words and Phrases

Cover design by Lori Raven Smith

Developed by

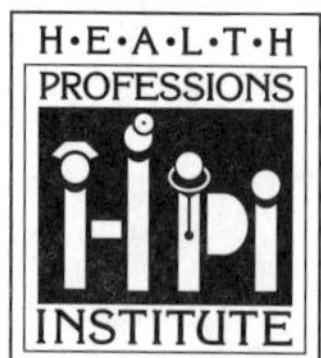

Sally C. Pitman
Editor & Publisher
Health Professions Institute
P. O. Box 801
Modesto, CA 95353-0801
Phone 209-551-2112
Fax 209-551-0404
Web site: http://www.hpisum.com
E-mail: hpi@hpisum.com

Printed by
Parks Printing & Lithograph
Modesto, California

ISBN 0-934385-37-8

Last digit is the print number: 9 8 7 6 5 4 3 2 1

With gratitude to

Diane S. Heath

Preface

In today's fast-paced, high-tech society, the quest to improve healthcare documentation is an ongoing challenge. Medical breakthroughs, new surgical techniques, and advances in pharmacology have given way to thousands of new medical terms. Every procedure must be documented in detail, each surgery described accurately, and every drug spelled correctly.

To stay abreast of the ever-changing world of healthcare documentation, it is vital to have direct access to the most accurate, comprehensive, up-to-date references. To this end we have produced *OB-GYN and Genitourinary Words and Phrases.*

OB-GYN and Genitourinary Words and Phrases is the first quick-reference guide to cover both male and female reproductive systems, urology, nephrology, and breast surgery. Every aspect of obstetrics is addressed, including prenatal care, genetics and genetic counseling, management of high-risk pregnancy, fetal surgery, multiple births, perinatology, and neonatology. The latest trends in infertility treatments and assisted reproductive technology, including medicolegal terminology related to surrogacy and egg donation, have been covered extensively. Renal diagnostic procedures and dialysis are covered in detail. Also included are transplantation surgery, sexual reassignment surgery, hormone replacement therapy, sexually transmitted diseases, and pertinent oncology.

OB-GYN and Genitourinary Words and Phrases is extensively cross-referenced to assure greater success in finding a desired word or phrase. Terms were gathered from thousands of actual obstetrics, gynecology, and genitourinary reports, from medical journals and textbooks, and through extensive research on the Internet.

Research for this quick-reference guide was done primarily by Linda C. Campbell, CMT; Georgia Green, CMT; and Diane S. Heath, CMT. Our warmest gratitude is also extended to those readers who called or wrote with comments and suggestions; this book is better because of their feedback.

Sally C. Pitman, M.A.
Editor & Publisher

Transcribing Genetic Terminology

Genetic terminology is important to a reference book on the male and female reproductive systems because it describes conditions that are passed through heredity as well as those caused by mutations, damage, or dysfunction in the genetic material of the developing fetus. The mapping of the genome is ongoing as this reference book goes to press, as is the discovery of a genetic basis for an increasing number of human diseases. Current estimates indicate there are between 70,000 and 100,000 human genes.

It would not be possible nor particularly useful to provide all this information in a single reference book. Instead, we have selected the widest possible variety of examples of genetic terminology as it is likely to be encountered in dictation, taken directly from discussions of genetic diseases and syndromes in current medical literature. An explanation of the naming of genes and chromosomes will illuminate your understanding of these examples and allow you to follow the same naming conventions as new genetic syndromes and genetic descriptions for existing diseases make their way into the lexicon.

Human somatic cells contain 46 chromosomes. These consist of 22 pairs of autosomes, numbered 1 through 22, plus two sex chromosomes—two X's in a normal female, an X and a Y in a normal male. A germ cell or gamete (ovum or spermatozoon) contains just one set of 23 chromosomes, enabling it to combine with another gamete during fertilization.

Chromosomes were originally described by their size, organized into groups A through G, and can still be referenced in this way, e.g., an "A group chromosome." Modern staining techniques reveal patterns of bands on a chromosome, and the banding designation refers to the staining method, e.g., "Q banding" indicates quinacrine staining. An arrayed set of banded chromosomes is called a karyotype. A karyotype is expressed as the total number of chromosomes per cell (including the sex chromosomes) followed by the individual sex chromosomes separated by a comma. A normal female karyotype is 46,XX. A normal male karyotype is 46,XY. A karyotype of 47,XXY indicates Klinefelter syndrome.

If multiple karyotypes are present, they are separated with a virgule, e.g., 45,X/46,XX. The absence of a complete chromosome is called monosomy. The presence of additional complete chromosomes of a particular type are referred to as trisomy, tetrasomy, or pentasomy.

Each pair of chromosomes is joined at the center by a centromere. The upper or short arm of a single chromosome is designated by a lowercase p. The lower or long arm is designated by a lowercase q. When the name of a chromosome includes an arm designation, it is transcribed with the chromosome number and the alpha character representing the arm. For example, the short arm of chromosome 18 is transcribed as 18p. The long arm of the X chromosome is transcribed as Xq. It is also correct to transcribe the phrase "chromosome arm 18p" or "chromosome arm Xq" but not "chromosome 18p" or "chromosome Xq."

To aid in identifying specific locations, or loci, on chromosomes, each arm is divided into regions numbered 1 through 4. Each region is further divided into bands and subbands. Regions and bands are appended directly to the chromosome arm designation. For example, 3p2 refers to region 2 on the short arm of chromosome 3. The location 13q22 refers to band 22 (or the second band of region 2) on the long arm of chromosome 13.

To identify a location with even greater precision, subbands and sub-subbands may be specified, separated by a period. In 18q12.14, we refer to band 12 (or the second band of region 1) on the long arm of chromosome 18, sub-subband 14 (or subband 1, sub-subband 4).

Abbreviations may be directly appended to the p or q, such as qter for the terminal end of the long arm. Other sets of abbreviations are separated by a space, as in "cht del" for chromatid deletion. A plus or minus sign may precede a chromosome, indicating a gain or loss of an entire chromosome. A minus sign appended to a chromosome arm indicates a loss of material from that arm, e.g., 5q- or 7p-.

A duplication or deletion of an area on the chromosome that results in a medical condition may be referred to in dictation as a duplication syndrome or deletion syndrome. For example, an 8p duplication syndrome is a duplication of the short arm of chromosome 8. An 8p23.1-8pter deletion syndrome refers to the deletion of the region on the short arm of chromosome 8 from band 23.1 to the terminal end of that arm. In dictation, the name of the arm may or may not be repeated, as in 8p12-p23 or 8p12-23.

Other structural abnormalities of chromosomes include ring chromosomes, reciprocal translocations, robertsonian translocations, insertional translocations, and inversions. A duplication may also be referred to as a partial trisomy. A triplication may be referred to as a partial tetrasomy.

A system of accepted abbreviations for these and other structural abnormalities is often employed in scientific literature but are more likely to be dictated in their expanded form. For example, t(11;22) refers to a robertsonian translocation of chromosomes 11 and 22, which is how a dictator would be most likely to describe it.

Chromosomes are actually made up of long strands of DNA (deoxyribonucleic acid). A gene is a portion of that DNA that contains the instructions for the proteins that form the structure of our cells and the enzymes needed for chemical reactions in our bodies. A human gene may be named for its DNA sequence, its biochemical constituents, or for the hereditary diseases or characteristics that it is found to influence. Human genes are abbreviated as gene symbols, which are combinations of letters or letters and numbers, with all letters capitalized. Animal genes may contain a combination of upper and lowercase letters and numbers. The entire term may be italicized, but this is *not* a universal practice, and gene symbols are not italicized in this book.

When a gene symbol is created from its formal name, Roman characters are converted to Arabic, and Greek letters are translated to their English equivalents. Numbers and Greek letter equivalents appearing at the beginning of a gene name are shown at or near the end in the associated genetic symbol. No subscripts or superscripts are used. No marks of punctuation are used, with the exception of hyphens for genes that encode for molecules of the HLA (human leukocyte antigen) system. An @ sign at the end of a genetic symbol indicates a gene family or cluster.

It is not necessary to expand a gene symbol, but keep in mind that just as with other abbreviations, there may be more than one expansion and/or meaning. The gene symbol EPO, for example, represents both the gene and the protein it codes for—erythropoietin, which is used therapeutically as recombinant human erythropoietin, and is also abbreviated EPO.

To learn more about the genetic basis for disease, gene testing, and new gene therapies, visit the Web sites for the Human Genome Project and the Mendelian Inheritance in Man. The current address for each of these sites can be located with any Internet search engine.

Georgia Green, CMT
Director of Education

How to Use This Book

The words and phrases in this book are alphabetized letter by letter of all words in the entry, ignoring punctuation marks and words or letters in parentheses. The possessive form ('s) is omitted from eponyms for ease in alphabetizing. Numbers are alphabetized as if written out, with the exception of subscripts and superscripts which are ignored.

Eponyms appear alphabetically as well as under the nouns they modify. For example, *OPERA* (outpatient endometrial resection/ablation) is found alphabetically in the O's under the acronym and its expansion as well as under the main entry *operation*. *Renografin-60* is found in the R's as well as under *imaging agent* and *medications*. The names of hundreds of medications used in obstetrics, gynecology, and genitourinary reports appear under the entry *medications*. Names of instruments appear under individual main entries like *catheter* and *forceps*, and in addition various kinds of technology are listed under the broad terms *device* and *system*.

In medical dictation physicians may arbitrarily refer to an operative procedure as an *approach*, *method*, *operation*, *procedure*, *repair*, or *technique*, or by the type of procedure, such as *hysterectomy* and *mastectomy*. Thus, all procedures are listed alphabetically by the eponym, such as *CASH (classic abdominal Semm hysterectomy)*, as well as under the type of procedure (*hysterectomy*) and the main entry *operation*.

Main entries with many subentries and phrases include the following:

bladder
breast
catheter
cervix
chemotherapy protocol
chromosome
contraceptive
cyst
deletion syndrome
device
dialysis
disease
duplication syndrome
endometrial
endoscope
erectile dysfunction
fertility
fetus
fistula
forceps
gene
glomerulonephritis
hormone
imaging
incontinence
infant
kidney
mammoplasty
medications
needle
neonatal
nephritis
operation
ovary
penis
placenta
pregnancy
prostate
renal
suture
syndrome
system
test
testes
therapy
tube
ureter
urethral
urinary
uterus
vagina

A, a

A (adenine)
Aagenaes syndrome
AA genotype
Aarskog-Scott syndrome
Aarskog syndrome
Aase-Smith syndrome
AAT (alpha$_1$-antitrypsin deficiency)
A&B (apnea and bradycardia) spells
Aastrom CPS (cell-production system)
AAWR (anti-androgen withdrawal response)
Ab, ab (abortion)
abarelix-depot-M
abatement of acute renal failure
Abbe-McIndoe vaginal construction
ABBI (advanced breast biopsy instrumentation) system
ABD pad dressing
abdomen
  acute
  pendulous
  protuberant
  scaphoid
  surgical
abdomen closed in anatomical layers
abdominal approach in surgery
abdominal apron
abdominal bloating
abdominal distention
abdominal endometriosis
abdominal endoscopic approach to hysterectomy
abdominal fat
abdominal hysterectomy
abdominal hysteropexy
abdominal hysterotomy
abdominal kidney
abdominal laparotomy
abdominal lymphatics
abdominal migraine
abdominal muscle deficiency syndrome
abdominal myomectomy
abdominal nephrectomy
abdominal obesity
abdominal panniculectomy
abdominal panniculus
abdominal part of ureter
abdominal pedicled inverted penile skin technique
abdominal pregnancy
abdominal sacral colpoperineopexy
abdominal sacrocolpopexy
abdominal salpingectomy
abdominal salpingotomy
abdominal testis
abdominal viscera

abdominocyesis
abdominocystic
abdominogenital
abdominohysterectomy
abdominopelvic CT scan
abdominopelvic procedure
abdominoperineal resection
abdominoscrotal
abdominal uterotomy
abdominovaginal hysterectomy
abdominovaginal palpation of uterus
abdominovesical
Aberdeen knot
aberrant goiter
aberrant vessel
aberration
abetalipoproteinemia
abetimus sodium
ability to attain orgasm
ablatio penis
Ablatherm HIFU (high intensity focused ultrasound) system
ablation
  EnAbl thermal
  endocrine
  endometrial
  endometrial laser
  Hydro ThermAblator (HTA) system
  laparoscopic uterine nerve (LUNA)
  laparoscopic uterosacral nerve (LUNA)
  NovaSure endometrial
  Opal R.F. tissue
  ovarian
  PEARL (physiologic endometrial ablation/resection loop)
  R.F. tissue
  radiofrequency interstitial tissue (RITA)
  rollerball endometrial
  T3 targeted transurethral thermoablation system
  transurethral needle (TUNA)

ablation *(cont.)*
  Urologic Targis transurethral thermoablation system
  VidaMed TUNA system
  Visica fibroadenoma cryoablation system
  visual laser ablation of the trigone (VLAT)
ablation of condyloma acuminatum
ablation of lesion
ablation of ovarian function
ablation of uterine lining
ablator (see *ablation*)
ablepharon macrostomia syndrome
ABMT (autologous bone marrow transplantation)
ABMTR (Autologous Bone Marrow Transplant Registry)
abnormal adherence of placenta
abnormal anion gap
abnormal bladder wall thickness
abnormal bleeding
abnormal buffering
abnormal carbohydrate metabolism
abnormal cerebral signs
abnormal cervical mucus
abnormal clotting
abnormal cystic growth inhibitors
abnormal exfoliate cells
abnormal gestational sac
abnormal hair growth
abnormality (pl. abnormalities)
  anatomic
  bleeding
  chromosomal
  fetal
  fetal chromosome
  fetal structural
  gestational sac
  intersex
  persistent breast
  testicular
abnormal lactation

abnormal mammographic findings
abnormal menses
abnormal phenotype
abnormal renal conservation of
  magnesium
abnormal renal excretion
abnormal serum chemistry
abnormal tubal function
abnormal tubular function
abnormal urine sediment
abnormal uterine bleeding (AUB)
abnormal vaginal bleeding
ABOG (American Board of Obstetrics
  and Gynecology)
ABO hemolytic disease of the newborn
ABO incompatibility
ABO isoimmunization
abort
aborted ectopic pregnancy
aborted pregnancy
aborter, habitual
aborticide
abortient
abortifacient
abortigenic
abortion (ab, AB)
  ampullar
  complete
  complete spontaneous
  criminal
  early
  elective
  failed induced
  first trimester
  habitual
  illegal
  illegally induced
  incomplete
  incomplete spontaneous
  induced
  inevitable
  infected
  late
  legal

abortion *(cont.)*
  legally induced
  menstrual extraction
  missed
  partial birth
  recurrent
  recurrent spontaneous (RSA)
  saline
  second trimester
  self-induced
  septic
  spontaneous
  suction curettage
  surgical
  therapeutic
  third trimester
  threatened
  tubal
abortionist
abortion method
  chemical
  digoxin induction
  dilation and curettage (D&C)
  dilation and evacuation (D&E)
  instrumental evacuation through
    vagina
  medical
  medical induction with stimulation
    of uterine contractions
  menstrual extraction
  methotrexate
  mifepristone (RU 486)
  misoprostol
  partial birth
  prostaglandin
  saline induction
  sharp curettage
  suction curettage
  surgical
  vacuum aspiration
abortion pill
abortion rate
abortive
abortus

abrupt anuria
abruption, placental
abruptio placentae
abscess
  areolar
  Bartholin gland
  bilateral tubo-ovarian
  bladder
  breast
  broad ligament
  bulbourethral gland
  coalescent multiple intrarenal
  corpus cavernosum
  Cowper gland
  Douglas
  fallopian tube
  fluctuant
  kidney
  Littré gland
  mammary
  medullary
  nipple
  nonpuerperal breast
  ovarian
  parametrial
  parametric
  pararenal
  pelvic
  penile
  perinephric
  perirectal
  perirenal
  periurethral
  pouch of Douglas
  premammary
  prostatic
  scrotal
  sperm
  subareolar
  submammary
  syphilitic
  testicular
  tubal rugae
  tubo-ovarian

abscess *(cont.)*
  urethral
  urethral gland
  vulvar
abscess drainage
abscess formation
Abscession fluid drainage catheter
abscess of pouch of Douglas
abscess of sperm in ejaculated semen
absence defect of limbs, scalp, and skull
absence of corpus callosum
absence of cranial vault
absence of eye tissue
absence of one or both kidneys
absence of sperm
absence of testes
absence of tubal rugae
absence of urine formation
absent cervix and adnexa
absent testicles
Absolok endoscopic clip applicator
absolute infertility
absolute normoglycemia
absorbable bovine gelatin
absorbable sponge
abstinence, sexual
abstain from sexual contact
abstain from sexual relations
abuse, sexual
Academy of Assisted Reproductive Technology Professionals (AARTP)
acanthocytosis
acanthosis nigracans
Accurette endometrial sampling device
acarbose
acardiacus, fetus
ACAT (automated computerized axial tomography)
acatalasemia
acatalasia
ACC (aplasia cutis congenita)
accessory atrioventricular pathways
accelerated hypertension

acceleration of fetal heart rate
Accelon Combi biosampler cervical
  cytology collecting device
Accel stopcock
access
  dialysis
  ipsilateral vascular
  long-term (for hemodialysis)
access blood flow
access flow measurement
Access Ostase test
access recirculation (AR)
access to circulation
  long-term
  temporary
accessory breast
accessory chromosome
accessory fallopian tube
accessory nipple
accessory placenta
accessory ureteral bud
access port
accidental hemorrhage
accouchement
accreditation
accreta, placenta
Accu-Chek Instant Plus blood glucose
  monitor
Accu-Chek II Freedom blood glucose
  monitor
Accucore II core biopsy needle
accuDEXA bone densitometer
Accu-Dx bladder cancer test
accumulation, residual urine
AccuPoint hCG Pregnancy Test Disc
AccuProbe 600 system cryotherapy
  probe
accurate DNA replication
Accuscope colposcope
AccuSite injectable gel
AccuSpan tissue expander
Accutane (isotretinoin)
ACE (angiotensin-converting enzyme)
  inhibitor
ACEI (angiotensin-converting enzyme
  inhibitor)
acellular ultrafiltrate
acentric chromosome
acephaly
acetaminophen
acetaminophen-codeine combination
acetic acid
acetoacetic acid
acetone
acetowhite epithelium
acetowhite reaction
acetylcholinesterase (AChE)
achalasia
  pelvirectal
  sphincteral
  ureteral
Achard syndrome
Achard-Thiers syndrome
AChE (acetylcholinesterase)
achondrogenesis
achondroplasia
achondroplasia tarda
achondroplastic dwarf
achondroplastic dwarfism
"achoo" syndrome
achromatopsia
acid
  acetic
  acetoacetic
  amino
  argininosuccinic
  beta-hydroxybutyric
  diethylenetriaminepentaacetic
    (DTPA)
  dimercaptosuccinic (DMSA)
  hippuric
  uric
acid-base balance
acid-base concentration
acid-base homeostasis
acid-base metabolism
acid ceramidase deficiency

acidemia
  fetal
  isoveric
  methylmalonic
  propionic
acid excretion, reduced
acidification
acidified urine specimen
acid load test
acid maltese deficiency
acidosis
  benign dietary
  diabetic
  dietary
  fetal
  hyperchloremic
  hyperchloremic metabolic
  ketoacidosis
  lactic
  metabolic
  perinatal
  primary renal tubular
  renal tubular (RTA)
  respiratory
  secondary renal tubular
  uremic
acid pH of vagina
acid phosphatase
aciduria
  glycolic
  orotic
  paradoxical
acid urine
Acier stainless steel suture
Acinetobacter lwoffi
ACIS (Automated Cellular Imaging System)
ACMI cystoscope
ACMI flexible cystoscope
ACMI nephroscope
ACMI rotating continuous flow resectoscope
ACMI ureteroscope
ACMI USA series endoscope
acne neonatorum
acne vulgaris
ACNM (American College of Nurse Midwives)
ACOG (American College of Obstetricians and Gynecologists)
AC137 analog of human amylin used with insulin
acorn cannula
acorn catheter tip
acorn-tipped catheter
acorn uterine manipulator
acoustical shadowing
acoustic cyst
acoustic neurilemoma
acoustic neuroma
acoustic stimulation test (AST)
ACPS (acrocephalopolysyndactyly)
acquired atrophy of ovary and fallopian tube
acquired cyst of kidney
acquired cystic disease
acquired diverticulum of bladder
acquired hydrocephalus
acquired immune derangement
acquired immunodeficiency immune reaction
acquired immunodeficiency syndrome (AIDS)
acquired mutations
acquired neurogenic bladder
acquired renal insufficiency
acquired syphilis
acquired tubular impairment
acquired vaginal enterocele
acquired vesicoureteral reflux
acquisition of head control
acral-lentiginous melanoma
acrocallosal syndrome, Schinzel-type
acrocentric chromosome
acrocephalic
acrocephalopolysyndactyly (ACPS)

acrocephalosyndactyly
type 1 (Apert syndrome)
type 2 (Crouzon disease)
type 3 (Saethre-Chotzen syndrome)
type 4 (Goodman syndrome)
type 5 (Pfeiffer syndrome)
acrocephaly
acrodermatitis enteropathica (AE)
acrodysostosis
acrodystrophic neuropathy
acrofacial dysostosis, Nager-type
acromegalic gigantism
acromegaly
acromelalgia, hereditary
acromesomelic dwarfism
acromesomelic dysplasia
acromicric dysplasia
acromicric skeletal dysplasia
acromion presentation
acro-osteolysis with osteoporosis and changes in skull and mandible
acroparesthesia
acrosome reaction
ACS (American Cancer Society)
ACS:180 BR breast cancer screening test
ACTH (adrenocorticotropic hormone)
ACTH deficiency
ACTH, exogenous
ACTH stimulation test
Acticoat burn dressing
actinomycosis
Action-II (pimagedine)
Actis VFC (venous flow controller)
activated complement (C3b)
activation and regulation of transcription
activation, egg
active bleeding
active fetal movement
active layer on membrane surface
active labor
active phase arrest of labor
active phase of labor
active urinary sediment
Activella (estradiol/norethindrone)
active, sexually
activin
activities of daily living (ADLs)
activity and diet as tolerated
activity, sexual
actocardiotocograph
Actonel (risedronate sodium)
Actos (pioglitazone)
Acucise endopyelotomy
Acucise retrograde ureteral procedure
acuminatum, condyloma (pl. condylomata acuminata)
Acuson computed sonography
Acuson transvaginal sonography
acute abdomen
acute bacterial prostatitis
acute bacterial pyelonephritis
acute cholangitis
acute circulatory decompensation
acute crescentic glomerulonephritis
acute cyclosporine nephrotoxicity
acute cystitis
acute drug intoxication
acute glomerulonephritis (AGN)
acute hemorrhagic cystitis
acute hemorrhagic glomerulonephritis
acute hydramnios
acute idiopathic polyneuritis
acute intoxication
acute inflammatory pelvic disease
acute intermittent porphyria (AIP)
acute interstitial nephritis
acute lobar nephrosis
acute metabolic decompensation
acute nephritic syndrome
acute nephritis
acute nephritis with lesion of necrotizing glomerulitis
acute nephropathy
acute nephrosis
acute noninfective tubulointerstitial nephritis

acute parametritis
acute peritonitis
acute-phase response
acute poststreptococcal glomerulonephritis (APGN)
acute proctitis
acute proliferative glomerulonephritis
acute prostatitis
acute pyelitis
acute pyelonephritis
acute pyonephrosis
acute renal failure (ARF)
acute renal failure and severe fluid overload
acute salpingitis
acute salpingitis and oophoritis
acute syphilitic meningitis
acute trigonitis
acute tubular injury
acute tubular necrosis (ATN)
acute tubulointerstitial nephritis
acute ureteral colic
acute urethral edema
acute yellow atrophy of liver in pregnancy
Acutrainer electronic bladder retraining device
acyclic bleeding
acyclic pelvic pain
acyclovir
acyl-CoA dehydrogenase deficiency
  long chain
  medium chain
  short chain
ADA (adenosine deaminase) deficiency
Adair breast clamp
ADAM (androgen decline in the aging male) syndrome
Adams-Oliver syndrome
adaptation
adapter, Check-Flo
Adaptic dressing
adaptive landscape
adaptive peak
adaptive radiation
adaptive surface
adaptive value
Adcon-L (carbohydrate polymer gel)
ADD (attention deficit disorder)
Add-A-Cath
Addison disease
Addison-Schilder disease
additive genetic variance
Add-On Bucky
adductor spasmodic dysphonia
adenine (A)
adenine, thymine, guanine, and cytosine (ATGC)
adenitis
  Skene gland
  vestibular
adenocanthoma, endometrial
adenocarcinoma
  acinar
  clear cell
  ductal
  endometrioid
  in situ
  invasive
  kidney
  mesonephric
  moderately well-differentiated
  poorly differentiated
  prostatic
  renal
  urachal
  well-differentiated
adenocarcinoma cyst
adenocarcinoma in situ (AIS)
adenocarcinoma in situ of cervix
adenocarcinoma in situ of endometrium
adenocystic carcinoma
adenofibroma (pl. adenofibromata)
adenofibromatous hypertrophy of prostate
adenohypophysis

adenoma
  aldosterone-producing
  benign liver
  fibroid
  lactating
  mammosomatotroph cell
  nephrogenic
  prolactin-producing
  prostatic
  renal cortical
adenoma-associated virilism
adenoma malignum
adenomatous polyposis of colon
adenomatous tissue enucleation
adenomatoid oviduct tumor
adenomatosis
  familial endocrine
  multiple endocrine
adenomatous goiter
adenomatous hyperplasia
adenomatous polyp of cervix
adenomyosis uteri
adenomyosis, uterine
adenomyotic nodule
adenosalpingitis
adenosine
adenosine deaminase (ADA) deficiency
adenosis
  sclerosing
  vaginal
adenovirus
adenylosuccinate lyase deficiency
Adept (icodextrin)
adequacy of depuration
adequacy of therapy
adequate caliber neovagina
adequate capacity urinary bladder
adequate length of urethra
ADH (antidiuretic hormone) deficiency
ADHD (attention deficit hyperactivity disorder)
adherence of viscera
adherent ovary
adherent placenta
adherent prepuce
adhesiolysis
adhesion
  amnionic
  bleb-like
  cervical
  dense
  filmy
  intra-abdominal
  intraluminal
  intrauterine
  kidney
  lysis of
  mesenteric
  omental
  pelvic
  peritoneal
  peritubal
  periureteral
  perivesical
  postradiation
  primary
  secondary
  takedown of
  tubo-ovarian
  ureter
adhesiotomy
adhesive bands of foreskin
adhesive cellulose tape test
adhesive endometriosis
adhesive plastic drape
adhesive vaginitis
Adie syndrome
Adie tonic pupil
Adipex-P (phentermine)
adipogenital-retinitis pigmentosa-polydactyly syndrome
adiposa dolorosa
adiponecrosis subcutanea neonatorum
adipose fossa of breast
adipose tissue
adiposogenital dystrophy
adiposuria
adjunctive hemodialysis

adjunctive suppressive medical therapy
adjustable saline breast implant
adjusted gestational age
adjustment of net fluid removal
adjustment to blood flow and ultrafiltrate recovery
adjuvant chemotherapy
adjuvant radiotherapy
adjuvant systemic therapy
adjuvant tamoxifen therapy
adjuvant therapy
ADNase (antideoxyribonuclease)
adnexa (pl. adnexa)
adnexa are normal
adnexa clear and nontender
adnexal area
adnexal areas are thickened
adnexal fullness
adnexal mass
adnexal space
adnexal structures
adnexal tenderness
adnexal torsion
adnexa, uterine
adnexa uteri
adnexectomy
adnexitis
adnexopexy
adolescence
adolescent
adoption, embryo
ADPHSP (autosomal dominant pure hereditary spastic paraplegia)
ADPKD (autosomal dominant polycystic kidney disease)
adrenal androgen
  dehydroepiandrosterone (DHEA)
  dehydroepiandrosterone sulfate (DHEAS)
adrenal androgen secretion
adrenal bed
adrenal cortex adenoma
adrenal cortical hyperfunction
adrenal cortical hyperplasia
adrenal cortical hypofunction
adrenal disease
adrenal gland
adrenal hemorrhage
adrenal hermaphroditism
adrenal hyperfunction resulting from pituitary ACTH excess
adrenal hyperplasia, congenital
adrenal hypoplasia
adrenal neoplasm
adrenal-retinitis pigmentosa-polydactyly syndrome
adrenal vein
adrenal virilism
adrenalectomy
adrenarche
adrenocortical hypofunction
adrenocortical insufficiency
  chronic
  primary
adrenocorticotropic hormone (ACTH) deficiency
adrenocorticotropin
adrenogenital syndrome
adrenoleukodystrophy
adrenomyeloneuropathy (AMN)
Adriamycin (doxorubicin)
ADS (anonymous donor sperm)
Adson forceps
adsorbent material
adult chronic immune thrombocytopenic purpura
adult onset diabetes mellitus
adult onset medullary cystic disease
adult polycystic kidney disease (APKD)
adult respiratory distress syndrome (ARDS)
adult spinal muscular atrophy (SMA)
advanced breast biopsy instrumentation (ABBI) system
advanced glycation end-products (AGE)
advanced maternal age

advanced ovarian cancer
adventitious albuminuria
adventitious sounds
adverse effects of radiotherapy
adverse outcome
adynamic ileus
adysplasia, hereditary renal
AE (acrodermatitis enteropathic) syndrome
AEC (ankyloblepharon-ectodermal defects-cleft lip/palate) syndrome
aerobic bacteria
AERx pulmonary drug delivery system
AESOP (automated endoscopic system for optimal positioning) 3000 surgical robot system
aesthetic donor-site defects
AFAFP (amniotic fluid alpha-fetoprotein)
afebrile
afetal
afferent arteriole
afferent glomerular arteriole
afferent vessels of kidney
affirmation of transgender identity
Affirm one-step pregnancy test
Affirm pregnancy test
AFI (amniotic fluid index)
afibrinogenemia, congenital
AFLP (amplified fragment length polymorphism)
AFM (Adriamycin, fluorouracil, methotrexate) chemotherapy protocol
AFP (alpha-fetoprotein), maternal serum
afterbirth
aftercoming head
aftercontraction
afterloading brachytherapy
afterloading radium sources
Ag (antigen)
AGA (appropriate for gestational age)
AGA (aspartylglycosaminuria)
AGA (average for gestational age)
agalactia
agammaglobulinemia, primary
agamogenesis
agamogenetic
agamogony
AGCUS (atypical glandular cells of undetermined significance)
age
  advanced maternal
  appropriate for gestational (AGA)
  childbearing
  developmental
  estimated gestational (EGA)
  fetal
  gestational
  large for gestational (LGA)
  menstrual
  small for gestational (SGA)
AGE (advanced glycation end-products)
age-creatinine clearance nomogram
age-dependent tetrasomy
agenesis
  gonadal
  mullerian
  ovarian
  renal
  vaginal
agenesis of commissura magna cerebri
agenesis of corpus callosum
age-related macular degeneration
age-specific PSA (prostate-specific antigen) testing
agglutination, labial
agglutination of the clitoral folds
aggregated human IgG (AHuG)
aggressive angiomyxoma
aglycosuria
AGN (acute glomerulonephritis)
agnosia, primary visual
agnosis
agranulocytosis
Agris-Dingman submammary dissector
AGT (aminoglutethimide)

AGU (aspartylglucosaminuria)
agyria
AHase (antihyaluronidase)
AHuG (aggregated human IgG)
Ahumada-del Castillo syndrome
AI (artificial insemination)
Aicardi-Goutieres syndrome
Aicardi syndrome
AID (artificial insemination-donor)
AIDS (acquired immunodeficiency syndrome)
AIDS-related complex (ARC)
AIDSvax
AIH (artificial insemination-husband)
AIH (artificial insemination, homologous)
AIHA (autoimmune hemolytic anemia)
AIP (acute intermittent porphyria)
air-bubble filling defect
air embolism
air-embolus protector
air entry
air-fluid level
air hunger
air leak
Airlift balloon retractor
AIS (adenocarcinoma in situ) of cervix
AIS (adenocarcinoma in situ) of endometrium
Aksys PHD hemodialysis system
ALACE (Association of Labor Assistants and Childbirth Educators)
alactasia
Alagille syndrome
alanine aminotransferase (ALT)
alaninuria
alar flaring
AlaSTAT latex allergy test
Alasulf (sulfanilamide and aminacrine)
Alatest Latex-specific IgE allergen test kit
Albarran deflecting level attached to cystoscope
alba, lochia
Albers-Schönberg syndrome
Albert-Smith pessary
albicans, corpus
albinism
Albright hereditary osteodystrophy (AHO)
Albright syndrome
albuginea plication
albumin
  human sonicated
  serum
albumin A
albumin B
albuminorrhea
albuminuria
  adventitious
  dietetic
Albunex (albumin, human sonicated)
Alcaligenes xylosoxidans
alcaptonuria
Alcock canal
alcohol embryopathy
alcohol related birth defects
alcoholic hypoglycemia
alcoholic ketoacidosis
ALD (adrenoleukodystrophy)
Aldara (imiquimod) cream
aldesleukin
aldosterone level
aldosterone-producing adenoma
aldosterone secretion
aldosterone test
aldosterone, urinary
aldosteronism
  primary
  secondary
aldosteronism with normal blood pressure
Aldridge-Studdiford urethral sling
Aldrich syndrome
Aldurazyme (iduronidase)
alendronate
Alesse (levonorgestrel/ethinyl estradiol) oral contraceptive pill

Alexagram breast lesion diagnostic test
Alexander disease
Alexa 1000 noninvasive breast lesion
  diagnostic system
alfacalcidol
Alferon LDO (interferon alfa-n3)
Alferon N (interferon alfa-n3)
Alferon N Gel
alfuzosin
ALG (antilymphocyte globulin)
algophilia
Alibra (alprostadil/prazosin)
alimentary glycosuria
alimentary hypoglycemia
alimentary pentosuria
Alimentum infant formula
Alista (alprostadil)
alkali
alkaline urine
alkalinization of urine
alkalosis
  metabolic
  respiratory
  saline-resistant
alkaptonuria
Alkeran (melphalan)
alkylating agent
Allan Herndon syndrome
allantoic sac
allantoinuria
allele
allele frequency
allele-specific associated primer
  (ASAP)
allele-specific oligonucleotide (ASO)
  testing
allele-specific polymerase chain
  reaction (AS-PCR)
allelic heterogeneity
allelic variants
Allen-Brown shunt
Allen-Doisy hormone evaluation test
allergic cystitis
allergic interstitial nephritis
allergic prostatitis
allergic tubulointerstitial nephritis
allergic tubulointerstitial renal disease
allergy, systemic iodine
all-fours maneuver
Allis clamp
Allis forceps
alloenzyme
alloerotism
allogamy
allogenic renal transplant
allograft
  dysfunctional
  functioning
  renal
alloimmune
AlloMune system
allopathic
alloploid
alloploidy
allopolyploid
allopolyploidy
allopurinol
AlloSling
allosome
allosyndesis
allotetraploidy
allotropism
allozygote
alobar holoprosencephaly
Aloe Vesta perineal foam
Aloka ultrasound
alopecia
  female pattern
  male pattern
  moth-eaten
  postpartum
  premature
alopecia androgenetica
alopecia areata
alopecia celsi
alopecia circumscripta
alopecia syphilitica
Alora (estradiol) transdermal patch

Alpers diffuse degeneration of cerebral gray matter with hepatic cirrhosis
Alpers syndrome
$alpha_1$ (also alpha-1-)
$alpha_1$-adrenergic blockers
$alpha_1$-adrenoceptor blockers
$alpha_1$-antitrypsin (AAT) deficiency
alpha-fetoprotein (AFP), maternal serum
alpha-fetoprotein levels
alpha-galactosidase deficiency
alpha helix
alpha high-density lipoprotein deficiency
alpha interferon
alpha liproteinemia
alpha mannosidosis
Alpha 1 penile implant
alpha-1,4-glucosidase deficiency
alpha satellite probe, chromosome-specific
alpha thalassemia
Alport post-transplant anti-GBM (glomerular basement membrane) disease
Alport syndrome
Alport syndrome, mental retardation, midface hypoplasia, ellipitocytosis (AMME syndrome)
alprostadil
alprostadil/prazosin for erectile dysfunction
Alprox-TD (alprostadil)
ALPS (autoimmune lymphoproliferative syndrome)
ALPS (autologous leukapheresis, processing, and storage)
Alredase (tolrestat)
ALS (amyotrophic lateral sclerosis)
Alsoy infant formula
Alström disease
Altemeier perineal rectosigmoidectomy
alteration of menses
altered collagen strands
altered hormone secretion
altered smooth muscle development
alternate form of contraception
alternate paternity
alternating hemiplegia
alternative pathway activation of complement system
Altra Flux hemodialyzer
ALT-RCC (autolymphocyte-based treatment for renal cell carcinoma)
altruism
Altra Nova hemodialyzer
altretamine
Altrex hemodialyzer
aluminum absorption and toxicity
aluminum, body burden of
aluminum carbonate gel
aluminum hydroxide gel
aluminum-related osteomalacia
alveolar hemorrhage
alveolar hydatid
alveolus (pl. alveoli)
Alzheimer disease (associated with ApoE)
AMA (antimalignan antibody)
Amadori intermediate pathway
Amaryl (glimepiride)
AMAS (antimalignan antibody in serum) test
amaurosis congenita of Leber
amaurotic familial idiocy
ambiguous external genitalia
ambiguous genitalia
ambulatory procedure
ambulatory surgery center
AMC (arthrogryposis multiplex congenita)
amebiasis
ameboid movement
amelogenesis imperfecta
Amen (medroxyprogesterone)
amenorrhea
    dietary
    dysponderal

amenorrhea *(cont.)*
  emotional
  exercise-induced
  hypergonadotropic
  hyperprolactinemic
  hypophysial
  hypothalamic
  jogger's
  lactation
  nutritional
  ovarian
  pathologic
  physiologic
  pituitary
  postpartum
  premenopausal
  primary
  relative
  secondary
  traumatic
amenorrhea-galactorrhea syndrome
amenorrheal
amenorrheic
amenstrual ovulation
Amerge (naratriptan)
American Association for Premature Infants (AAPI)
American Board of Obstetrics and Gynecology (ABOG)
American Cancer Society (ACS)
American College of Nurse Midwives (ACNM)
American College of Obstetricians and Gynecologists (ACOG)
American Society for Reproductive Medicine (ASRM)
American Fertility Society
American Fertility Society Classification of Endometriosis, Revised
  stage I (minimal)
  stage II (mild)
  stage III (moderate)
  stage IV (severe)
American Fertility Society scoring sheet for adnexal adhesions
American Fertility Society scoring sheet for endometriosis
American Urological Association (AUA)
AMF (autocrine motility factor)
amifostine
amiloride
aminacrine
Amin-Aid diet supplement
amino acid
amino acid-based formula
amino acid disorders
amino acid translation
amino acid infusion
amino acid metabolic disorder
aminoaciduria
amino acid valine
aminobenzoate potassium
aminobiphosphonates
Amino-Cerv pH 5.5 cervical cream
aminoglutethimide
aminoglycoside
aminophylline
Amko vaginal speculum
AML (angiomyolipoma) solid renal tumor
AMMECR1 gene
AMME syndrome (Alport syndrome, mental retardation, midface hypoplasia, ellipitocytosis)
ammonia
ammoniacal odor
ammoniacal urine
ammoniuria
amnii, hydrops
amniocele
amniocentesis for lecithin/sphingomyelin (L/S) ratio
amniocentesis needle (see *needle*)
amniocentesis, ultrasonic guidance for
amniochorial

amniochorionic
amniocytes
amniogenesis
amniography
amniohook
amnioinfusion
amnion
amnion graft
amnionic (see *amniotic*)
amnion nodosum
amnion ring
amnion rupture
amnionitis, febrile
amniorrhea
amniorrhexis
amnioscope
amnioscopy
AmnioStat-FLM test
amniotic adhesion
amniotic band
amniotic band syndrome
amniotic cavity
amniotic cyst
amniotic duct
amniotic fluid
  escape of
  meconium-stained
amniotic fluid alpha-fetoprotein (AFAFP)
amniotic fluid embolism
amniotic fluid index (AFI)
amniotic fluid location
amniotic fluid syndrome
amniotic fluid volume
amniotic fold
amniotic instillation
  prostaglandin
  saline
  urea
amniotic membrane, rupture of
amniotic raphe
amniotic sac
  infection of
  intact

amniotic sac *(cont.)*
  transabdominal aspiration of fluid from
amniotome, Beacham
amniotomy
Amoena breast prosthesis
amorphous debris
amorphous fetus
amorphous silicon filmless digital x-ray detection technology
amp (ampule)
"amp and gent" (ampicillin and gentamicin)
amphidiploidy
amphimixis
Amphojel (aluminum hydroxide gel)
ampicillin
ampicillin and gentamicin ("amp and gent")
amplification
amplified fragment length polymorphism (AFLP)
Amplatz Teflon-coated guidewire
amplicon
Amplicor Chlamydia Assay
Amplicor CT/NG test
amplification
  gene
  genetic
ampule (amp)
ampulla of ductus deferens
ampulla of uterine tube
ampulla, rectal
ampullar abortion
ampullar pregnancy
ampullary folds of uterine tube
ampullary tubal pregnancy
amputation
  clitoral
  cervical
  penile
AMS (ablepharon macrostomia syndrome)
AMS (American Medical Systems)

AMS Ambicor penile prosthesis
AMS endoview camera
AMS ProstaJect ethanol injection system
AMS reservoir
AMS 200CX inflatable penile prosthesis
AMS 600 malleable penile prosthesis
AMS 600M malleable penile prosthesis
AMS 650 malleable penile prosthesis
AMS 700CX inflatable penile prosthesis
AMS 700CXM inflatable penile prosthesis
AMS 800 sphincter urinary prosthesis
Amsel criteria for bacterial vaginosis
AMS Securo-T urinary prosthesis
Amsterdam dwarf syndrome
amylase
amyloid disease
amyloid fibril
amyloid kidney
amyloid nephrosis
amyloidosis
  acquired
  dialysis
  hereditary
  idiopathic
  primary
  reactive
  renal
  secondary
amylo-1,6-glucosidase deficiency
amylopectinosis
amyoplasia
amyotrophic lateral sclerosis (ALS)
AN (acanthosis nigricans)
AN (acoustic neuroma)
ANA (antinuclear antibody)
anabolic steroids
anaerobe
anaerobic bacteria
anaerobic cocci
anaerobic infection
anagestone
anagenesis
anal atresia
anal condyloma
anal EMG PerryMeter sensor
anal erotism
analgesia
analgesia and hydration
analgesic nephritis
analgesic nephropathy
analgesic nephrotoxicity
anal intercourse
anal mucosa tear
analphalipoproteinemia deficiency
analphoid inverted duplicated marker
anal procidentia
anal prolapse
anal protrusion
analrectal malformation
anal stenosis
anal sex
anal sphincter laceration
anal triangle
anal verge
analysis (pl. analyses)
  BRACAnalysis
  chemical
  crystallographic
  cytogenic
  Diacyte DNA ploidy
  DNA ploidy analysis
  estrogen-receptor
  progesterone-receptor
  quantitative
  semen
analyzer
  automated blood cell
  ChromaVision digital
  oxygen
anamnionic
anamniotic
Anandron (nilutamide)
anaphase
anaphylaxis

anaplasia of cervix
anaplastic cervix
anaplastic spindle cells
anasarca, fetoplacental
anastomosis (pl. anastomoses)
  arteriovenous
  Clado
  Coffey ureterointestinal
  cystocolic
  end-to-end
  end-to-side
  glomeriform arteriovenous
  glomeriform arteriovenular
  hand-sewn
  heel-toe
  Higgins ureterointestinal
  LeDuc (for ureteral reimplantation)
  nonobstructed
  pyeloureterovesical
  radial artery to cephalic vein
  right internal mammary
  side-to-side
  splenorenal
  transureteroureteral
  transureteroureterostomy
  tubal
  ureterocaliceal
  ureteroileal
  ureteroileocutaneous
  ureterosigmoid
  ureteroureteral
  urethroileal
  vascular
  ventral strip
  vesicourethral
anastrozole
anatomic abnormality
anatomic barriers
anatomical layers
anatomically shaped silicone breast implant
anatrophic nephrolithotomy
anatrophic nephrotomy
anazoturia
ANCA (antineutrophil cytoplasmic antibody)
ANCA-associated glomerulonephritis
ancephaly
ancestral organs
anchor
  AxyaWeld bone
  In-Tac bone
  Mainstay urologic soft tissue
  Ogden soft tissue
  Precision Tack transvaginal
  Precision Twist transvaginal
  UMB-E umbilical catheter
anchored carrier
anchor in the pubic bone
anchor mastopexy
Andersen disease
Anderson Fabry syndrome
Anderson-Warburg syndrome
Ande syndrome
andogenesis
Andractim (dihydrotestosterone gel)
Androcur (cyproterone)
Androderm testosterone transdermal patch
AndroGel (testosterone gel 1%; formerly Androgel-DHT)
androgen
  adrenal
  androstenedione
  attenuated
  circulating
  testosterone
androgen ablation therapy
androgen-controlled homeostasis
androgen decline in the aging male (ADAM)
androgen deprivation therapy
androgenic control
androgenic side effects
androgen independence
androgen-independent cell clones
androgen-independent cells
androgen insensitivity

androgen measurement
androgen-producing neoplasm
androgen receptors (AR)
androgen-secreting tumor
androgen target tissue
androgen withdrawal, intermittent
androgen withdrawal therapy
androgyny
android distribution of body fat
android obesity
android pelvis
andrology
andromorphous
andropathy
andropause
Androsorb
androstanedione
androsterone
anejaculation
anejaculatory male under anesthesia
anembryonic gestation
anemia
  angiopathic hemolytic
  aplastic
  Blackfan-Diamond
  congenital
  congenital hypoplastic
  Cooley
  cow's milk
  Fanconi
  fetal
  folic acid deficiency
  goat's milk
  hemolytic, of newborn
  hereditary nonspherocytic
    hemolytic
  hereditary spherocytic hemolytic
  hypoplastic
  hypoproliferative
  iron deficiency
  iron-resistant microcytic
  late
  macrocytic, of pregnancy

anemia *(cont.)*
  megaloblastic
  microangiopathic hemolytic
  microcytic
  milk
  neonatal
  normochromic normocytic
  posthemorrhagic
  traumatic
anemia-congenital triphalangeal thumb
anemia neonatorum
anemia of chronic disease
anemia of prematurity
anemia of renal failure
anemia with basophilic stippling
anencephaly
anephric
anesthesia
  caudal
  CLA Kit continuous regional
  epidural
  general
  general endotracheal
  general mask
  intravenous sedation
  lidocaine
  local
  lumbar epidural
  Marcaine
  Nesacaine
  paracervical block
  pudendal
  Raplon
  regional
  saddle block
  spinal
  Xylocaine
  Xylocaine with epinephrine
anesthesiologist
anestrous ovulation
aneuploid chromosome complement
aneuploid tumor
aneuploidy, partial

aneurysm
  pararenal aortic
  renal artery
  rerupture
  suprarenal
  suprarenal extension of
  syphilitic
  uterine cirsoid
aneurysmal lesion
AneuVysion assay
Angelman syndrome
angina
Angiocath catheter
angioedema, hereditary
angiogenesis
angiogenic protein
angiogram, angiography
  digital subtraction
  preoperative renal
  renal
  selective renal artery
AngioJet rapid thrombectomy system
AngioJet Rheolytic thrombectomy
  system
angiokeratoma corporis diffusum
AngioMark MRI contrast medium
angiomatosis retina
angiomyolipoma (AML) solid renal
  tumor
angiomyxoma, aggressive
angioneurotic anuria
angio-osteohypertrophy syndrome
angiopathic hemolytic anemia
angioplasty
  percutaneous transluminal
  percutaneous transluminal renal
    (PTRA)
angiotensin-converting enzyme (ACE)
  inhibitors
angiotensin-converting enzyme inhibitor
  (ACEI)
angiotensin II
angle
  costovertebral (CVA)
  posterior urethrovesical

angle *(cont.)*
  urethrovesical (UVA)
  vesicourethral
angle of bladder
angle of inclination of urethra
angle of vagina
angle sutures
angle-tip catheter
angry erythema
angulation of bladder
angulation of ureter
angulation, postoperative
aniline dye
animal model
anion-exchange membrane
anion gap, abnormal
anion, intracellular
aniridia
aniridia-cerebellar ataxia-mental
  deficiency
anisomastia
anisotropic crystals
ankylosing spondylitis
annamycin
anneal
annual examination
annular grooves
annular hymen
annual mammogram
annular placenta
anoderm
anodontia
anogenital band
anogenital raphe
anogenital skin
anomalous dysplasia of dentin
anomalous uterus
anomaly (pl. anomalies)
  branchial cleft
  congenital
  developmental
  DiGeorge
  fetal
  fetal cardiac
  gross fetal

anomaly *(cont.)*
  intersex
  kidney transport
  müllerian duct
  multiple congenital (MCA)
  renal
  urinary tract
  urogenital sinus
  uterine
anomaly of gonadal differentiation
anonymous donor
anonymous donor of genetic material
anonymous donor sperm (ADS)
anophthalmia
anorchia
anorchism
anorectal malformation
anorectal ring
anorectovaginoplasty
anorexia
anorexia nervosa
anorexic
anorgasmia
anorgasmic
anosmia
anovesical fistula (AVF)
Anovlar oral contraceptive
Anovulatorio oral contraceptive
anovular menstruation
anovular ovarian follicle
anovulation
  chronic
  functional
anovulational menstruation
anovulatory bleeding
anovulatory cycle
anovulatory masculinization
anovulatory nonfertile patient
anoxia
  antepartum
  cerebral
  fetal
  intrapartum
anoxia neonatorum

Answer pregnancy test
Antagon (ganirelix)
antecubital fossa
anteflexed uterus
anteflexion
antegrade cystography
antegrade endopyelotomy
antegrade pyelogram
antegrade pyelography
antegrade scrotal sclerotherapy
antegrade ureteral stent
antegrade urography
antenatal diagnosis
antenatal events
antepartum care
antepartum complications
antepartum deep-vein phlebothrombosis
antepartum events
antepartum hemorrhage
antepartum risk factors
antepartum surveillance
antepartum tamponade
anteprostatic gland
anterior and posterior (A&P) repair
anterior axillary line
anterior border of testis
anterior colporrhaphy
anterior colporrhaphy with plication
anterior fibroid
anterior fontanelle
anterior fornix of vagina
anterior leaf of broad ligament
anterior lip of cervix
anterior lip of external os of uterus
anterior lobe disorder
anterior part of fornix of vagina
anterior pelvic exenteration
anterior pelvic wall
anterior pituitary hyperhormonotropic
  syndrome
anterior pituitary gonadotropin
anterior plication incontinence
  procedure
anterior-posterior plane

anterior rectus fascia
anterior rectus sheath overlying bladder
anterior repair
anterior superior iliac spine (ASIS)
anterior surface of lower uterine segment
anterior urethra
anterior urethral valve
anterior urethritis
anterior urethropexy
anterior uterovesical pouch
anterior vaginal colporrhaphy
anterior vaginal fornix
anterior vesicourethropexy
anterior wall of rectum
anterior wall of urinary bladder
anterior wall of vagina
anterolateral fontanelle
anteroposterior
antestrogen or antiestrogen drug
anteversion
anteversion of uterus
anteverted uterus
anteverted, anteflexed uterus
anthracycline therapy
anthracyclines
anthropoid pelvis
antiandrogen withdrawal response (AAWR)
antiandrogens
anti-angiogenesis
antibacterial Foley catheter
Antibacterial Personal Catheter
antibiotic, prophylactic intravenous
antibiotic prophylaxis
antibiotic therapy
antibodies as cause of amyloid and myeloma
antibodies to streptococcal antigenic products
antibody (pl. antibodies)
    ANCA (antineutrophil cytoplasmic)
    anti-glomerular basement membrane (anti-GBM)

antibody *(cont.)*
    anti-D
    antideoxyribonuclease (ADNase)
    antiendometrial
    anti-GBM
    anti-HER2 humanized monoclonal
    antihyaluronidase (AHase)
    antiphospholipid
    antineutrophil cytoplasmic (ANCA)
    antiphospholipid
    anti-Rh
    antisperm
    antistreptokinase (ASKase)
    antistreptolysin-O (ASO)
    atypical maternal
    BrevaRex monoclonal
    carcinoma-specific monoclonal
    CEA-Cide (^{131}I-labeled humanized antibody against carcino-embryonic)
    cervicovaginal
    CytoTAb purified monoclonal
    dacliximab (also daclizumab)
    daclizumab (also dacliximab)
    daclix
    fluorescein-labeled specific
    huHMFG1
    islet cell
    maternal
    monoclonal
    OKT3
    polyclonal
    Prostascint (CYT-356 radiolabeled with indium-111 chloride) monoclonal
    syphilitic
    Therex (huHMFG1) humanized monoclonal
antibody excess
antibody-mediated attack
antibody-mediated immune reaction
antibody-mediated immunity
antibody molecules
antibody response

antibody screen
anticholinergic drugs
anticipation (genetic)
anticoagulant
anticoagulant therapy
anticoagulation, systemic
anticodon
anticonvulsant hypersensitivity syndrome
anti-D antibodies
antidiuresis
antidiuretic hormone (ADH)
antidysuric
antiembolic stockings
antiendometrial antibody
antiestrogen or antestrogen drug
antiestrogenic effect
antiestrogen, oral
antifungal vaginal ointment
anti-GBM (anti-glomerular basement membrane) antibody
anti-GBM disease
anti-GBM glomerulonephritis
anti-GBM nephritis
anti-GBM RPGN
antigen (Ag)
  CA27.29
  CA-125 (cancer antigen-125)
  carcinoembryonic (CEA)-^{99m}Tc
  CEA-Tc 99m carcinoembryonic
  DR
  endogenous
  exogenous
  foreign
  free PSA (prostate-specific antigen)
  group A betahemolytic streptococcal antigens
  hepatitis-associated
  hepatitis B surface antigen (HBsAg)
  histocompatibility
  histocompatibility leukocyte (HLA)
  human leukocyte
  human lymphocyte (HLA)
  IgA

antigen *(cont.)*
  nonrenal
  oncofetal
  Pathfinder DFA (direct fluorescent)
  prostate-specific (PSA)
  prostate-specific membrane (PSMA)
  renal
  streptococcal
  streptococcal cell wall
  tissue polypeptide-specific (TPS)
  tumor peptide (TPA)
antigen-antibody complex
antigen-antibody ratio
antigenemia
antigenically dissimilar RBCs
antigenic stimulation, deposition of
antigenic triggering of immune inflammation
antigen load
antigen specific
anti-glomerular basement membrane (anti-GBM) antibody
anti-glomerular basement membrane glomerulonephritis
anti-glomerular basement membrane nephritis
antigonorrheic
anti-HER2 humanized monoclonal antibody
antihormones
anti-human thymocyte immunoglobulin, rabbit
antihypertensives
anti-kidney serum nephritis
antilymphocyte globulin (ALG)
antimalignan antibody (AMA)
antimalignan antibody in serum (AMAS) test
antimesenteric border
antimetabolite
antimicrobial prophylaxis
antimicrobial therapy
antimicrobial treatment
anti-MPO (antimyeloperoxidase)

antimyeloperoxidase (anti-MPO)
antineoplastic drugs
antineutrophil cytoplasmic antibody (ANCA)
antinuclear antibody (ANA), speckled pattern
antiphospholipid antibodies
antirejection medications
anti-Rh antibody
antischistosomal drugs
antisense
antisense strand
antisepsis
antiseptic
antispasmodic medication
antisperm antibody
Anti-Surrogate Mother Act
anti-Tamm-Horsfall protein in interstitial cystitis
anti-TBM disease
antithrombin III
antithrombin III deficiency
antithymocyte globulin (ATG), rabbit
antiviral agents
Antizol (fomepizole)
Antley-Bixler syndrome
Antopol-Goldman lesion
antrum, follicular
anular placenta
anulus ovalis
anulus urethralis
anuresis
anuria
- abrupt
- angioneurotic
- calculous
- irreversible
- obstructive
- persistent
- postrenal
- prerenal
- renal
- suppressive

anuria/extreme oliguria
anuric renal failure
anus, imperforate
anus vesicalis
anxietas tibialis
anxiety regarding future pregnancy
AODM (adult onset diabetes mellitus)
AO genotype
aorta, coarctation of
aortic atheromatous plaque, ruptured
aortic nipple
aorticorenal ganglion
aortic plexus
aortic stenosis (AS)
aortitis, syphilitic
aortography
aortorenal-saphenous vein bypass graft
apareunia
aparoschisis
APC tumor suppressor gene
APD (automated peritoneal dialysis)
APECED (autoimmune polyendocrinopathy, candidiasis, ectodermal dysplasia) syndrome
aperistaltic distal ureteral segment
Apert syndrome
apex (pl. apices)
- bladder
- prostate
- prostatic
- vaginal

Apgar score at 1 and 5 minutes
Apgars
APGN (acute poststreptococcal glomerulonephritis)
aphallia
aphasia
apheresis
Aphrodyne (yohimbine)
APIB (Assessment of Preterm Infant's Behavior)
apical tissue
APKD (adult polycystic kidney disease)
A.P.L. (chorionic gonadotropin)
aplacenta

aplasia
  congenital thymic
  congenital uterine
  congenital vaginal
  germinal
  germinal cell
  gonadal
  pure red cell
  uterine
  vaginal
aplasia cutis
aplasia cutis congenita (ACC)
aplastic anemia
aplastic uterus
apnea
  central
  initial
  mixed
  obstructive
  sleep
apnea and bradycardia (A&B) spells
apnea neonatorum
apnea of prematurity
apneic spells
apocrine metaphysis of breast
apocrine metaplasia
ApoE (apolipoprotein E) gene
apogamy
apolipoprotein E (ApoE)
Apollo triple-lumen papillotome
apomixis
apomorphine
aponeurosis of external oblique
aponeurosis of internal oblique
apoplexy
  neonatal
  uteroplacental
apoptosis
apoptotic index
apoptotic potential
aposthia
apparatus
  genitourinary
  juxtaglomerular

apparatus *(cont.)*
  urinary
  urogenital
apparent rejection factor
AP-PCR (arbitrarily primed
  polymerase chain reaction)
appearance
  bouquet-of-carnations
  moth-eaten
  spidery
appearance of urine
appendage
  testicular
  uterine
appendage of fetus
appendectomy, incidental
appendiceal endometriosis
appendicovesicostomy
appendicovesicotomy
appendix (pl. appendices)
  endometriosis of
  epididymal
  epiploic
  fetal
  healthy
  ovarian
  retrocecal
  ruptured
  testicular
  tubal
  uterine
  vermiform
appendix epididymidis
appendix of testis
appendix of uterine tube
appendix testis
appendix vermiformis
apple-core configuration
apple peel syndrome
apple shape
application of tamponade
applicator
  Falope ring
  Fletcher

applicator *(cont.)*
  Fletcher-Suit
  Hulka clip
  MCAS (modular clip application system)
  multiple-site perineal applicator (MUPIT)
  radium
applier, MultApplier clip
apposition of device
Appraise blood glucose monitoring system
appreciable dilation
approach (see also *maneuver, operation, technique*)
  combined abdominoperineal
  extraperitoneal abdominal
  inframammary
  Seldinger
  takedown abdominal
  transabdominal
  transperineal
  transperitoneal
  transvaginal
  transvesicle
appropriate for gestational age (AGA)
appropriate urea clearance values
approximate (verb)
approximation
  skin
  tissue
Apra (CT-2584 mesylate)
apraxia
Apri (desogestrel and ethinyl estradiol) tablets
apron
  abdominal
  fatty
  pudendal
APSGN (acute poststreptococcal glomerulonephritis)
Apt-Downey alkali denaturation process
Apt test
aquaporin-1 protein
aqueous procaine penicillin G
aqueous vasopressin
AR (access recirculation)
AR (aortic regurgitation), syphilitic
arachnodactyly
arachnoid cysts
Aran-Duchenne syndrome
Aranesp (darbepoetin alfa)
arbitrarily primed polymerase chain reaction (AP-PCR)
arbitrary primer
arborization of cervical mucus
ARC (AIDS-related complex)
arcade, ileocolic
arching-type diaphragm
arcuate artery of kidney
arcuate uterus
ARDS (adult respiratory distress syndrome)
area
  adnexal
  pretibial
  sclerotic
area of irregularity
area of mosaicism
area of mucosal irregularity
area of punctation
area of whitened epithelium
Aredia (pamidronate)
areola (pl. areolae)
areolar abscess
areolar gland
areolar lesion
areolar mastopexy
areolar tissue
ARF (acute renal failure), post-transplant
arginase deficiency
argininemia
argininosuccinic acid
argininosuccinic acid synthetase deficiency
argininosuccinic aciduria
argon beam coagulator

argon laser lysis of adhesions
Argyle umbilical vessel catheter
Aries-Pitanguy correction of mammary ptosis
Arimidex (anastrozole)
arm
ipsilateral
prolapsed fetal
ARM, AROM (artificial rupture of membranes)
arm abducted to 90 degrees
arm and leg recoil
arm board
Armanni-Ebstein kidney
Armenian syndrome
Army-Navy retractor
Arnold-Chiari deformity
Arnold-Chiari malformation
Arnold-Chiari syndrome
AROM (artificial rupture of membranes)
Aromasin (exemestane)
aromatase enzyme
aromatase inhibitor, aminoglutethamide
Aroplatin
ARPKD (autosomal recessive polycystic kidney disease)
arrayed library
Arrequi laparoscopic knot pusher ligator
arrest
active phase
deep transverse
incomplete spermatogenic
spermatogenic
transverse
arrested dilation
arrest disorder
arrest of active phase dystocia
arrest of descent
arrest of descent dystocia
arrest of labor
arrhinencephaly
arrhythmogenic right ventricular dysplasia
Arrow-Trerotola PTD
ARS (autonomous replication sequence)
ART (assisted reproductive technology)
ART cycle
Artegraft
arterial and venous circulations
arterial hypertension
arterialized forearm veins
arterial nephrosclerosis
arterial pole of corpuscle
arteries were skeletonized
arteriogram
arteriograph
arteriography, renal
arteriohepatic dysplasia
arteriolar nephrosclerosis
arteriole
afferent glomerular
efferent glomerular
spiral
arteriolosclerotic kidney
arteriosclerotic kidney
arteriosclerotic nephritis
arteriosclerotic nephrosclerosis
arteriosus, persistent truncus
arteriovenous (AV)
arteriovenous anastomosis
arteriovenous bridging via filter
arteriovenous fistula (AVF)
arteriovenous hemofiltration
arteriovenous malformation (AVM) of uterus
arteriovenous shunt
arterioventricular (AV) canal defect
arteritis
systemic necrotizing
Takayasu
artery (pl. arteries)
ascending branch of uterine
ascending uterine
brachial

artery *(cont.)*
  common iliac
  cord of umbilical
  external iliac
  external mammary
  fetal umbilical
  hypogastric
  inferior mammary (IMA)
  inferior vesical
  interlobar
  internal iliac
  internal pudendal
  internal spermatic
  intrarenal
  left internal mammary (LIMA)
  middle suprarenal
  ovarian
  penile
  perforating
  perineal
  posterior labial
  pudendal
  renal
  segmental
  single umbilical
  superficial and deep external pudendal
  superior segmental
  superior suprarenal
  superior vesical
  testicular
  umbilical
  ureteric branches of inferior suprarenal
  ureteric branches of ovarian
  ureteric branches of patent part of umbilical
  ureteric branches of renal
  ureteric branches of testicular
  urethral
  uterine
  vaginal
  vesical
artery of superior segment of kidney
artery to ductus deferens
artery to vas deferens
arthralgia
arthritis
  blennorrheal idiopathic
  gonococcal
  gonorrheal
  juvenile
  rheumatoid
  venereal
arthritis urethritica
arthrogryposis multiplex congenita (AMC)
arthro-onychodysplasia
arthro-ophthalmopathy
articular cartilaginous proliferation
artifact (see also *imaging artifacts*)
artifact, breast
artificial embryonation
artificial erection
artificial insemination (AI)
artificial insemination-donor (AID)
artificial insemination, homologous (AIH)
artificial insemination-husband (AIH)
artificial insemination surrogacy
artificial insemination with donor sperm
artificial kidney, Gambro Lundia Minor
artificial kidney machine
artificial rupture of membranes (ARM or AROM)
artificial sphincter device
artificial sphincter muscle
artificial urinary sphincter
artificial vagina
arylsulfatase-B deficiency
arzoxifene
Asahi AM dialyzer
Asahi AM-K dialyzer
ASAP (allele-specific associated primer)
ascending branch of uterine artery
ascending paralysis
ascending pyelonephritis

ascending thick limb of loop of Henle
ascending upper urinary tract infection
ascending uterine artery
Aschheim-Zondek pregnancy reaction
Asch intrauterine catheter
ascites
  dialysis-related
  fetal
  nephrogenic
ascitic fluid
ASCUS (atypical squamous cells
  of undetermined significance)
ASD (atrial septal defect)
AS-800 artificial urinary sphincter
aseptic myocarditis of newborn
aseptic technique
asexual dwarfism
asexual generation
asexual reproduction
Asherman syndrome
ASIS (anterior superior iliac spine)
ASKase (antistreptokinase)
Ashkenazi Jew
Ask-Upmark kidney
ASO (allele-specific oligonucleotide)
  testing
ASO (antistreptolysin-O)
ASO and complement titers
aspartylglycosaminuria
AS-PCR (allele-specific polymerase
  chain reaction)
Aspen laparoscopy electrode
Aspen ultrasound system
Asperger syndrome
aspermatogenic sterility
aspermia
asphyxia
  birth
  fetal
  perinatal
asphyxiating thoracic dystrophy
Aspiracath catheter
aspiration
  endocervical
  fine-needle

aspiration *(cont.)*
  meconium
  needle
  percutaneous
  percutaneous epididymal sperm
  pipelle uterine
  sperm
aspiration and drainage of pelvic cyst
aspiration cannula
aspiration catheter (see *catheter*)
aspiration curettage
aspiration needle (see *needle*)
aspiration of ovarian cyst
aspiration of uterine distention medium
aspirator
  Cavitron ultrasonic
  Pedi vaginal
  Vabra
asplenia syndrome with cardiovascular
  anomalies
ASRM (American Society for
  Reproductive Medicine)
assay (see also *test*)
  Amplicor chlamydia
  AneuVysion
  Auto-Lyte cotinine EIA (enzyme
    immunoassay)
  bacterial inhibition (BIA)
  bladder tumor (BTA)
  BTA TRAK bladder tumor
  CT (*Chlamydia trachomatis*)
  Elecsys total PSA immunoassay
  Emit 2000 cyclosporine specific
  enzyme-linked immunosorbent
  estrogen-receptor immunochemical
    (ER-ICA)
  FastPack PSA
  Gen-Probe amplified CT
  Immulite third-generation PSA
  leukocyte hexosaminiside
  radioimmunoassay
  sperm penetration (SPA)
  steroid-binding
  Truquant BR RIA

assay *(cont.)*
Virgo ANCA (antineutrophil cytoplasmic antibodies)
Virgo cANCA
Virgo pANCA
assessment
APIB (Assessment of Preterm Infant's Behavior)
Ballard gestational
urodynamic
assignment, sex
assisted breech delivery
assisted cephalic delivery
assisted hatching
assisted reproduction
assisted reproductive technology (ART)
assisted vaginal delivery
assisted zonal hatching (AZH)
assortative mating
assumption of parental responsibility
AST (acoustic stimulation test)
asthenospermic
asthma
Astroglide personal lubricant
asymptomatic
asymmetrical breast prosthesis
asymmetric membrane
asymmetry in breast size
asymmetry, breast
asymptomatic bacteriuria
asymptomatic hematuria
asymptomatic neurosyphilis
asymptomatic proteinuria
asymptomatic urinary tract infection (AUTI)
AT (ataxia telangiectasia)
ataxia
Friedreich
hereditary
locomotor
Marie
spinocerebellar
ataxia telangiectasia (AT)
ataxia with lactic acidosis
atelectasis
partial
primary
secondary
ATG (antithymocyte globulin)
Atgam (antithymocyte globulin)
ATGC (adenine, thymine, guanine, and cytosine)
ATGC (genetic code)
atheroemboli
atheroembolic renal disease
atheromatous embolization
atheromatous material
atherosclerosis, pararenal aortic
atherosclerotic renovascular disease
atherosclerotic stenosis of renal artery
athlete's pseudonephritis
athVysion HER-2 DNA probe kit
AtLast blood glucose monitoring system
ATN (acute tubular necrosis)
atonic bladder
atonic segment
atonic ureter
atonic uterus
atony
bladder
muscular
postpartum
sphincter
ureter
uterine
atrasentan
atraumatic forceps
atresia
biliary
choanal
follicular
urethral
vaginal
atresia folliculi
atresia of cervix
atresia of esophagus (with or without tracheoesophageal atresia)

atretic cells
atretic ovarian follicle
atretic ovary
atrial septal defect (ASD) (also atrioseptal)
atrial septal defect secundum
atriodigital dysplasia
atrioseptal (also atrial septal)
atrioventricular septal defect
atrophia bulborum hereditaria
atrioseptoplasty
atrioventricular septal defect (AVSD)
atrophic breasts
atrophic changes
atrophic endometrium
atrophic glomeruli
atrophic kidney
atrophic ovary
atrophic pyelonephritis
atrophic testicle
atrophic vaginitis
atrophic vulvar dystrophy
atrophied ovary
atrophy
  acute yellow
  cervical
  focal tubulointerstitial
  labia majora
  Landouzy-Dejerine
  mammary
  ovarian
  Parrott
  renal
  vaginal
  vulvar
atrophy of cervix
atrophy of corpus cavernosum
atrophy of kidney
atrophy of penis
atrophy of prostate
atrophy of testicle
atrophy of vulva
Atrosept (methenamine)
attachments, bladder
attacks, cyanotic
ATT (alpha$_1$-antitrypsin) deficiency
attempted arrest of labor
attention deficit disorder (ADD)
attention deficit-hyperactivity disorder
(ADHD)
attenuated androgen
attenuated umbilical cord
attenuation, breast
attenuation by breast tissue
atypia
  nuclear
  reactive
  reparative
atypical achondroplasia
atypical adenomatous hyperplasia
atypical endometrial hyperplasia
atypical endometrium
atypical glandular cells of undetermined
significance (AGCUS)
atypical hyperphenylalaninemia
atypical hyperplasia
atypical maternal antibodies
atypical squamous cells of uncertain
significance (ASCUS)
atypical squamous cells of undetermined significance (ASCUS)
atypical vessels
atypical vulvar dystrophy
atypism, cervical
AUA (American Urological Association) Symptom Score
AUB (abnormal uterine bleeding)
Auchincloss modified radical mastectomy
auditory canal atresia
augmentation
  breast
  labor
  oxytocin
  penile
  Pitocin
  Polytef
  transumbilical breast (TUBA)

augmentation cystoplasty
augmentation mammoplasty
augmentation mastopexy
augmentation of anesthesia
augmentation of labor
auramine-stained buffy coat smear
AuraTek FDP (fibrin/fibrinogen degradation products)
AuraTek FDP rapid cancer test
aureus, Staphylococcus
auriculo-oculovertebral syndrome
Aurora MR breast imaging system
AUR-7 flexible ureteroscope
Austin syndrome
AUTI (asymptomatic urinary tract infection) (pronounced "ah-dee")
autism
autoantibody, islet cell
autoaugmentation of bladder
Autocath 100 bladder-control device
Autoclix finger stick device for blood glucose testing
autocrine mediator of bone metastasis
autocrine motility factor (AMF)
autocystoplasty
autodetoxification
autoerotic
autoerotism
autogamy
autogenous saphenous vein graft
autoimmune disease
autoimmune disorders
autoimmune hepatitis
autoimmune hypoglycemia
autoimmune lymphoproliferative syndrome (ALPS)
autoimmune thyroiditis
autoinoculation
autologous blood
Autologous Bone Marrow Transplant Registry (ABMTR)
autologous leukapheresis, processing, and storage (ALPS)
autologous rectus abdominis fascia
autologous transfusion
autologous tumor cells
autologous urethral sling
autolymphocyte-based treatment for renal cell carcinoma (ALT-RCC)
Auto-Lyte cotinine EIA (enzyme immunoassay)
automated blood cell analyzer
Automated Cellular Imaging System (ACIS)
automated computerized axial tomography (ACAT)
automated-cycler intermittent peritoneal dialysis (IPD)
automated endoscopic system for optimal positioning (AESOP)
automated peritoneal dialysis (APD)
automated urinalysis
automatic bladder
automatic insufflator
autonomic nerves
autonomic neurogenic bladder
autonomous replication sequence (ARS)
AutoPap 300 QC automatic Pap screener
autopolyploidy
autoradiography
autosomal chromosome aberration
autosomal dominant
autosomal dominant genetic disorder
autosomal dominant genetic trait
autosomal dominant inheritance
autosomal dominant polycystic kidney disease (ADPKD)
autosomal recessive
autosomal recessive disorder
autosomal recessive genetic trait
autosomal recessive mutations
autosomal recessive polycystic kidney disease (ARPKD)
autosomes
AutoSonix system
autostapler, TA-55

Auto Suture
Auto Suture ABBI system
autotransplantation of kidney
autozygote
Auvard laser weighted speculum
Avandia (rosiglitazone)
avascular necrosis
AVA 3Xi advanced venous access device
AVC vaginal cream
average for gestational age (AGA)
AV (arteriovenous) fistula
AVF (anovesical fistula)
AVF (arteriovenous fistula)
Aviane-28 (levonorgestrel and ethinyl estradiol)
Avicidin
Avicine therapeutic cancer vaccine
Avina female urethral plug
Avitene microfibrillar collagen hemostatic material
AVM (arteriovenous malformation)
AVPR2 gene
AV shunt
avulsion injury
avulsion of inner symphyseal cartilage
avulsion of scrotum
axilla (pl. axillae, axillas)
axillary and femoral vessels
axillary approach in augmentation mammoplasty
axillary contents
axillary dissection
axillary envelope
axillary fat pad
axillary fossa
axillary line
axillary lymphadenopathy
axillary lymph nodes
axillary node dissection
axillary node dissection mastectomy
axillary node sampling
axillary tail
axillary vein
axis
  HPA (hypothalamic-pituitary-adrenal)
  renal
axis of pelvis
AxyaWeld Bone Anchor System
Aygestin (norethindrone)
Ayre cervical spatula
Ayre spatula-Zelsmyr Cytobrush technique
azathioprine
AZH (assisted zonal hatching)
azidothymidine (AZT)
azodicarbonamide
Azo-Gantrisin (sulfisoxazole; phenazopyridine)
azoospermia
  irreparable obstructive
  nonobstructive (NOA)
  obstructive
  persistent
  virtual
azorean disease
Azo-Sulfisoxazole (sulfisoxazole)
azotemia
  nonrenal
  obstructive
  postrenal
  prerenal
  renal
azotemic nephritis
azotemic osteodystrophy
azothioprine sodium
AZT (azidothymidine)
azurophilic neutrophil granules
azygos artery of vagina

B, b

Babcock clamp
Babcock forceps
BABE ultrasound
Babinski reflex
baby (see also *infant; newborn*)
  blue
  blueberry muffin
  breast-fed
  breech
  breech-born (with delayed fetal activity)
  collodion
  crack
  jittery
  test-tube
BABYbird II respirator
BABYbird II ventilator
"baby blues" (postpartum depression)
BabyFace 3-D surface rendering
Babyflex ventilator
babyscope
BabyShades eye protector
BabyStart ovulation prediction kit
baby Tischler cervical biopsy forceps
BAC (bacterial artificial chromosome)
bacille Calmette-Guérin (BCG)
bacille Calmette-Guérin instillation therapy
bacilli, intracytoplasmic
bacilli in urine
bacilluria
bacillus
  Calmette-Guérin (BCG)
  Döderlein (Doederlein) bacillus
  intravesical
bacitracin ointment
backache, sacral
back-cross
backflow
  pyelotubular
  pyelovenous
backflow phenomenon
backflush
background risk
Backhaus towel clamp
back labor
Bacon-Babcock correction of rectovaginal fistula
bacteremia
  community-acquired
  persistent
  polymicrobial
  transient
bacteria (see also *pathogen*)
  Acinetobacter
  aerobic

bacteria *(cont.)*
  anaerobic
  Calymmatobacterium granulomatis
  Campylobacter
  Candida
  corynebacteria
  Cryptococcus
  Enterobacter
  gas-forming
  gram-negative
  gram-positive
  Haemophilus ducreyi
  Klebsiella
  lactobacilli
  Nocardia
  occasional
  Proteus
  Pseudomonas
  Salmonella
  Serratia
  Shigella
  Toxoplasma
bacteria-impervious seal of catheter
bacterial artificial chromosome (BAC)
bacterial casts
bacterial culture
bacterial cystitis
bacterial epididymitis
bacterial infection
bacterial inhibition assay (BIA)
bacterial prostatitis
bacterial pyelonephritis
bacterial urethritis
bacterial vaginosis (BV)
bactericidal antibiotics
Bacterioides
bacteriophage
bacteriospermia
bacteriostatic water
bacteriotoxic endometritis
bacterium (pl. bacteria)
bacteriuria
  asymptomatic
  covert renal

Bactrim; Bactrim DS (trimethoprim; sulfamethoxazole)
Bactroban (mupirocin)
BAER (brain stem auditory-evoked response) test
bag
  dialysate
  douche
  Endobag laparoscopic specimen retrieval
  Endo Catch specimen retrieval
  EndoMate Grab Bag endoscopic specimen retrieval
  Endopouch Pro specimen retrieval
  Endosac specimen collection
  eXtract specimen
  multiprong administration manifold and drainage
  Ponsky Endo Sock retrieval
  urinary drainage
bag and mask ventilation
bag exchange method
Baggish aspiration catheter
Baggish contact panoramic hysteroscope
Baggish injection tube
bag method of continuous ambulatory peritoneal dialysis
bag of waters
Bair Hugger warmer blanket
Bakelite
Baker amniocentesis needle
Bakes common
duct dilator
baking soda and vinegar douche
baking soda douche
balance
  acid-base
  electrolyte
  fetal acid-base
balanced electrolyte solution
balanced salt solution (BSS)
balanced translocations
balanic hypospadias

balanitic epispadias
balanitis diabetica
balanitis, plasma cell
balanitis xerotica obliterans
balanoplasty
balanoposthitis, candidal
balantidiasis
balanus
Baldy-Webster correction of uterine retrodisplacement
Balfour retractor
Balkan nephritis
Balkan nephropathy
Ball operation for treatment of pruritus ani
Ballantine clamp
Ballard exam
Ballard gestational assessment
Baller-Gerold syndrome
balloon
  Extractor three-lumen retrieval
  Kaye tamponade nephrostomy
  Origin
  ThermaChoice uterine
  traction
  ureteral dilation
balloon catheter
balloon catheterization (to stop uterine bleeding)
balloon dilation catheter
balloon dilation of prostate
balloon dilation of prostatic urethra
balloon dissector
balloon inflation
ballooning of tube
balloon tuboplasty to open blocked fallopian tubes
balloon uterine stent
ballottable vertex
ballottement
  abdominal
  renal
ball-tip electrode
BAMBI (breast augmentation mammoplasty by injection)
banana sign of fetal cerebellum
band
  adhesive
  amniotic
  anogenital
  chromosome
  Clado
  frenular
  snap gauge
  ventral frenular
bandage
  Band-Aid
  Snugs mastectomy
  tumescent absorbent (TAB)
bandage scissors
Band-Aid bandage
banding pattern
band intensity
band level
Bandl ring
band of uterus
bandolier cord
bands of cervix
banjo curet
bar
  leading
  median
bar of bladder
barbiturate
Barcat hypospadias repair
Bard Biopty gun
Bard BTA test for detection of recurrent bladder cancer
Bardet-Biedl syndrome
Bardex I.C. catheter
Bard flexible endoscopic injection system
Bard Safety Excalibur peripherally inserted catheter (PIC) introducer
Bard Sperma-Tex preshaped mesh
Bard Visilex mesh

barium hydroxide using Giemsa (CBG) chromosome staining method
Barlow disease
Barlow maneuver
barotrauma
Barraquer syndrome
Barr body
barrel chest
Barrett placenta forceps
barrier
  blood-brain
  blood-testis
  charge-selective
  incest
  placental
  size-selective
  Splash-Shield endoscopic
  SprayGel adhesion
barrier contraceptive
Barr sex chromatin bodies
Bartholin abscess
Bartholin abscess of vulvovaginal gland
Bartholin cystectomy
Bartholin cyst, marsupialization of
Bartholin duct
Bartholin duct cyst
Bartholin gland
Bartholin gland abscess
Bartholin gland secretion
bartholinitis
Bartholin, urethral, and Skene (BUS) glands
Barth hernia
Barth syndrome
Barton bladder blade
Barton obstetrical forceps
Bartter syndrome
basal body temperature (BBT)
basal body temperature measurement
basal cell
basal cell carcinoma
basal lamina
basal prolactin level
baseball stitch
Basedow disease
Basedow goiter
base excess
baseline fetal heart rate
baseline irritability
baseline mammogram
baseline mammography
baseline variability
basement membrane
  expanded
  glomerular capillary
  glomerular (GBM)
  pulmonary alveolar
  subendothelial side
  subepithelial side
  tubular (TBM)
basement membrane thickening
base of bladder
base of penis
base of prostate
base of tumor
base pair (bp)
base pair substitution
base sequence
base sequence analysis
base substitution
bas-fond ("bah-fawn") obstruction
basic fibroblast growth factor (bFGF)
basket (see also *stone basket*)
  Ellik kidney stone
  Segura stone
  stone
  SurLok
basket extraction, cystoscopic
basket extraction of stones
basketing, stone
basophilic stippling
Bassen-Kornzweig syndrome
Basset en-bloc radical vulvectomy
Bassini hernia repair
BAT (B-mode acquisition and targeting) system

bath
  lithotripsy
  Sitz
bathe
bathing tumor tissues
Batten disease
Batten-Mayou syndrome
Batten-Spielmayer-Vogt disease
Batten-Vogt syndrome
battledore placenta
Baudelocque maneuver
Baumrucker resectoscope
Bayer HER-2/neu serum test
Baylor amniotic perforator
bayonette forceps
BBD (benign breast disease)
BBT (basal body temperature)
BCC (benign cellular changes)
BCG (bacillus Calmette-Guérin)
BCI-Immune Activator
Bc1-2 oncogene
BCT (breast-conserving therapy)
B-D Basal Thermometry Kit
BD Insyte Autoguard-P shielded IV catheter
BD Insyte Autoguard shielded IV catheter
BD Sensability breast self-examination aid
BDProbeTec ET system
Beacham amniotome
Beacon incontinence surgical device
Beacon Technology System (BTS)
beading of tube
Beals-Hecht syndrome
Beamer injection stent system
Bean syndrome
Bear Cub infant ventilator
bearing-down efforts
bearing-down pain
Bear NUM-1 tidal volume monitor
Bear respirator
beat-to-beat variability
BEBIG iodine-125 seed implant
Becker breast implant
Becker muscular dystrophy (BMD)
Becker nevus
Becker tissue expander
Beckwith-Wiedemann syndrome
beclomethasone
bed
  adrenal
  bladder
Bednar aphthae
bed of breast
bed of prostate
bed-wetting
beef lung heparin
beeturia
behavioral genetics
behavior, maladaptive coping
Behçet disease
Behçet syndrome
Bell-Buettner hysterectomy
bell-clapper deformity
Belle-Amie breast prosthesis
Bellini duct carcinoma
Bell palsy
"belly button" augmentation mammoplasty
Belzer organ preservation unit
Belzer solution
BEMP (bleomycin, Eldisine, mitomycin, Platinol) chemotherapy protocol
Benadryl (diphenhydramine)
Bence Jones protein
Bence Jones proteinuria
Benderev bone fixation procedure for stress urinary incontinence (SUI)
benefits of chemotherapy
Benelli lollipop mastopexy
Benelli pursestring mastopexy
Benenenti rotation of bulbous urethra
benign adenoma of prostate
benign adenomatous hyperplasia of prostate
benign breast condition

benign breast disease (BBD)
benign cellular changes (BCC)
benign cranial nerve tumors
benign cyst
benign dietary ketoacidosis
benign enlargement of prostate
benign essential blepharospasm (BEB)
benign essential hypertension
benign essential tremor
benign familial polymyopathy
benign fibrocystic disease of breast
benign fibroids
benign glycosuria
benign liver adenoma
benign mammary dysplasia
benign neoplasm
benign nephroangiosclerosis
benign nephrosclerosis
benign nodular hyperplasia of prostate
benign paroxysmal peritonitis
benign postural proteinuria
benign prostate
benign prostatic hyperplasia (BPH)
benign prostatic hypertrophy (BPH)
benign recurrent hematuria
benign reflux nephropathy
benign secretory endometrium
benign tertiary syphilis
benign variant
benzathine penicillin G
benzidine stain
BEP (bleomycin, etoposide, Platinol) chemotherapy protocol
beractant
Berger disease
Berger focal glomerulonephritis
beriberi, infantile
Berkeley suction
Berkson-Gage breast cancer survival calculation
Berlind-Auvard weighted vaginal speculum
Bernard-Soulier syndrome
Bertin, renal column of
Berwick dye
Be Sure One Step pregnancy test
beta-adrenergic blocking drugs
beta-blockers
beta core fragment of hCG
betacyaniuria
Betadine (povidone-iodine)
Betadine douche
Betadine gel
Betadine scrub
Betadine solution
beta-endorphin
beta gene
beta-globin gene
beta-glucuronidase deficiency
beta hCG (human chorionic gonadotropin)
beta-hemolytic streptococci
beta-hydroxybutyric acid
betaine anhydrous
betalipoprotein deficiency
betamethasone
betamethasone suspension
betamethasone sodium phosphate
BetaSorb hemodialysis treatment
betastarch solution
beta subunit of hCG
beta testing centrifuge
bethanechol chloride
Bethesda classification
Bethesda rating scale
Bethesda system for reporting cervical and vaginal cytologic diagnoses
Betke stain
Betke-Kleihauer test
Beuren myopathy
bezoar
BFP (biologic false-positive)
BGF (bridge-graft fistula)
BH4 deficiency
bias stockinette wrap
biaxial fluoroscopy
bicalutamide
bicameral uterus

Bicarbolyte bacteriostatic solution
bicarbonate (HCO_3)
bicarbonate buffer system
bicarbonate precursors
  acetate
  lactate
bicarbonate titration test
Bicitra (sodium citrate; citric acid)
BiCOAG 3-mm bipolar forceps
bicornate uterus
bicornuate uterus
bicuspid aortic valve
bidet
bidiscoidal placenta
Bierer ovum forceps
Biesenberger technique of mastopexy
bifid cranium
bifid pelvis
bifid scrotum
bifid ureter
bifid uterus
bifida, spina
biforate uterus
bifurcate
bifurcation of iliac vessels
bifurcation, ureteral bud
bigeminal pregnancy
Bihrle dorsal clamp
Bihrle needle holder
BiLAP bipolar cutting and coagulating probe
BiLAP bipolar needle electrode
bilateral acoustic neuroma
bilateral adnexal masses
bilateral descended testes
bilateral hermaphroditism
bilateral hypertrophy
bilateral incomplete ureteral injury
bilateral inguinofemoral lymphadenectomies
bilaterality of ureteral duplication
bilaterally descended testicles
bilateral mammogram
bilateral mastectomy
bilateral nephrectomy
bilateral oophorectomy
bilateral orchiectomy
bilateral orchidectomy
bilateral reflux nephropathy
bilateral right-sidedness
bilateral salpingectomy
bilateral salpingo-oophorectomy (BSO)
bilateral small kidneys
bilateral tubal coagulation
bilateral ureteral obstruction (BUO)
bilateral vasectomy
bilateral vulvectomy
bile duct, congenital obstruction of
bile extravasation
bile plug syndrome
bilharzial fibrosis
bilharziasis
biliary atresia
Biliband phototherapy mask
bili lights (slang for bilirubin lights)
Bili mask
biliary atresia
Bilibed phototherapy system
Biliblanket phototherapy system
BiliBottoms phototherapy diapers
BiliChek
bilirubin
bilirubin encephalopathy
bilirubinometer, Colormate TLc.Bili-Test system
bilirubinuria
bilirubin, urine
biliuria
bilobate placenta
bilocular uterus
bimanual abdominorectal palpation of uterus, fallopian tubes, and ovaries
bimanual abdominovaginal palpation of uterus, fallopian tubes, and ovaries
bimanual examination of pelvis
bimanual palpation of adnexa
bimanual palpation of uterus to assess consistency, mobility, position, size, surface contour, and tenderness

bimanual pelvic examination
bimanual version
Bimexes
binder
  breast
  Expand-a-Band breast
  obstetrical
binder syndrome
binding, breast
binding site
binocular fiberoptic colposcope
binovular twin
bioabsorbable urethral sling
Biocell RTV saline-filled breast implant
Biocept-5 pregnancy test
Biocept-G pregnancy test
biochemical assay
biochemical characteristics
biochemical genetics
biochemical relapse-free survival (bRFS)
biocompatible
biocompatible membranes
biocompatible ultrafilters
BioDimensional breast implant
biofeedback for incontinence
Biofield diagnostic system
Biofield test
biofilm of organisms
Bio-Flex CS catheter
bioinformatics
biologic false-positive (BFP)
biological fatherhood
biologically inert
biological offspring
biological response modifiers
  interferons
  interleukin-2
  lymphocyte-activated killer cells
  monoclonal antibodies
  tumor necrosis factors
biometry
biophysical profile (BPP) monitoring
biopirimine

biopsy (pl. biopsies)
  Biopty cut needle for breast
  Cell Recovery System (CRS) brush
  cervical
  cervical cone
  cervical punch
  chorionic villi (CVB)
  cold cup bladder
  cold knife
  cold knife cone
  colposcopically directed
  colposcopically directed punch
  cone
  confirmatory needle
  directed
  embryo
  endocervical
  endometrial
  excision
  excisional
  fetal
  fine-needle aspiration
  four-quadrant cervical
  guided needle
  hot
  incision
  incisional
  Keyes punch
  laser cone
  mammogram-guided
  mammogram-guided core
  Mammotest breast
  Mammotest Plus breast
  MIBB breast
  mirror image breast
  MRI-guided breast
  needle core
  negative breast
  open
  open renal
  para-aortic node
  percutaneous
  percutaneous excisional breast (PEBB)

biopsy *(cont.)*
  percutaneous renal
  punch
  renal
  sentinel node
  SiteSelect percutaneous breast
  Sonopsy 3-D ultrasound breast
  stereotactic needle breast
  stereotaxic core needle (SCNB)
  testicular
  transrectal prostatic ultrasonographic
  transurethral
  wedge
biopsy forceps (see *forceps*)
biopsy needle (see *needle*)
biopsy needle depth marker
biopsy of breast, needle core
biopsy of cervix
biopsy of kidney
Biopty cut needle for breast and prostate biopsy
BioSling urethral sling
BioSorb resorbable urologic stents
Biospal dialyzer
Biosyn suture
biotechnology
biotinidase deficiency
Bio-Vascular remodelable tissue urethral sling
BIP (bleomycin, ifosfamide, Platinol) chemotherapy protocol
biparietal diameter (BPD)
bipartite diamnionic twins
bipartite uterus
bipartite vagina
biphosphonate therapy
biphosphonates
biplane sector probe for transrectal prostatic ultrasonographic biopsy
bipolar Adson forceps
bipolar cautery
bipolar coaptation forceps
bipolar Cushing forceps
bipolar cutting loop
bipolar electrovaporization technology
bipolar Gerald bayonette forceps
bipolar grasping forceps
bipolar Hardy bayonette forceps
bipolar Jansen bayonette forceps
bipolar jeweler forceps
bipolar Malis forceps
bipolar McPherson forceps
bipolar membrane
bipolar Semkin forceps
bipolar surgical technique
bipolar Tenzel forceps
bipolar urological loop
bipolar version
BI-RADS (Breast Imaging and Reporting Data System) of the American College of Radiology
Bird cup
Bird OP cup
Bird vacuum extractor
Birtcher Medical Systems argon beam coagulator
birth
  cesarean
  complete
  cross
  dead
  head
  live
  multiple
  over-term
  post-term
  premature
  pre-term
  term
  vaginal
birth asphyxia
birth attendant, traditional
birth canal
birth control
birth control device (see *contraceptive device*)
birth control pills

birth defects
- chromosomal
- mendelian
- multifactorial
- NTD (neural tube defects)
- teratogenic

birthing
birthing ball
birthing center
birthing chair
birthing room
birth injury
birthmark, port wine
birth of malformed fetus
birth rate
birth trauma
birth weight
- average for gestational age (AGA)
- extremely low (ELBW)
- high
- large for gestational age (LGA)
- low
- micropreemie
- small for gestational age (SGA)
- very low (VLBW)

bisection of ovary
bisexual
Bishop score for cervical ripening
Bissinger detachable bipolar coagulation forceps
Biswas Silastic pessary
bites of tissue
bites, suture
Bittorf reaction
bivalent chromosome
bivalve
bivalved
Bjornstad syndrome
Blackfan-Diamond syndrome
black urine
bladder
- abscess of
- acquired diverticulum of
- adequate capacity urinary

bladder *(cont.)*
- anterior wall of urinary
- apex of urinary
- atonic
- automatic
- autonomic neurogenic
- bar of
- base of
- body of
- calcified
- centrally uninhibited
- contracted
- contraction of
- distended
- distended urinary
- dome of urinary
- dropped
- endometrectomy of
- endometriosis of
- external blow over a full
- false diverticulum of
- fistulectomy of
- flaccid
- fundus of urinary
- high capacity
- high compliance
- hourglass
- hyperemia
- hyperreflexic
- hypertrophic
- hyporeflexive
- hypotonic
- ileal conduit
- ileal neobladder
- inflammation of
- laceration of
- lateral wall of urinary
- low capacity
- low pressure, adequate capacity
- low pressure urinary
- malfunctioning urinary
- motor paralytic
- mucosa of urinary
- muscular layer of urinary

bladder *(cont.)*
  neck of urinary
  neurogenic
  neurogenic dysfunction of
  neuropathic
  nonemptying
  non-neurogenic
  nontraumatic rupture of
  overactive
  palpable
  panmural fibrosis of
  papilloma of
  paralysis
  posterior wall of urinary
  reflexic neurogenic
  refluxing spastic neurogenic
  removal of urinary
  ruptured
  sensory paralytic
  serosa of urinary
  "shock"
  spastic
  thickened
  traumatic rupture of
  trigone of urinary
  uninhibited
  uninhibited neurogenic
  unstable
  urethral orifice of
  urinary
  uvula of
  wedge resection of
bladder advancement
bladder atony
bladder attachments
bladder bed
bladder blade
bladder blisters
bladder calculus
bladder cancer
bladder capacity
bladder carcinoma
bladder carcinoma classification
bladder cavity
bladder chips
bladder compliance
bladder contour
bladder contractility study
bladder contraction
bladder control
bladder debris
bladder decompression
bladder detritus
bladder detrusor
bladder displaced inferiorly
bladder distention
bladder diverticulum (pl. diverticula)
bladder dome
bladder drainage
bladder dysfunction
bladder dyssynergia
bladder elasticity
bladder emptying
  complete
  incomplete
bladder endometriosis
bladder exstrophy
bladder fistula
bladder flap
bladder flap dissection
bladder flap was reflected
bladder floor
bladder fundus
bladder hyperactivity
bladder hypertrophy
bladder hypotonicity
bladder incontinence
bladder inertia
bladder infection
bladder injury
bladder innervation disruption
bladder irrigation
bladder irritant
bladder journal
bladder laceration
bladder lavage
BladderManager ultrasound device
bladder mucosa

bladder neck
bladder neck contracture
bladder neck elevation procedure
bladder neck fibers
bladder neck obstruction
bladder neck reconstruction
bladder neck resected circumferentially
bladder neck spreader
bladder neck stabilization, percutaneous (PBNS)
bladder neck stenosis
bladder neck support prosthesis
bladder neck suspension, laparoscopic
bladder orifice
bladder outlet
bladder outlet competence
bladder outlet obstruction (BOO)
bladder outlet obstructive symptoms
bladder paresis
bladder pathology
bladder perforation
bladder pheochromocytoma
bladder pillar
bladder pressure
bladder prolapse
bladder reflection
bladder reflex
bladder retraining
BladderScan
bladder scissors
bladder sling
bladder sound
bladder spasm
bladder spatula
bladder stasis
bladder stone
bladder storage
bladder suspension
bladder tear
bladder trabeculation
bladder trigone
bladder tumor
Bladder Tumor Assay (BTA) for monitoring urinary specimens
bladder wall
bladder wall compliance
bladder wall contour
bladder wall hemorrhage
bladder wall pathology
bladder wall, posterior
bladder washout technique
bladder was mobilized
bladder was reflected
blade (see also *knife*)
  Barton bladder
  Doyen vaginal retractor
  guillotine
  LaserSonics EndoBlade
  LaserSonics Nd:YAG LaserBlade
  LaserSonics SurgiBlade
  UltraCision ultrasonic knife
Blaivas classification of urinary incontinence
Blake drain
Blalock-Taussig clamp
Blalock-Taussig shunt
blanch and flush of skin
blanket
  Bair Hugger warmer
  Biliblanket
Blassuchi curved catheter tip
blastocyst cavity
blastocyst, human
blastomycosis
bleb, submucosal
bleeder
bleeding
  abnormal uterine (AUB)
  abnormal vaginal
  acyclic
  breakthrough
  cervical
  concomitant
  dysfunctional uterine (DUB)
  estrogen breakthrough
  first trimester
  genital
  heavy vaginal

bleeding *(cont.)*
  inappropriate uterine
  intermenstrual
  intra-abdominal
  intraperitoneal
  menopausal
  postcoital
  postmenopausal
  retroplacental
  scanty vaginal
  second trimester
  third trimester
  unilateral renal
  uterine
  vaginal
  withdrawal
bleeding abnormality
bleeding diathesis
bleeding from navel due to endometriosis
bleeding from nipple
bleeding from urinary tract due to endometriosis
bleeding points
bleeding ulceration of vaginal tissues
bleed, withdrawal
blennorrheal idiopathic arthritis
blenuria
blepharophimosis, ptosis, epicanthus inversus syndrome
blepharospasm, benign essential
blepharospasm-oromandibular-dystonic syndrome
Blessig cyst
Blessig embryonal groove
blighted ovum
blind needle insufflation
blindness
blind vaginal pouch
blink reflex
blisters in bladder
bloated
bloating, abdominal

block
  epidural
  intercostal nerve
  paracervical
  penile
  pudendal
  saddle
  Wenckebach heart
blockade
  alpha-adrenergic
  intrarenal tubular
  total estrogen
blockage from cellular debris
blockage in ureter
blockage of ureters
blockage, tubal
blocked fallopian tube
blocked urethra
blockers
  adrenergic
  beta
  calcium channel
Block-Siemens-Sulzberger disease
Block-Sulzberger disease
blood
  autologous
  cord
  dialyzed
  extravasated
  shunted
  swallowed maternal
  urinary
blood cast
blood extravasation
blood flow
  access
  occlusion of testicular
blood flow in CAVH
blood gas
blood glucose, fasting
blood glucose monitor
  Accu-Chek InstantPlus
  Accu-Chek II Freedom
  Appraise

blood glucose monitor *(cont.)*
  AtLast
  CFC BioScanner System implantable
  Chemstrip MatchMaker
  Companion 2
  Diasensor 1000
  ExacTech
  ExpressView
  Glucochek Pocketlab II
  Glucometer DEX
  Glucometer Elite R
  Glucometer II
  Gluco-Protein OTC self-test
  GlucoWatch
  Medisense Pen 2
  One Touch
  One Touch Basic
  One Touch FastTake
  One Touch Profile
  One Touch II hospital
  Select GT
  Sof-Tact
  Supreme II
  SureStep
  TD Glucose
  Tracer
blood glucose tolerance test
Bloodgood syndrome
blood in cul-de-sac
blood in pouch of Douglas
blood in urine
blood loss, fetal
blood outflow line
blood pressure (BP)
blood pump
blood purification
blood pressure, orthostatic
blood substitute, Hemolink
blood-testis barrier
blood-tinged urine
blood urea nitrogen (BUN)
blood vessel necrosis
blood volume expansion
bloody discharge
bloody nipple discharge
bloody semen
bloody show
bloody urine
Bloom syndrome
blotting
blue baby
blueberry muffin baby
blue diaper syndrome
blue dome breast cyst
blue dome syndrome
blue dot sign for infarcted appendix epididymidis
blue ring pessary
blue rubber bleb nevus syndrome
Bluestein Table
bluish discoloration around umbilicus
bluish discoloration of cervix in pregnancy
bluish discoloration of vaginal mucosa in pregnancy
Blumer rectal shelf
blunt and sharp dissection
blunt dissection
Bluntport disposable trocar
blunt trauma to kidney
blush, tumor
BMD (Becker muscular dystrophy)
BMI (body mass index)
B-mode acquisition and targeting (BAT)
BMT (bone marrow transplant)
BMT (bone marrow transplantation)
BNBAS (Brazelton Neonatal Behavioral Assessment Scale)
Bochdalek hernia
body (pl. bodies)
  Barr
  Barr sex chromatin
  Call-Exner
  Döhle (Doehle)
  Donovan
  doubly refractile fat
  intraluminal foreign

body *(cont.)*
  juxtaglomerular
  mamillary
  oval fat
  paranephric
  perineal
  polar
  suprarenal
body burden of aluminum
body habitus
body mass index (BMI)
body of bladder
body of breast
body of mammary gland
body of penis
body of uterus
body stalk
body surface area (BSA)
boggy prostate
boggy uterus
Bohr effect
boil of corpus cavernosum
boil of penis
bolster
  cotton
  Dacron velour
bolus of contrast medium
Bonanno suprapubic catheter
Bondek absorbable suture
bonding, mother-infant
bone-anchor bladder suspension technique
bone-anchoring of sutures
bone demineralization
bone densitometer, accuDEXA
bone density measurement
bone locator
bone marrow transplant (BMT)
bone marrow transplantation (BMT)
  autologous
bone mass measurement
BonePlast bone void filler
bone tumor-epidermoid cyst-polyosis
Bonnevie-Ulrich syndrome
Bonney abdominal hysterectomy
Bonney test for stress urinary incontinence
bony landmarks
bony metastasis
bony pelvis
bony spicule embolization
BOO (bladder outlet obstruction)
Bookler swivel-ball laparoscopic instrument holder
Bookwalter self-retaining retractor
BOP (bleomycin, Oncovin, Platinol) chemotherapy protocol
border, antimesenteric (not ante-)
borderline ovarian tumor
borderline pelvis
border of uterus
Bordetella pertussis
Borjeson syndrome
BOR (branchio-otorenal) syndrome
Bosniak classification of renal cystic mass
boss (pl. bosses)
bosselated appearance
"bother" score of prostatic symptoms
botryoid sarcoma
bottle-feeding
bottle repair of hydrocele
"bottoming-out" of breast following reduction
botulinum-A toxin injection
bougie (see also *sound*)
  EndoLuminan
  ureteral
  Van Buren urethral
bougie á boule
bound carrier
bound down with adhesions
"bouquet of carnations" appearance
Bourneville disease
Bovie cautery
Bovie cautery unit
Bovie electrosurgical unit
Bovie 1250 electrosurgical device

Bovie 2100 electrosurgical device
bovine carotid xenograft
bovine fistula autogenous vein graft
bovine heterograft
bowel and bladder dysfunction
bowel contents
bowel function
bowel laceration
bowel packed out of the way
bowel retractor
Bowen disease of anal canal
Bowen Hutterite syndrome
bowenoid papulosis
Bowman capsule
Bowman space
bow "T" IUD
Boyle uterine elevator
Bozeman operation for uterovaginal fistula
Bozeman uterine dressing forceps
bp (base pair)
BP (blood pressure)
BPD (biparietal diameter)
BPD (bronchopulmonary dysplasia)
BPH (benign prostatic hyperplasia)
BPH (benign prostatic hypertrophy)
BPP (biophysical profile)
bra
  Caromed postaugmentation
  postaugmentation mammoplasty
  The Bandeau postaugmentation
Braasch bulb with whistle catheter tip
BRACAnalysis genetic susceptibility test
brachial palsy
brachial plexus injury
brachiosubclavian bridge graft fistula (BSGF)
Brachmann-de Lange syndrome
Bracht maneuver
brachycephaly
brachypellic pelvis
BrachySeed iodine-125 (^{125}I seeds
BrachySeed palladium-103 (^{103}Pd) seeds
brachytherapy
  afterloading
  CT-guided
  episcleral plaque
  intraoperative high dose rate (IOHDR)
  palladium 103 (^{103}Pd) implantation
  permanent
  remote afterloading
  Syed-Neblett
  Symmetra ^{125}I seed
BrachyVision software for brachytherapy
brackish water
Bradley method
bradycardia
  fetal
  intrapartum fetal
  marked fetal
  maternal
  mild fetal
bradyspermatism
bradyuria
brain stem death
Bralon braided nylon suture
branch
  lateral mammary
  ureteral
  ureteric
branched calculus
branched chain ketonuria
brancher deficiency
branchial cleft anomaly
branchio-oculofacial syndrome
branchio-otorenal (BOR) syndrome
Brandt-Andrews maneuver
Brandt syndrome
brandywine-type dentinogenesis imperfecta
Branham sign
Brantley-Scott penile implant
Braun episiotomy scissors
Brava breast enhancement system
Braxton Hicks contractions

Brazelton Neonatal Behavioral
  Assessment scale
BRCA (breast cancer [gene]) mutation
BRCA1 breast cancer susceptibility
  gene
BRCA2 breast cancer susceptibility
  gene
breakdown of perineum
breaking water
breakpoint
breakthrough bleeding
breast
  accessory
  areola of
  atrophic
  bed of
  body of
  caked
  Cooper ligaments of
  crablike lesion of
  cystic
  cystic disease of
  dense
  ductal ectasia of
  estrogen-dependent adenocarcinoma
    of
  fat necrosis of
  fibroadenoma of
  fibroadenosis of
  fibrocystic
  fibrocystic disease of
  fibrosclerosis of
  hypertrophy of
  induration of
  inferior pedicle of
  infiltrating ductal carcinoma of
  ipsilateral
  irritable
  isolated clustered calcifications of
  lactating
  linguine sign in
  lobular carcinoma of
  lumpectomy of
  lumpiness in

breast *(cont.)*
  lymphangitis of
  male
  massive pubertal hypertrophy of
  medullary carcinoma of
  microcalcifications of
  mobilization of
  neoplasm
  nonpuerperal abscess of
  peau d'orange appearance of
  pendulous
  periodic fibroadenosis of
  periprosthetic capsulectomy of
  proemial
  ptosis of
  puerperal abscess of
  retraction of skin of
  sagging of
  scirrhous carcinoma of
  sclerosing adenosis of
  sebaceous cyst of
  segmental fibroadenosis of
  shoemaker's
  shotty
  solitary cyst of
  subinvolution of
  superficial infection of the
  suspensory ligaments of
  tail of
  thickening in
  thrombophlebitis of
breast abscess
  nonpuerperal
  puerperal
BreastAlert differential temperature
  sensor (DTS)
breast artifact
breast asymmetry
breast atrophy
breast attenuation
breast augmentation (see *mammoplasty*)
breast augmentation mammoplasty by
  injection (BAMBI)

breast binder, Expand-A-Band
breast binding
breast biopsy
  Lorad StereoGuide stereotactic
  Mammotest
  MIBB
  mirror image
  MRI-guided
  negative
  percutaneous excisional (PEBB)
  SiteSelect percutaneous
  Sonopsy 3-D ultrasound
  stereotactic needle
breast bolster
breast bone or breastbone
breast budding
breast calcifications
breast cancer
  cystosarcoma phyllodes
  family history of
  hormone-sensitive metastatic
  inflammatory
  in situ
  intraductal
  invasive
  male
  metastatic
  neovascularization in human
  Paget disease
  sigmaS serum tumor marker for
breast cancer genes
  BRCA1
  BRCA2
breast cancer metastasis
Breast Cancer Prevention Trial
breast cancer survival rates, Berkson-Gage calculation of
breast cancer tumor marker (see *tumor marker*)
breast carcinoma (see *breast cancer*)
BreastCheck device for breast examination
BreastCheck handheld electronic device
breast contour
breast core biopsy specimen
breast cyst
breast degeneration
breast diagnostic system, Alexa 1000 noninvasive breast
breast duct, stenosis of
breast engorgement in newborn
BreastExam device for breast cancer detection
breast examination
breast-fed baby
breast-feed
breast-feeding
breast fibroadenoma
breast fibrocystic disease
breast form (see *breast implant*; *prosthesis*)
breast fullness
breast hyperplasia
breast hypertrophy
breast hypoplasia
breast imaging
  Aurora MR system
  diffraction-enhanced
  Miraluma nuclear
Breast Imaging and Reporting Data System (BI-RADS) of the American College of Radiology
breast implant (see also *prosthesis*)
  adjustable saline
  Amoena
  asymmetrical
  Becker
  Becker tissue expander
  Belle-Amie
  Biocell RTV saline-filled
  BioDimensional
  calcified
  Contour Profile
  Cronin breast
  custom
  Discrene
  Dow Corning

breast implant *(cont.)*
encapsulated
explantation of
filled
gel-filled
Hartley
Leading Lady
McGhan
Mentor
moulage for custom
Nearly Me
NovaGold (PVP-hydrogel-based)
NovaSaline inflatable saline
NovaSaline pre-filled
Perras-Papillon
saline
silicone
silicone gel
Siltex silicone gel
Spectrum
Spenco
subcutaneous
submuscular
subpectoral
symmetrical
teardrop
3M
Trilucent
Trulife silicone
Yours Truly
breast implant insertion, delayed
breast induration
breast inflammation
breast lesion localizing grid device
breast lesion, needle localization of
breast-lift mastopexy
breast localizer
breast lump
breast marking system, Sadowsky
breast mass
benign
fat necrosis
fibroadenoma
malignant

breast mass *(cont.)*
painless
resected
sclerosing adenosis
solid
breast mass lesion with poorly defined margins
breast maturation
breast microcalcifications
breast milk jaundice
breast neoplasm
breast open periprosthetic capsulotomy
breast pain
breast parenchyma
breast prosthesis (see *breast implant*; *prosthesis*)
Amoena
asymmetrical
Becker tissue expander
Belle-Amie
CUI gel
CUI saline
Nearly Me
Perras
subpectoral
breast pump
Egnell
The Whittlestone Physiological Breastmilker
vacuum-type
breast reconstruction
fleur de lis pattern
free flap
Kiricuta
lateral transverse thigh flap or "saddle bags"
latissimus dorsi myocutaneous flap
rectus abdominis flap
Rubens flap
transverse rectus abdominis myocutaneous flap
breast reconstruction donor sites
breast reconstruction during mastectomy

breast reconstruction pocket
breast reduction (see *operation*)
  Lejour-type
  short-scar technique
  tumescent technique
  vertical pedicle technique
  wet technique
  wet technique with liposuction
breast reduction technique
breast self-examination (BSE)
breast self-examination aid, BD Sensability
breast shadow
breast skin changes
breast skin satellite metastasis
breast-sparing mastectomy
breast support dressing
breast surgery (see *operations*)
  BAMBI (breast augmentation mammoplasty by injection)
  "belly button" augmentation mammoplasty
  Kiricuta breast reconstruction
  L.I.F.T. (laser-assisted internal fabrication) technique
  lumpectomy
  Rubens flap for breast reconstruction
  SAMBA (simultaneous areolar mastopexy and breast augmentation)
  TUBA (transumbilical breast augmentation)
  WAMBA (Wise areola mastopexy breast augmentation)
breasts without masses or nipple discharge
breast symmetry
breast tenderness
breast thickened, without masses
breast thickening
breast thrombophlebitis
breast tissue, attenuation by
breast tumor
breast ultrasound
breech
  complete
  double-footling
  footling
  frank
  incomplete
  single-footling
breech baby
breech-born babies with delayed fetal activity
breech delivery
breech delivery total extraction
breech extraction
breech presentation of the fetus:
  sacroanterior (SA) position
  sacroposterior (SP) position
  sacrotransverse (ST) position
breed
breeding line
bregmatic fontanelle
Breisky-Navratil retractor
Brennen biosynthetic surgical mesh
Brenner tumor of ovary
brephoplastic
brephotrophic
Brescio-Cimino arteriovenous fistula for hemodialysis access
Brescia-Cimino shunt
Brethine (terbutaline)
BrevaRex monoclonal antibody
Brevicon oral contraceptive
Brevi-Kath epidural catheter
Brevinor 21 or 28 oral contraceptive
bRFS (biochemical relapse-free survival)
Bricanyl (terbutaline)
brick dust urine
Bricker ileal conduit
Bricker operation
Bricker ureteroileostomy
bridge-graft fistula (BGF)
Bridge X3 renal stent system
bridging cross

bridging, intrafimbrial
Bright disease
brim, pelvic
brim sign
bring the stone down
bris *or* briss
Brissaud infantilism
Brite-Life One Step pregnancy test
brittle bone disease
brittle diabetes mellitus
broad beta disease
broad casts
broad ligament abscess
broad ligament cyst
broad ligament endometriosis
broad ligament fibroid
broad ligament hematocele
broad ligament laceration syndrome
broad ligament polyp
broad ligament pregnancy
broad thumb-hallux syndrome
broad thumb syndrome
Broca pouch
brokering of a surrogacy arrangement
bromocriptine mesylate
bronchiectasis, congenital
bronchiolitis
bronchopulmonary dysplasia (BPD)
bronchospasm
bronze baby syndrome
bronze diabetes
bronze disease
Bronze-Schilder disease
Broviac catheter
brown baby syndrome
Brown-Buerger cystoscope
brown discharge
brown enamel, hereditary
brown pigmented granular casts
Brown-Sequard syndrome
Brown syndrome, congenital
brow presentation
Broxidine (broxuridine)
broxuridine
Brueghel syndrome
Bruel-Kjaer transvaginal ultrasound probe
Bruel-Kjaer ultrasound scanner
Bruhat maneuver for CO_2 laser surgery neosalpingostomy
bruising of cord
Brunn nests
Brunschwig total pelvic exenteration
brush
  Cragg hemodialysis thrombolytic
  Detect cytology
  endocervical
  OTW Thrombolytic
  Sklar Cervex (*not* Cervix)
  Zelsmyr Cytobrush
brush biopsy, Cell Recovery System (CRS)
Brushfield spots
bryostatin
BSA (body surface area)
BSE (breast self-examination)
BSGF (brachiosubclavian bridge graft fistula)
BSO (bilateral salpingo-oophorectomy)
BSU (Bartholin, Skene, and urethral) glands
BTA (bladder tumor assay)
BTA stat bladder tumor assay
BTA TRAK bladder tumor assay
BTK gene
bubble point
bubo (pl. buboes), fluctuant
buccal smear
Buck fascia
bud
Budd-Chiari syndrome
budding yeast cells
Buerger-Gruetz syndrome
buffer agents
buffer system
buffy coat smear

Bugbee electrode
bulbar stricture
bulbar urethra
bulbar urethral sling
bulbar urethral stricture
bulb, mucus aspiration
bulbocavernosus muscle
bulbocavernosus reflex
bulb of penis
bulbomembranous urethral stricture
bulbospongiosus muscle of penis
bulbourethral gland
bulbourethral gland abscess
bulbourethral gland duct
bulbourethral sling procedure
bulbous urethra
bulbous urethral stricture
bulb suctioning
bulb syringe
bulb-tip catheter
bulbus corporis spongiosi
bulbus urethrae
bulbus vestibuli vaginae
bulging anterior fontanel
bulging bag of waters
bulging membranes
bulimia
bulked segregant analysis
bulk laxatives
bulk selection
bulky dressing
bulky tumor
bulldog clamp
bulldog syndrome
bullet tip forceps
bullous appearance
bullous CIE (congenital ichthyosiform erythroderma)
bullous cystitis
bullous edema
bullous edema vesicae
bullous impetigo of newborn
bumetanide
Bumex (bumetanide)
Bumm uterine curette
BUN (blood urea nitrogen)
BUN/creatinine ratio
bundle
  neurovascular
  vascular
BUO (bilateral ureteral obstruction)
Burch bladder neck suspension procedure
Burch colposuspension for stress incontinence
Burch iliopectineal ligament urethrovesical suspension.
Burch laparoscopic procedure
Burch retropubic urethropexy
Burhenne steerable catheter
burial of testes
buried penis
buried testis
buried vaginal island
Burke cervical biopsy punch forceps
Burkitt lymphoma
burned-out endometriosis
burning
  urethral
  urinary
  vaginal
burning on urination
burning or pain on voiding
burning vulvar syndrome
burning when urine hits labia
burying of fimbriae in uterine wall
Buselmeier vascular access shunt for hemodialysis
BUS (Bartholin, urethral, and Skene) glands
BUS normal
Bush CL ureteral illuminating catheter
busulfan
butoconazole nitrate
butterfly breast shadow
butterfly rash

buttonhole puncture technique for hemodialysis needle insertion
buttonhole the skin
button, polypropylene
BV (bacterial vaginosis)
Byler disease
bypass mode of dialysis machine

C, c

C (complement)
C (cytosine)
Ca (calcium)
CA (cellulose) dialyzer
CAB (combined androgen blockade)
CAB (complete androgen blockade)
cabergoline
cable, FlexStrand
Cabot cystoscope
CAC (cervical access catheter)
cachectic-appearing
cachexia, primary
CADASIL (cerebral autosomal dominant arteriopathy with subcortical infarcts and leukoencephalopathy)
cadaver donor
cadaveric donation
cadaveric donor
cadaveric kidney
cadaveric transplant
CAF (Cytoxan, Adriamycin, fluorouracil) chemotherapy protocol
Cafcit (caffeine citrate) oral solution
café au lait spots
caffeine
caffeine citrate oral solution
CA 15-3 RIA (radioimmunoassay) serum tumor marker
CA 19-9 ovarian cancer test
CAFTH (Cytoxan, Adriamycin, fluorouracil, tamoxifen, Halotestin) chemotherapy protocol
CAH (congenital adrenal hyperplasia)
CAHP hemodialyzer
caked breast
cake kidney
cake layer
calcaneal vargus
calcaneovalgus
calcareous metastasis
calcariuria
calcification
  breast
  clustered
  linear
  malignant-type
  questionable
  suspicious
calcific density
calcified bladder
calcified bladder mass
calcified breast implants
calcified fetus

calcified mass
calcified outline of cyst
calcified phleboliths in pelvis
calcified uterine fibroid
Calcijex (calcitriol injection; vitamin D)
calcinosis
calcinosis circumscripta
calcinosis universalis
calcinuric diabetes
calciotropic hormones
calcitonin
  human
  piscine
  porcine
  salmon
calcitriol (serum 1,25-dihydroxyvitamin D3)
calcitriol injection
calcitriol production
calcium (Ca)
calcium carbonate
calcium, extraosseous deposit of
calcium gluconate
calcium homeostasis
calcium nephrolithiasis
calcium oxalate urolithiasis
calcium set point
calcium-vitamin D therapy
calciuria
calculation, Berkson-Gage
calculous anuria
calculous pyelitis
calculous pyelonephritis
calculus (pl. calculi) (see also *stone*)
  bladder
  branched
  dislodged
  encysted
  fibrin
  hard nodular urinary
  infection
  kidney
  mammary
  mulberry

calculus *(cont.)*
  nephritic
  nonopaque
  opaque
  oxalate
  primary renal
  primary vesical
  prostatic
  radiopaque vesical
  renal
  secondary renal
  staghorn renal
  stonelike
  ureteral
  urethral
  urinary tract
  uterine
  vesical
calculus colic
calculus disease
calculus in diverticulum of bladder
Calcutript lithotriptor
calendar rhythm method
CALF-E (Cytoxan, Adriamycin, leucovorin calcium, fluorouracil, ethinyl estradiol) chemotherapy protocol
Calgiswab calcium alginate swab
caliber of urinary stream
calibration, urethral
caliceal (also, calyceal)
caliceal deformity
caliceal dilation
caliceal diverticulum
caliceal drainage system
caliceal system
calicectomy
calices (also calyces)
  dilation of
  dilated
  major
  minor
  obstructed
calices tube
calicoplasty

calicotomy
caliectasis
calioplasty
caliorrhaphy
calix, calyx (pl. calices, calyces)
Call-Exner body
callosal agenesis
CALM II (computer-assisted labor monitoring)
calusterone
calyceal
Calymmatobacterium granulomatis
calyx (pl. calyces)
camera
  AMS endoview
  Endoview endoscopy
  Enview
  one-chip
  OptiVu HDVD (high definition video display)
  Stryker endoscopy one-chip
  Stryker endoscopy three-chip
  three-chip
Camey continent reservoir
Camey ileocystoplasty
Camey reservoir
Camey urinary pouch
cAMP (cyclic adenosine monophosphate)
  nephrogenous
  plasma
  urinary
Campath monoclonal antibody
Campbell radical retropubic prostatectomy
Campion forceps
camptodactyly-cleft palate-clubfoot
camptodactyly, facultative-type
camptodactyly-limited jaw excursion
camptodactyly-trismus syndrome
camptomelic dysplasia
Camurati-Englemann disease
Camptosar (irinotecan)
Campylobacter
Canadian Urology Oncology Group (CUOG) trials
canal
  Alcock
  birth
  cervical
  cervicouterine
  deferent
  endocervical
  fallopian
  inguinal
  Nuck
  obstetric
  pudendal
  vesicourethral
canalization, wire guide
canal of Nuck
Canasa (mesalamine)
Canavan disease
C-ANCA, cANCA (cytoplasmic staining pattern of ANCA)
canceled cycle
cancer (see *carcinoma*)
Candida albicans
Candida glabrata
Candida test
candidal balanoposthitis
candidal vulvovaginitis
candidate gene
candidiasis
  disseminated
  hematogenously disseminated
  genital
  neonatal
  primary renal
  vaginal
  vulvovaginal
candiduria, covert asymptomatic
Candistat-G
Candistroy (herbal remedy for candidiasis)
candle, vaginal
C&S (culture and sensitivity)
candy-cane stirrups

cannula (see also *catheter*)
  acorn
  aspiration
  Cohen
  Cohen/Jarcho
  Core cannula system
  DeRoyal surgical
  EndoTIP
  evacuating
  Gyne-Flo Leventhal
  Hasson
  Hasson blunt-end
  Hasson intrauterine
  Hasson laparoscopy
  Hasson SAC (stable-access cannula)
  Humi inflatable uterine
  Iotec flexible
  Jacobs
  Jarcho
  LaparoSac single-use
  Leventhal Gyne-Flo
  Margolin HSG (hysterosalpingography)
  MultAport
  Reuter
  Rubin
Cantrell-Haller-Ravich syndrome
Cantrell pentalogy
Cantrell syndrome
CA-125 (cancer antigen-125)
CA-170 (cellulose) dialyzer
cap
  CranioCap for infants
  endoscopic
  Oves cervical
  Oves conception
  Oves fertility
capacitation
capacity, functional bladder
CaP CURE (association for cure of prostate cancer)
CaP CURE Gene and Family Studies Consortium
CAPD (continuous ambulatory peritoneal dialysis)
capecitabine
capillary epithelial cell
capillary fill
capillary flow dialyzer
capillary sludging
Capio CL transvaginal suture-capturing device
Capoten (captopril)
CAPS (cleaved amplified polymorphic sequence)
capsula glomeruli
capsular contracture following breast reconstruction
capsular fibers of prostate
capsular flap pyeloplasty
capsular tear
capsule
  Bowman
  breast implant
  fatty renal
  glomerular
  multicystic ovaries with thickened
  prostatic
CapSure continence shield
captopril renography
Capture-S test for syphilis
caput medusae
caput succedaneum
carbamyl phosphate synthetase (CPS) deficiency
carbohydrate deficient glycoprotein syndrome (CDGS)
carboxylase deficiency, multiple
carbimazole
carbohydrate depletion
carbon dioxide gas (CO_2)
carbon dioxide pressure
carboplatin/docetaxel chemotherapy regimen
carbuncle of corpus cavernosum
carbuncle of kidney

carbuncle of penis
carbuncle of vulva
carcinoembryonic antigen (CEA)
carcinogen, urinary
carcinoma (also *cancer, sarcoma, tumor*)
  adenocystic
  angiosarcoma of vulva
  Bartholin gland
  Bellini duct
  bladder
  breast
  cervical
  "chimney sweep's" of skin of scrotum
  cutaneous metastatic breast
  cystic
  ductal transitional cell of prostate
  Dukes (*not* Duke's)
  embryonal
  endometrial
  endometrioid
  epidermoid
  epithelial ovarian
  familial breast
  genital
  glans
  hereditary papillary renal
  hereditary prostate
  hormone-sensitive breast
  hypernephroid
  infiltrating duct
  inflammatory breast
  intraductal
  intraepithelial endometrial
  invasive
  invasive bladder
  invasive squamous cell
  kidney
  large cell
  leiomyosarcoma vulvar
  liposarcoma vulvar
  lobular
  malignant fibrous histiocytoma vulvar

carcinoma *(cont.)*
  malignant melanoma vulvar
  mucinous
  node-negative breast
  noninfiltrating lobular
  noninvasive
  nonpapillary renal cell (RCC)
  occult cervical
  ovarian
  pelvic
  penile
  prostate
  prostatic
  renal
  renal cell
  renal pelvic urothelial
  rhabdomyosarcoma vulvar
  schistosomal bladder
  spiculated breast
  squamous cell
  superficial bladder
  testicular
  urethral
  urothelial
  uterine cervix
  uterine corpus
  vaginal
  vulvar
carcinoma in situ (CIS)
  ductal (DCIS)
  lobular (LCIS)
  squamous cell
  urothelial
carcinoma in situ of cervix
carcinoma in situ of penis
carcinoma-specific monoclonal antibody
carcinosarcoma
cardiac apnea monitor
cardiac decompensation
cardiac diuretic
cardiac hemodynamics, altered
cardinal ligament
cardioauditory syndrome

cardiofaciocutaneous syndrome
cardiomegalia glycogenica diffusa
cardiomyopathy
cardiomyopathy-neutropenia syndrome
cardiomyopathy, postpartum
cardionephric
cardiorespiratory distress syndrome
cardiovascular stress
cardiovascular syphilis
CARDS Q.S. hCG serum/urine
care, kangaroo
Carignan syndrome
Carlesta skin treatment for urinary incontinence
CARMEN (cryoablation reduction of menstruation) procedure
C-arm fluoroscope
Carnation Follow-Up Formula
Carnation Good Start infant formula
carneous degeneration
carneous mole
carnitine deficiency, hereditary
carnitine palmitoyl transferase deficiency (CPT)
carnosinemia
Caroli disease
Caromed postaugmentation bra
carotene
carotenemia
carpal tunnel syndrome
carpenter syndrome
CarraVex injectable
carrier
carrier complexation
carrier complexation coefficient
carrier deactivation
carrier detection
carrier frequency
carrier leaching
carrier-mediated (facilitated) separations
carrier-mediated (facilitated) transport
carrier protein
carrier screening
carrier status
carrier testing
carryover of tumor cells in marrow inoculum
Carson endo-electrosurgical set
Carter-Thomason suture passer
cartilage
    avulsion of inner symphyseal
    inner symphyseal
    symphyseal
cartilage-derived inhibitor (CDI)
cartilage-hair hypoplasia
caruncle of labia
caruncle, urethral
cascade, metastatic
cascade of events
casein hydrolysate infant formula
CASH (classic abdominal Semm hysterectomy)
Casodex (bicalutamide)
Casser fontanelle
castration
    female
    functional prepubertal
    male
    medical
    radiotherapeutic
    surgical
castration complex
castration plus anti-androgen therapy
casts
    bacterial
    blood
    broad
    brown pigmented granular
    coma
    decidual
    endometrial
    epithelial cell
    fatty
    granular
    hemoglobin
    hyaline
    miscellaneous
    mixed

casts *(cont.)*
- pigmented
- plain
- RBC (red blood cell)
- red blood cell (RBC)
- red cell
- renal
- tube
- tubular cell
- urinary
- waxy
- WBC

casts in urine
catabolism
- endogenous protein
- increased protein

Cataflam (diclofenac)
catamenia
cataplexy
cat cry syndrome
catecholamines
Catel-Manzke syndrome
cathepsin D lysozoma enzyme
catheter (see also *cannula*)
- Abscession fluid drainage
- acorn-tipped
- Angiocath
- angle-tip
- antibacterial Foley
- Antibacterial Personal Catheter
- Argyle umbilical vessel
- Asch intrauterine
- Aspiracath
- Baggish aspiration
- balloon
- Bardex I.C.
- BD Insyte Autoguard shielded IV
- BD Insyte Autoguard-P shielded IV
- Bio-Flex CS
- Bonanno suprapubic
- Brevi-Kath epidural
- bulb-tip
- Burhenne steerable
- Bush DL ureteral illuminating

catheter *(cont.)*
- CathLink 20 port system with ChronoFlex
- Caud-A-Kath epidural
- ChronoFlex polyurethane
- coaxial
- color-coded
- Comfort Cath I or II
- Conceptus fallopian tube
- Conceptus Soft Seal cervical
- Conceptus Soft Torque uterine
- Conceptus VS (variable softness)
- cone-tip
- ContiCath
- Cook-Cope loop suprapubic
- Cook cystotomy
- Cook hysteroscopic
- Cook silicone balloon HSG
- Cook tissue morcellator
- coudé
- Councill
- Cystocath
- cystotomy
- Dale Foley
- Deltec long-term dual-lumen hemodialysis
- DeOrio intrauterine insemination
- Derrick intrauterine insemination
- Dewan intrauterine insemination
- dialysis
- DiMattina laparoscopic
- directable coaxial
- Dorros brachial internal mammary guiding
- double-cuff dialysis
- double-J indwelling
- double-J ureteral
- double-lumen femoral vein
- double-lumen subclavian vein
- double-lumen venous umbilical
- double-pigtail ureteral
- Duo-Flow dual-lumen
- Du Pen epidural
- E-cath tunneled epidural

catheter *(cont.)*
- Echosight Jansen-Anderson intrauterine
- Echosight Patton coaxial
- Embryon GIFT transfer
- Embryon HSG (hysterosalpingography/hysterosonography)
- epidural
- epididymal aspiration
- female
- Feth-R-Kath epidural
- Firlit-Sugar intermittent
- Flexi-Tip ureteral
- Flexxicon Blue dialysis
- Flexxicon dialysis
- Foley
- Foley three-way
- Foley ureteral
- F-series insemination
- Garceau tapered
- Gazelle balloon dilation
- Gesco umbilical
- Gleicher salpingography
- Goldstein sonohysterography
- Groshong
- GyneSys cervical access
- GyneSys Dx diagnostic
- GyneSys guidewire
- GyneSys uterine cornual access
- GyneSys uterine ostial access
- Haas intrauterine insemination
- HealthShield wound drainage
- heat-transmitting balloon
- Hemo-Cath
- Hickman
- HSG (hysterosalpingography)
- HUMI uterine
- Hurwitz dialysis
- hysterosalpingography/hysterosonography (H/S or HSG)
- I-Cath
- illuminating
- indwelling urinary bladder
- In-Flow intraurethral valved

catheter *(cont.)*
- Insemi-Cath
- Intran disposable intrauterine pressure management
- intrauterine
- intrauterine injection
- intrauterine pressure
- Jansen-Anderson intrauterine
- Katayama hysteroscopic
- KDF-2.3 intrauterine
- Kish urethral illuminated
- KISS (kidney internal splint/stent)
- Koala intrauterine pressure
- Labcath
- Lawrence SupraFoley
- Leung coaxial
- Loc-Sure single-pass
- Malecot
- MammoSite RTS (radiation therapy system)
- Marrs intrauterine
- Marrs laparoscopic
- Meostar hemodialysis
- nephrostomy balloon
- nephrostomy-type
- Niagara temporary dialysis
- nitrofuran delivery
- Norfolk intrauterine
- Novy cornual cannulation
- Oligon Foley
- olive-tipped
- On-Command
- open-end ureteral
- Opticon
- Opti-Flow
- Opti-Plast XT balloon
- Oreopoulos-Zellerman peritoneal dialysis
- Ott intrauterine
- paracervical instillation
- Patton laparoscopic
- PBN hysterosalpingography
- P.D. Access over-the-needle
- peripherally inserted central (PICC)

catheter *(cont.)*
PermaCath dual-lumen
Philips
pigtail ureteral
Pipelle endometrial suction
Pollack open-end Flexi-Tip ureteral
PolyFlo peripherally inserted central
polyurethane pail-handle coiled-tip peritoneal dialysis
porous polyethylene dialysis
Port-A-Cath
Privet coaxial
prostatic
Quinton
Quinton Mahurkar dual-lumen hemodialysis
Quinton PermCath vascular access
rectal pressure
red Robinson
red rubber
Release-NF (nitrofurazone Foley)
Reliance urinary control insert
Rentrop infusion
retrograde urethrogram
Robinson straight urethral
Rosch-Thurmond fallopian tube
Royal women's coaxial
Rutner percutaneous suprapubic balloon
self-retaining
Seroma-Cath wound drainage
S.E.T. hemodialysis
Shapiro intrauterine insemination
Shepard intrauterine insemination
Sholkoff balloon hysterosalpingography
Silastic
Silber aspiration
silicone
silicone Foley
silicone Malecot
single-cuff dialysis
single-lumen femoral vein
single-lumen subclavian vein

catheter *(cont.)*
SMS coaxial
Sof-Flex loop suprapubic
Soft-Cell
soft coaxial
Soft-Pass laparoscopic
Soft Seal cervical
Soft Seal transcervical balloon
soft silicone rubber dialysis
Soft Torque uterine
Solera thrombectomy
Soules intrauterine insemination
Spectrum silicone Foley
SPI-Argent II peritoneal dialysis
spiral-tip
Spirtos coaxial
Stamey-Malecot
Stargate falloposcopy
SupraFoley
suprapubic
suprapubic urodynamic
surgically implanted hemodialysis
Swan-Ganz
Talon balloon dilation
Targis
Tefcat intrauterine
Tenacath HSG (hysterosalpingography)
Tenckhoff peritoneal dialysis
Tenckhoff silicone
Tesio hemodialysis access
three-way
Tis-U-Trap endometrial suction
transcervical
transcervical tubal access (T-TAC)
triple-lumen umbilical
T-TAC (transcervical tubal access)
UCAC (uterine cornual access)
Uldall (*not* Udall) subclavian hemodialysis
UMB-E umbilical
umbilical artery (UAC)
Umbili-Cath Tecoflex umbilical
UOAC (uterine ostial access)

catheter *(cont.)*
Ureflex ureteral
Ureflex urethral
ureteral (with an olive-shaped tip)
urethral
urodynamic loop
UroLume flow-directed
UroMax II urethral balloon
UroQuest On-Command
uterine cornual access (UCAC)
uterine ostial access (UOAC)
van Andel
Vas-Cath
Vas-Cath Flexxicon II
Vas-Cath Opti-Flow long-term dual-lumen hemodialysis
Vas-Cath Soft-Cell permanent dual-lumen hemodialysis
Vector
Vector X
Werlin-Ishida coaxial
whistle-tip ureteral
Xpeedior
catheter à demeure
catheter-associated urinary tract infection (CAUTI)
catheter drainage
catheter guide, Mandrin
catheter holder, Dale Foley
catheter insertion set, Neo-Sert umbilical vessel
catheter introducer
Bard Safety Excaliber
Foley
catheterization
clean intermittent bladder (CIC)
Foley
hysteroscopic selective
intermittent self-catheterization
periodic intermittent
retrograde ureteral
self
straight
suprapubic
catheterize
catheterized urine
catheterized urine specimen
catheter plug
catheter-related infection
catheter tip
acorn
Blassuchi curved
Braasch bulb with whistle
cone
flexible filiform
olive
round
ureteral
whistle
CathLink 20 port system with ChronoFlex catheter
CathTrack catheter locator system
cation-exchange membrane
cation-exchange resin
CAT (computerized axial tomography) scan
CA27.29 antigen (breast cancer) tumor marker
CA-210 (cellulose dialyzer)
cauda equina syndrome with neurogenic bladder
caudad
Caud-A-Kath epidural catheter
caudal anesthesia
caudal dysgenesis
caudal regression syndrome
cause
constitutional
exciting
necessary
precipitating
predisposing
proximate
specific
sufficient
cauterization
cauterization of cervix
cauterize

cautery
  BiLAP
  bipolar
  cryocautery
  electrocautery
  Electroloop
  SingleBAR electrode
  wet-field
cautery conization
CAUTI (catheter-associated urinary tract infection)
Caverject (prostaglandin E1, PGE1, alprostadil)
CaverMap surgical device
cavernitis
cavernosa, corpora
cavernosal dilation
cavernosphenous shunt
cavernoso spongiosum shunt
cavernosography
cavernosometry
cavernosum, corpus (pl. corpora cavernosa)
cavernotome
cavernous body of clitoris
cavernous body of penis
cavernous hemangioma
cavernous nerves of clitoris
cavernous nerves of penis
CAVH (continuous arteriovenous hemofiltration)
CAVHD (continuous arteriovenous hemodialysis)
cavitary mass
Cavitron ultrasonic aspirator (CUSA)
cavity (pl. cavities)
  abdominal
  amnionic
  amniotic
  bladder
  blastocyst
  endometrial
  epamniotic
  pelvic
cavity *(cont.)*
  peritoneal
  pyramidal
  uterine
  vaginal
  wound
cavity prostatitis
cavography
Cayler syndrome
CBC (complete blood count)
CBG (cord blood gases)
C-bloc continuous nerve block system
CBP (chronic bacterial prostatitis)
CBP (cyclophosphamide, cisplatin, carmustine) chemotherapy protocol
CC (creatinine clearance)
CCAAT box (a genetic sequence)
CCMS (cerebrocostomandibular syndrome)
CCPD (continuous cycler peritoneal dialysis)
CCPD (continuous cyclical peritoneal dialysis)
CCUP (colpocystourethropexy)
CDAC (*Clostridium difficile*-associated diarrhea)
CDC (The Centers for Disease Control and Prevention)
Cdc2L1-2 gene
CDGS (carbohydrate deficient glycoprotein syndrome)
CDH (congenital diaphragmatic hernia)
CDK (congenital dislocation of knee)
CDI (cartilage-derived inhibitor)
CDL1 gene region
CdLS (Cornelia de Lange syndrome)
cDNA (complementary DNA)
cDNA library
CDP (continuous distending pressure)
CDUS (color-flow Doppler ultrasound)
CEA (carcinoembryonic antigen)
CEA-Cide (^{131}I-labeled humanized antibody against carcinoembryonic antigen)

CEA-Tc 99m carcinoembryonic antigen
CEB (carboplatin, etoposide, bleomycin) chemotherapy protocol
cebocephaly
Cecil urethroplasty
cecoureterocele
cecum
CEF (Cytoxan, epirubicin, fluorouracil) chemotherapy protocol
cefadroxil
cefazolin sodium
cefepime
Cefobid (cefoperazone)
cefpodoxime proxetil
ceftazidime
ceftriaxone
celiac disease
celiac ganglion
celiac plexus
celiac sprue
celioblastoma
celiotomy, vaginal
cell
    anaplastic spindle
    androgen-independent
    atretic
    budding yeast
    ciliated
    clue
    collecting duct
    convoluted tubular
    cytotoxic T
    cytotrophoblast
    dead
    desquamated
    dysmorphic red blood
    egg
    exfoliated
    fetal squamous
    fetouterine
    genital tract
    germ
    glomerular capillary endothelial
    glomerular epithelial

cell *(cont.)*
    granulosa
    HeLa
    helper T
    hilus
    insulin-secreting
    interstitial
    islet (*not* eyelet)
    Leydig
    male germ
    mast
    mesangial
    mesenchymal core
    nucleated
    nurse
    parafollicular
    perivascular decidualized stromal
    phagocytic
    polymorphonuclear leukocyte
    primordial germ
    renal
    Sertoli
    shedding of
    syncytial
    T
    theca
    thyroid "C"
    trophoblast
    tubular
    umbrella
    universal donor
    vascular endothelial
    von Hansemann
    well-differentiated, with keratinization
CellCept (mycophenolate mofetil [MMF])
cell contact
cell cycle
cell division
cell energetics
cell-mediated (delayed) immune reaction
cell-mediated immune inflammation

Cell Recovery System (CRS) brush biopsy
cell surface markers
cellular components and plasma
cellular debris, blockage from
cellular defense mechanisms
cellular inclusion bodies
cellular invasion
cellular proliferation
cellular senescence in vitro
cellular swelling
cellule formation
cellules and diverticula
cellulitis
  corpus cavernosum
  pelvic
  penile
  periurethral
  seminal vesical
  vaginal
  vaginal cuff
  vulvar
cellulose-based filters
cellulose-based intermittent hemodialysis filters
Celsior organ preservation solution
Cenestin (synthetic conjugated estrogen)
Cenogen-OB prenatal formula
Centara (priliximab)
Centers for Disease Control and Prevention, The (CDC)
centimorgan (cM)
central apnea
central cone technique reduction mammoplasty
central core disease
central dogma
central hypoventilation syndrome, congenital
central laceration
centrally uninhibited bladder
central neurofibromatosis (NF2)
central nervous system (CNS)
central pelvic pain
central placenta previa
central technique of mastopexy
central venous catheter (CVC)
central venous line
central venous pressure (CVP) line
centrifuge
centrifuged urine sediment
centromere interference
Centrysystem 3 hemodialyzer
CEP (congenital erythropoietic porphyria)
cephalad
cephalhematoma (also cephalohematoma)
cephalhydrocele (also cephalohydrocele)
cephalic delivery
cephalic disorders
cephalic pole
cephalic presentation
cephalic presentation of the fetus
  frontoanterior (FA) position
  mentoanterior (MA) position
  mentoposterior (MP) position
  mentotransverse (MT) position
  occipitoanterior (OA) position
  occipitotransverse (OT) position
cephalic vein
cephalic version
cephalopelvic disproportion (CPD)
cephalosporin
cephalotome
cephalotomy
cephalotribe
CEPRATE SC (stem cell) concentration system
Ceprate TCD T-cell depletion system
c-erb B-2 oncogene
cerclage
  cervical
  McDonald cervical
  Shirodkar cervical
  transabdominal cervicoisthmic (TCIC)

cerclage cabling system, Tylok
cerclage of incompetent cervix uteri
cerclage of isthmus uteri
cerebellar agenesis
cerebellar aplasia
cerebellar hemiagenesis
cerebellar hypoplasia
cerebellar hypoplasia
cerebellar syndrome
cerebellomedullary malformation syndrome
cerebello-oculocutaneous telangiectasia
cerebellopontive angle tumor
cerebelloretinal hemangioblastomatosis
cerebral anoxia
cerebral depression
cerebral diplegia
cerebral edema
cerebral gigantism
cerebral hemorrhage
cerebral hernia
cerebral infarction
cerebral irritability in newborn
cerebral palsy (CP)
cerebral venous thrombosis
cerebrocostomandibular syndrome (CCMS)
cerebrohepatorenal syndrome (CHRS)
cerebro-oculofacioskeletal (COFS) syndrome
cerebro-oculorenal dystrophy
cerebroside lipidosis
cerebrospinal fluid (CSF)
cerebrovascular accident (CVA)
cerebrovascular ferrocalcinosis
Certican (everolimus)
Certified Nurse Midwife (CNM)
Cerveillance cervical scope
Cerveillance vaginal scope
Cervex-Brush
cervical amputation
cervical atrophy
cervical atypism
cervical biopsy
cervical bleeding
cervical bleeding on contact
cervical canal
cervical cancer
cervical cancer test, ThinPrep and ThinPrep 2000
cervical cancer treatment,
cervical cap
cervical cerclage
  McDonald
  Shirodkar
  transabdominal cervicoisthmic (TCIC)
cervical change
cervical collar
cervical cone biopsy
cervical congestion
cervical conization
cervical cryoconization
cervical cryosurgery
cervical culture
cervical cytology
cervical cytology collecting device, Accel Combi biosampler
cervical dilation
cervical dilation with laminaria
cervical dilator
cervical dysplasia
cervical dysplasia to exocervical margins
cervical edema
cervical effacement
cervical endometriosis
cervical erosion
cervical eversion
cervical fibroid
cervical fistula
cervical ganglion
cervical gel
cervical glands of uterus
cervical Gram stain
cervical hypoplasia
cervical incompetence
cervical incompetency

cervical intraepithelial neoplasia (CIN)
cervical isthmus
cervical laceration
cervical malignancy
cervical motion tenderness
cervical mucus, abnormal
cervical mucus penetration test
cervical mucus viscosity
cervical neoplasia
cervical os, incompetent
cervical polyp
cervical pregnancy
cervical punch biopsy
cervical ripening, Bishop score of
cervical smear
cervical spasm
cervical stenosis
cervical stump
cervical tearing
cervical tissue obtained by scrapings
cervical vascularity
cervicectomy
cervicitis
    chlamydial
    chronic
    gonorrheal
    granulomatous
    hypertrophic
    nongonococcal mucopurulent
    recurrent
    traumatic
cervicitis with ectropion
cervicography
cervico-oculoacoustic syndrome
cervicoplasty
cervicosigmoid fistulectomy
cervicotomy
cervicouterine canal
cervicovaginal antibody
cervicovaginal fistula
cervicovaginal junction
cervicovaginal ridge
cervicovesical fistula
Cervidil (dinoprostone)
cervigram
cervitome
cervix (pl. cervices)
    adenocarcinoma in situ (AIS) of
    adenomatous polyp of
    adhesions of
    anaplasia of
    anterior lip of
    atresia of
    atrophy of
    bands of
    carcinoma in situ of
    carcinoma of
    cicatricial
    cicatrix of
    closed
    cockscomb
    conization of
    contracture of
    dilation of
    dysplasia of
    effacement of
    elongated
    elongation of
    eversion of
    hypertrophic
    hypertrophic elongation of
    incompetent
    long
    mucous polyp of
    multiparous
    nulliparous
    occlusion of
    open
    parous
    posterior lip of the
    rigid
    stenosis of
    stenotic
    strawberry
    stricture of
    supravaginal part of
    tapiroid
    unfavorable

cervix *(cont.)*
  uterine
  vaginal part of
  well-epithelialized
  cervix clean
cervix closed
cervix exquisitely tender to palpation
cervix fingertip dilated
cervix 4+ tender to motion
cervix grasped and retracted
cervix is clean
cervix is closed and long
cervix is well epithelialized
cervix of uterus
cervix protrudes through the os
cervix reaches the introitus
cervix serially dilated
cervix showing radiation changes
cervix uteri
  cerclage of incompetent
  excision of
cervix vesicae
cesarean birth
cesarean hysterectomy
cesarean operation
cesarean section (C-section) delivery
  classical
  "crash"
  corporeal
  elective
  extraperitoneal
  Latzko
  low cervical
  lower segment
  lower uterine segment transverse
  low transverse
  low vertical
  Munro Kerr
  Porro
  primary
  repeat
  supravesical
  transperitoneal
  transperitoneal classical

cesarean section *(cont.)*
  transverse
  vaginal
  Walters extraperitoneal
cesium
cesium application to cervix
cesium implant
cessation of menses
cessation of urinary output
cetrorelix
Cetrotide (cetrorelix)
CF (cystic fibrosis)
CFC (cardiofaciocutaneous) syndrome
CFTR gene associated with cystic fibrosis
CFC BioScanner System implantable blood glucose monitor
C567 (chemotactic factor)
c-fos oncogene
CFU (colony-forming unit)
CG (chorionic gonadotropin)
CGA (chromogranin A)
CGP (chorionic growth hormone-prolactin)
CH (crown-heel) length
Chadwick sign of pregnancy
chair, birthing
Chamberlen forceps
chancre, extragenital
chancroid
chandelier sign
change (pl. changes)
  atrophic
  cervical
  fatty
  pelvicaliceal
  harlequin color
  hormone-stimulated endometrial
  nipple
change in baseline temperature
change of life (menopause)
channel, lymphatic
char
character

characteristics
  primary sex
  secondary sex
charcoal
Charcot-Marie-Tooth (CMT) disease
CHARGE (coloboma of the eye, heart defects, atresia of the choanae, retardation of growth and development, genital and urinary anomalies, ear anomalies) association
charge nurse
charge-selective barrier
Charnin-Dorfman syndrome
Chaussier sign
CHAV (continuous arteriovenous hemodiafiltration)
Cheatle syndrome
Check-Flo adapter
Check-Flo valve
Check-Flo suprapubic urinary probe
Chediak-Higashi syndrome
cheesy discharge
cheesy material
cheilitis granulomatosa
Chemet (succimer)
chemical abortion
chemical analysis of stone
chemical base
chemical composition of ECF
chemical dissolution of uric acid calculi
chemically distinct layers
chemical luminescent testing
chemically multifunctional material
chemical pregnancy
chemstrip
chemolysis
chemoprevention
chemopreventive agent
chemotactic factor (C567)
chemotherapy
  adjuvant
  combination
  multi-drug
  multi-drug systemic

chemotherapy *(cont.)*
  nuclear matrix-based
  preoperative
  primary
  systemic
  ThermoChem-HT system
chemotherapy protocol
  AFM (Adriamycin, fluorouracil, methotrexate)
  BEMP (bleomycin, Eldisine, mitomycin, Platinol)
  BEP (bleomycin, etoposide, Platinol)
  BIP (bleomycin, ifosfamide, Platinol)
  BOP (bleomycin, Oncovin, Platinol)
  CAF (cyclophosphamide, Adriamycin, fluorouracil)
  CAF (Cytoxan, Adriamycin, fluorouracil)
  CAFTH (cyclophosphamide, Adriamycin, fluorouracil, tamoxifen, Halotestin)
  CAFTH (Cytoxan, Adriamycin, fluorouracil, tamoxifen, Halotestin)
  CALF-E (Cytoxan, Adriamycin, leucovorin calcium, ethinyl estradiol)
  CEB (carboplatin, etoposide, bleomycin)
  CEF (cyclophosphamide, epirubicin, fluorouracil)
  CEF (Cytoxan, epirubicin, fluorouracil)
  CMFP (cyclophosphamide, methotrexate, fluorouracil, prednisone)
  CMFPT (cyclophosphamide, methotrexate, fluorouracil, prednisone, tamoxifen)
  CMFPTH (Cytoxan, methotrexate, fluorouracil, prednisone, tamoxifen, Halotestin)

chemotherapy protocol *(cont.)*
- CMFVP (cyclophosphamide, methotrexate, fluorouracil, vincristine, and prednisone)
- CMFVP (Cytoxan, methotrexate, fluorouracil, vincristine, and prednisone)
- COF/COM (Cytoxan, Oncovin, fluorouracil + Cytoxan, Oncovin, methotrexate)
- CTCb (Cytoxan, thiotepa, carboplatin)
- E-MVAC (escalated methotrexate, vinblastine, Adriamycin, cisplatin or Cytoxan)
- FCAP (fluorouracil, cyclophosphamide, Adriamycin, Platinol)
- FCAP (fluorouracil, Cytoxan, Adriamycin, Platinol)
- FEC (fluorouracil, epirubicin, cyclophosphamide)
- FNM (fluorouracil, Novantrone, methotrexate)
- H-CAP (hexamethylmelamine, Cytoxan, Adriamycin, Platinol)
- MCV (methotrexate, cisplatin, vinblastine)
- MVAC or M-VAC (methotrexate, vincristine, Adriamycin, cisplatin)
- MVF (mitoxantrone, vincristine, fluorouracil)
- STAMP V (cyclophosphamide, thiotepa, carboplatin [CTCb])
- TEMP (tamoxifen, etoposide, mitoxantrone, Platinol)
- VAB-6
- VAC (vinblastine, actinomycin D, Cytoxan)
- VACA (vinblastine, actinomycin D, Cytoxan, Adriamycin)
- VACAD (vincristine, Adriamycin, Cytoxan, actinomycin D, dacarbazine)

chemotherapy protocol *(cont.)*
- VACP (VePesid, Adriamycin, Cytoxan, Platinol)
- VAD (vincristine, Adriamycin, dexamethasone)
- VAD/V (vincristine, Adriamycin, dexamethasone, verapamil)
- VAI (vincristine, actinomycin D, ifosfamide)
- VALOP-B (etoposide, doxorubicin, cyclophosphamide, vincristine, prednisone, and bleomycin)
- VAM (VP-16, Adriamycin, methotrexate)
- VBMCP (vincristine, BCNU, melphalan, Cytoxan, prednisone)
- VBMF (vincristine, bleomycin, methotrexate, fluorouracil)
- VBP (vinblastine, bleomycin, cisplatin)
- VeIP (vinblastine, ifosfamide, Platinol)
- VIC (vinblastine, ifosfamide, CCNU)
- VIE (vincristine, ifosfamide, etoposide)
- VIP (VePesid, ifosfamide, Platinol)
- VIP (VePesid, ifosfamide [with mesna rescue], Platinol)
- VIP-B (VP-16, ifosfamide, Platinol, bleomycin)
- VPCA (vincristine, prednisone, Cytoxan, ara-C)

chemotherapy regimen
Chemstrip bG
Chemstrip MatchMaker blood glucose monitor
Cheron dressing forceps
CHESS (comprehensive health enhancement support system) for breast cancer patients
chest physiotherapy
Cheung BPH (benign prostatic hypertrophy) treatment system

chevron incision
Chiari-Frommel syndrome
Chiari malformations
Chiari types 1-2
chiasma interference
Chiba biopsy needle
chickenpox vaccine
chief complaint
chignon from vacuum extraction
CHILD (congenital hemidysplasia with ichthyosiform erythroderma and limb defects) syndrome
childbearing
childbearing age
childbirth, difficult
childbirth education classes
childbirth phobia
chills and fever
chills, shaking
chimera
chimerism
chimney sweep's cancer of skin of the scrotum
chips
  bladder
  evacuation of
  prostatic
Chirocaine (levobupivacaine)
Chiron Diagnostics ELISA assay
CHL (crown-heel length)
Chlamydia
Chlamydia enzyme test
Chlamydia pelvic inflammatory disease
Chlamydia slide test
Chlamydia trachomatis
chlamydial cervicitis
chlamydial infection
chlamydial ophthalmia neonatorum
chlamydial salpingitis
chloroplast DNA (cpDNA)
chloasma occurring in pregnancy
chlorambucil
chloramphenicol administration in newborn
chlorotrianisene (TACE)
chlorpropamide
choanal atresia
chocolate cyst of ovary
cholelithiasis
cholemic nephrosis
cholestasis
  hereditary Norwegian-type
  intrahepatic, of pregnancy
cholestatic hepatitis
cholesterinuria
cholesterol ester storage disease
cholesteroluria
cholestyramine
choluria
chondrocalcinosis
chondrodystrophia fetalis
chondrodystrophy
chondrodysplasia
chondrodysplasia punctata
chondrodystrophic calcificans congenita
chondrodystrophy, epiphyseal
chondrodystrophy with clubfeet
chondroectodermal dysplasia
Chondrogel tissue augmentation vesicoureteral reflux treatment
chondrosarcoma, uterine
chordee
  isolated
  ventral
chorea gravidarum
choreoathetosis
Chorex-5 (chorionic gonadotropin)
Chorex-10 (chorionic gonadotropin)
chorioadenoma destruens
chorioallantoic placenta
chorioamnionic placenta
chorioamnionitis
chorioamniotic placenta
chorioangioma
chorioangiosis
choriocarcinoma
chorioepithelioma
choriogenesis

choriogonadotropin
chorioepithelioma
chorion
chorionic adrenocorticotropin
chorionic gonadotropic hormone
chorionic gonadotropin
chorionic growth hormone-prolactin (CGP)
chorionic membrane
chorionic plate
chorionic sac
chorionic tissue samples
chorionic villi
chorionic villi biopsy (CVB)
chorionic villus sampling (CVS)
  transabdominal
  transcervical
  transvaginal
choristoma
choroidal sclerosis
choroideremia
chorioretinal anomalies
Choron-10 (chorionic gonadotropin)
Chotzen syndrome
Christchurch chromosome
Christensen-Krabbe
Christmas disease
Christmas tree syndrome
Chromagen OB prenatal vitamins
chromatid
chromatin
chromatographic urinalysis
chromatography, thin-layer
chromaturia
ChromaVision digital analyzer
chromic progressive chorea
chromic suture
chromogens
chromogranin A (CGA)
chromohydrotubation
chromolaparoscopy (LSC)
chromomere
chromonema
chromopertubation
chromosomal aberration
chromosomal abnormality (see *chromosome abnormality*)
chromosomal abnormality with stigmata of Turner syndrome
chromosomal address
chromosomal analysis
chromosomal anomaly (see *chromosome abnormality*)
chromosomal banding
chromosomal breakage
chromosomal defect (see *chromosome abnormality*)
chromosomal deletion (see *deletion syndrome*)
chromosomal inversion
chromosomal irregularity causing mental retardation
chromosomal marker
chromosomal mosaicism
chromosomally mediated resistant *Neisseria gonorrhoeae* (CMRNG)
chromosomal nondisjunction during meiosis
chromosomal pattern
chromosome (pl. chromosomes)
  accessory
  acentric
  acrocentric
  bivalent
  centromere of
  Christchurch
  derivative
  dicentric
  double minute
  8
  18
  11
  15
  5
  4
  14

chromosome *(cont.)*
- fragile X
- giant
- heterotypical
- homologous
- lampbrush
- late replicating
- marker
- metacentric
- mitochondrial
- 9
- 19
- nonhomologous
- nucleolar
- odd
- 1
- Philadelphia
- polytene
- reduction of
- ring
- 7
- 17
- sex
- 6
- 16
- submetacentric
- supernumerary marker
- telocentric
- 10
- 13
- 3
- translocation
- 12
- 20
- 21
- 22
- 2
- unpaired
- W
- X
- Y
- yeast artificial
- Z

chromosome abnormality (see *deletion syndrome; duplication syndrome; gene; monosomy; pentasomy; syndrome; tetrasomy; trisomy*)
- bivalent (II)
- break (b)
- constitutional (c)
- deletion (del)
- de novo mutation
- duplication (dup)
- fragile site (fra)
- gonadal dysgenesis
- insertion (ins)
- inversion (inv
- mixed
- monosomy
- mosaic (mos)
- mutation
- pentasomy
- pure
- quadrivalent (IV)
- quadruplication (qdr)
- rearrangement (rea)
- reciprocal (rcp)
- recombinant (rec)
- ring syndrome (r)
- robertsonian translocation (rob)
- tandem (tan)
- terminal (ter)
- tetrasomy
- translocation (t)
- triplication (trp)
- triploidy
- trisomy
- trivalent (III)
- univalent (I)
- variant (v)

chromosome arm
- long (q)
- p (short)
- q (long)
- short (p)

chromosome bands: C, CBG, G, NOR, Q, QF, QFQ, R, T

chromosome group (A-G)
chromosome jumping
chromosome mapping
chromosome mosaicism
chromosome pair
chromosome puffs
chromosome-specific alpha satellite probe
chromosome-specific painting probe
chromosome staining method
  barium hydroxide using Giemsa (CBG)
  constitutive heterochromatin (C)
  fluorescence (QF)
  fluorescence using quinacrine (QFQ)
  Giemsa (G)
  nucleolar organizing region (NOR)
  quinacrine (Q)
  reverse Giemsa (R)
  telomeric (T)
chromosome walking
chromotubation
chronic active hepatitis
chronic alcoholic cirrhosis
chronic alcoholic hepatic cirrhosis
chronic alcoholic liver disease
chronic anovulation
chronic anovulation of suprapituitary origin
chronic atrophic vulvitis
chronic bacterial prostatitis (CBP)
chronic bacterial pyelonephritis
chronic cervicitis
chronic cystic mastitis
chronic dialysis therapy
chronic diuretic administration
chronic dyspareunia
chronic fatigue immune dysfunction syndrome (CFIDS)
chronic fatigue syndrome
chronic glomerulonephritis
chronic granulomatous disease
chronic home dilation
chronic hydramnios
chronic hydrocephalus
chronic hypertrophic vulvitis
chronic hypocomplementemic glomerulonephritis
chronic incontinence
chronic inflammation of bladder
chronic interstitial cystitis
chronic interstitial salpingitis
chronic intestinal pseudo-obstruction (CIP)
chronic kidney failure
chronic laxative abuse
chronic lead syndrome
chronic lung disease (CLD)
chronic lymphocytic thyroiditis
chronic nephritic/proteinuric syndrome
chronic nephritis
chronic nephritis with lesion of necrotizing glomerulitis
chronic nephropathy
chronic nephrosis
chronic nonbacterial prostatitis
chronic parametritis
chronic pelvic pain (CPP)
chronic progressive external ophthmoplegia syndrome (CPEO)
chronic progressive renal insufficiency
chronic sinobronchial disease and dextrocardia
chronic prostatitis
chronic pyelitis
chronic pyelonephritis
chronic pyonephrosis
chronic renal allograft rejection
chronic renal dialysis
chronic renal failure (CRF)
chronic renal failure with uremia
chronic salpingitis and oophoritis
chronic spasmodic dysphonia (CSD)
chronic suppressive therapy
chronic trigonitis
chronic tubulointerstitial nephritis
chronic uremia

ChronoFlex polyurethane catheter
CHT (combined hormonal therapy)
chylocele of tunica vaginalis
chylous hydrocele
chylous urine
chyluria
Cialis (IC351)
CIC (clean intermittent catheterization)
cicatricial cervix
cicatricial kidney
cicatrix of cervix
Ciclovulan oral contraceptive
cidofovir gel
CIE (congenital ichthyosiform erythroderma)
  bullous
  nonbullous
ciliated cells
cimetidine
Cimino shunt
CIN (cervical intraepithelial neoplasia) staging
  grade CIN-1 (mild dysplasia)
  grade CIN-2 (moderate dysplasia)
  grade CIN-3 (severe dysplasia)
Cinobac (cinoxacin)
cinoxacin
CIP (chronic intestinal pseudo-obstruction)
Cipro (ciprofloxacin)
ciprofloxacin
Circon-ACMI electrohydraulic lithotriptor probe
Circon Cryomedics colposcope
circular hymen
circular self-retaining retractor
circular sulci
circulating androgen level
circulating antiphospholipid antibodies
circulating gonadal steroids
circulation
  fetal
  fetal hemorrhage into mother's
  hyperdynamic of pregnancy
circulation *(cont.)*
  maternal
  persistent fetal
  placental
  primordial uteroplacental
  uteroplacental
circulatory collapse
circulatory decompensation
circulatory overload
circumareolar incision
circumareolar mastopexy
circumcaval ureter
circumcised
circumcision
  female
  male
  pharaonic female genital
  Sunna
circumference, head
circumferential incision
circumferentially suture ligated
circumferential running stitch
circumoral cyanosis
circumrenal
circumvallata placenta
cirrhosis
  renal
  syphilitic
cirsoid placenta
CIS (carcinoma in situ)
cis configuration
cisplatin (formerly cis-platinum)
cis-trans configuration
cistron
citrate, urinary
Citrobacter amalonaticus (formerly *C. freundii*)
citrullinemia
citrus pectin, modified
citta
CK (creatine kinase)
CKPT (combined kidney and pancreas transplant)
clade

Clado anastomosis
Clado band
cladogenesis
Claforan (cefotaxime)
CLA Kit continuous regional anesthesia
clamp (see also *clip*)
  Adair breast
  Allis
  Babcock
  Backhaus towel
  Ballantine
  Bihrle dorsal
  Blalock-Taussig
  bulldog
  Clark
  cord
  Cunningham
  cut, and suture technique
  Dardik
  Goldstein Microspike approximator
  Gomco circumcision
  Gusberg hysterectomy
  Guyon-Pean kidney
  Heaney
  Herrick kidney
  Kelly
  Kitner (also Kittner)
  Klintmalm
  Kocher
  Lahey
  laser Backhaus towel
  laser wand
  Mayo-Guyon kidney pedicle
  McDougal prostatectomy
  M.D. Anderson
  Microspike approximator
  Mogen circumcision
  mosquito
  Muculicz peritoneal
  Pean
  right-angle
  Shirodkar
  Sweetheart
  tonsillar

clamp *(cont.)*
  towel
  vascular
  Veridien umbilical
clamped, cut, and ligated
clamped, cut, and sutured
clam shell
"clap" (gonorrhea)
Clark clamp
Clark classification of vulvar melanoma
Clarke-Reich knot pusher
Clark perineorrhaphy
classic abdominal Semm hysterectomy (CASH)
classic uterine incision
classical cesarean section
classical genetics
classification
  Berkson-Gage breast cancer survival calculation
  Bethesda
  bladder carcinoma
  Blaivas urinary incontinence
  Bosniak renal cystic mass
  Clark vulvar melanoma
  diabetes mellitus
  Dubin and Amelar varicocele
  Jewett bladder carcinoma
  Priscilla White diabetes
  selective estrogen receptor modulator (SERM)
  van Heuven diabetic retinopathy
  White diabetes mellitus
  Wolfe breast carcinoma
class of Pap smear
Claus breast cancer model
clavicotomy of fetus
clavipectoral fascia
clavulanate potassium
CLD (chronic lung disease)
clean-catch specimen
clean-catch urinalysis
clean-catch urine
clean-catch urine specimen

clean, cervix is
clean intermittent catheterization (CIC)
clean midstream voided urine
Clean Seals waterproof bandage
cleansing acid secretion of vagina
clean-voided midstream urine
clean-voided urine
clearance iothalamate
clearance of small solutes
clearance, urea
ClearBlue Easy pregnancy test
ClearBlue Easy One-Step pregnancy test
clear cell adenocarcinoma of vagina and cervix
clear cell carcinoma
clear cell of kidney
clear discharge
clear efflux of urine
clear margins of tumor
ClearPlan Easy pregnancy test
ClearPlan fertility monitor
clear tap
ClearView CO_2 laser
cleavage of C3 to active C3b
cleaved amplified polymorphic sequence (CAPS)
"cleavoplasty" augmentation mammoplasty
cleft
  pudendal
  urogenital
cleft lip and palate
cleft palate
cleidocranial dysplasia
Clemetson forceps
Cleocin vaginal cream or ovules
click, hip
climacteric menorrhagia
Climara (estradiol transdermal system) patch
Climara Pro estrogen replacement patch
climax
clindamycin
clinical diagnosis
clinical genetics
clinically indicated
clinically significant organ edema
clinical pregnancy
clinical relapse
clip (see also *clamp*)
  Filshie female sterilization
  Hemoclip
  Hulka
  Hulka ligating spring-loaded
  Lapro-Clip ligating
  Ligaclip
  Secu ("C-Q")
  skin
  surgical steel skin
  Sutured-Clip
  Weck
clip applicator, MCAS (modular clip application system)
clip applier, MultApplier clip
Clirans dialyzer
clitoral amputation
clitoral folds, agglutination of the
clitoral hood
clitoral hypertrophy
clitoral lesion
clitoral prepuce
clitoral recession
clitoral reduction
clitoral therapy device
clitoridean
clitoridectomy
clitoridis
clitoriditis
clitoridotomy
clitoris (pl. clitorides)
  cavernous body of
  cavernous nerves of
  corpus cavernosum of
  crus of
  deep artery of
  deep dorsal vein of

clitoris *(cont.)*
  deep veins of
  dorsal artery of
  enlarged
  frenulum of
  glans of
  hypertrophy of
  oral stimulation of
  painful erection of
  prepuce of
  prolonged erection of
  superficial dorsal veins of
  suspensory ligament of
clitorism
clitoritis
clitoromegaly
clitoroplasty
cloacal exstrophy
clockwise direction
clodronate
clofibrate
Clomid (clomiphene citrate)
clomiphene citrate
clone
clone bank
clonidine
cloning
cloning vector
clonus, muscle
closed cervix
closed crib
closed-drainage system
closed hydronephrosis
closed-space infection
closed-wound suction drainage
CloseSure wound closure device
clostridial infection
Clostridium difficile-associated diarrhea (CDAC)
Clostridium perfringens
Clostridium tetani
closure
  primary
  water-tight
clot
  blood
  fibrin
  large
  uterine
Clot Buster Amplatz thrombectomy device
clotrimazole vaginal cream
clotted forearm fistula
clotted shunt
clotting, abnormal
clotting deficiency
cloudy urine
Clq binding
clubbed end of fallopian tube
clubbed fallopian tube
clubbed penis
clubfeet
clubfoot
clue cells
clumped urates
clustered calcifications on mammogram
clustered microcalcifications
cluster of ulcers
Clutton bladder sound
cM (centimorgan)
CMBC (cutaneous metastatic breast cancer)
CMF (cyclophosphamide, methotrexate, and 5-FU) chemotherapy protocol
CMFP (cyclophosphamide, methotrexate, fluorouracil, prednisone) chemotherapy protocol
CMFP (Cytoxan, methotrexate, fluorouracil, prednisone) chemotherapy protocol
CMFPT (cyclophosphamide, methotrexate, fluorouracil, prednisone, tamoxifen) chemotherapy protocol
CMFPT (Cytoxan, methotrexate, fluorouracil, prednisone, tamoxifen) chemotherapy protocol

CMFPTH (Cytoxan, methotrexate, fluorouracil, prednisone, tamoxifen, Halotestin)
CMFVP (cyclophosphamide, methotrexate, fluorouracil, vincristine, and prednisone)
CMFVP (Cytoxan, methotrexate, fluorouracil, vincristine, prednisone) chemotherapy protocol
CMG (cystometrogram)
CMI/Mityvac cup
CMI/O'Neil cup for vacuum-assisted vaginal deliveries
CMI vacuum pump
CMRNG (chromosomally mediated resistant *Neisseria gonorrhoeae*)
CMT (Charcot-Marie-Tooth) disease
CMV (cytomegalovirus)
CMV titers
CNM (Certified Nurse Midwife)
CNS (central nervous system)
CNS-hypothalamic-pituitary unit
CO_2 (carbon dioxide)
  CO_2 gas
  CO_2 Guard gas filter for laparoscopy
  CO_2 laser
  CO_2 laser surgery
  CO_2 laser vaporization
  CO_2 medium
coagulated dissolved polymer
coagulase-negative staphylococci
coagulation
  bipolar
  confirmatory checks of
  diffuse intravascular (DIC)
  disseminated intravascular
  electrocoagulation
  ILC (interstitial laser)
  intrarenal
coagulation defect
coagulation disorder
coagulation factor
coagulator
  argon beam
  BiLAP bipolar

coagulator *(cont.)*
  Birtcher Medical Systems argon beam
  Bissinger detachable bipolar
  Bovie
  Coaguloop
  Cosman
  Endopath EZ-RF linear
  LaparoSonic
  LigaSure vessel-sealing
  Modulap
  VersaPoint
Coagulin-B gene therapy
Coaguloop resection electrode
Coaguloop system
coagulopathy
  consumption
  disseminated intravascular
coagulum pyelolithotomy
coalescent multiple intrarenal abscesses
coaptation of muscularis
coaptation of serosa
coarctation of aorta
coat, buffy
Coats disease
coaxial catheter (see *catheter*)
coaxial uterine sound
Cobalt Knife
Cobalt Scalpel
Coban dressing
cobblestone appearance
cobblestoning
Cobb-Ragde needle
Coca-Cola urine
coccidioidomycosis
coccygeal discomfort
coccygeus muscle
coccyx
Cochin Jewish disorder
cochleate uterus
Cockcroft-Gault equation/formula for calculating renal function
cockscomb cervix
cockscomb deformity

cocktail
  immunosuppressant
  renal
co-current flow
code
coding region
coding sequence
codominance
codominant gene
codon
coefficient of coancestry
coefficient of inbreeding
coefficient of parentage (COP)
coefficient of relationship
coelom, extraembryonic
coelomic epithelium
coelomic metaplasia
coexisting fetus
COF/COM (Cytoxan, Oncovin, fluorouracil + Cytoxan, Oncovin, methotrexate) chemotherapy protocol
Coffey ureterointestinal anastomosis
Coffin-Lowry syndrome
Coffin-Siris syndrome
cognitive development
Cohen cannula
Cohen/Jarcho cannula
Cohen syndrome
coil
  double breast
  Intercept prostate microcoil
  Intercept urethra microcoil
  intraurethral
  Surgi-Vision prostate MRI microcoil
  Surgi-Vision urethral MRI microcoil
coiling of stent
coil IUD
coil-spring diaphragm
coinheritance
coital headache
coitophobia
coitus incompletus
coitus, interrupted
coitus interruptus
COL2A1 gene
Colaris molecular diagnostic test
colchicine poisoning
cold cup bladder biopsy
cold injury syndrome of newborn
cold knife biopsy
cold knife cone biopsy
cold knife conization of cervix
colfosceril
colic
  acute ureteral
  calculus
  gallbladder
  gallstone
  left-sided ureteral
  menstrual
  nephritic
  ovarian
  renal
  ureteral
  uterine
colicky pain
coliform gram-negative bacilli
colitis
  ulcerative
  uremic
collagen hemostatic material, Avitene
collagen implant/injection
  Contigen
  Contigen Bard
  Contigen glutaraldehyde cross-linked
  glutaraldehyde cross-linked
  periurethral
  transurethral
collagen-vascular disease
collapse
  circulatory
  pressure
  pulmonary
collapsible polyvinyl chloride dialysate bags
collapsing glomerulopathy
collapsing glomerulosclerosis

collar, cervical
collateral lymph channels
collateral vessels
collecting duct cells
collecting ducts
collecting system
  inferior
  renal
  upper pole
collecting tubule
collection
  egg
  oocyte
  sperm
  24-hour urine
collection cannister
collection of sperm for artificial insemination
colliculectomy
colliculus (pl. colliculi), seminal
colli, hygroma
collimator (radiation oncology)
  high resolution multileaf
  Millennium MLC-120
Collin pelvimeter
Collin vaginal speculum
Collings electric knife
collision dyspareunia
collodion
collodion baby
collodion dressing
colloid goiter
Collyer pelvimeter
coloboma
colocolponeopoiesis, Kun
colon
  endometriosis of
  rectosigmoid
colon aganglionosis
colon conduit
colonic involvement of endometriosis
colonoscopy
colon segments
colony count
colony-forming unit (CFU)
colony-stimulating factor (CSF)
colony survival assay (CSA)
color blindness or color deficit
color-coded catheter
color Doppler
color-flow Doppler ultrasound (CDUS)
Colorgene DNA Hybridization Test
Colormate TLc.BiliTest bilirubinometer system
colorectal cancer
colorimetric analysis
colosplenic ligament
colostomy, loop
colostrorrhea
colostrous
colostrum
colovaginal fistula
colovesical fistula
colpocele
colpocephaly
colpocleisis, LeFort
colpocystitis
colpocystocele
colpocystoplasty
colpocystotomy
colpocystoureterotomy
colpocystourethropexy (CCUP)
colpodynia
colpohysterectomy
colpohysteropexy
colpohysteroscope
colpohysterotomy
colpomicroscope
colpomicroscopy
colpomycosis
colpomyomectomy
colpoperineopexy, abdominal-sacral or abdominosacral
colpoperineoplasty
colpoperineorrhaphy
  Manchester
  posterior
colpopexy, sacral

colpoplasty
colpopoiesis
colpoptosis
colporectopexy
colporrhagia
colporrhaphy, anterior vaginal
colporrhexis
colposcope (see also *endoscope*)
  Accuscope
  binocular fiberoptic
  Circon Cryomedics
  Cryomedics
  Gyne-Tech B101-D
  KryMed FO-101
  Leica
  Seiler
  video
  Wallach ColpoStar
  Wallach PentaScope
  Wallach TriScope
  Wallach ZoomScope Quantum
  Welch Allyn
  Welch Allyn Video Path
  Zeiss
  Zoomscope
colposcopically directed punch biopsy
colposcopist
colposcopy
colpospasm
colpostat
colpostenosis
colpostenotomy
colposuspension, Burch
colposuspension needle
colposuspension suture
colpotomizer, KOH
colpotomy incision
colpotomy, posterior
colpoureterotomy
colpourethropexy
colpoxerosis
columnar epithelium
column
  renal
  vaginal
coma
  diabetic
  nonketotic hyperglycemic-hyperosmolar (NKHHC)
  uremic
coma cast
Combidex (ferumoxtran)
combination argon beam coagulator-bipolar-unipolar cautery system
combination chemotherapy
combination oral contraceptive
combined abdominoperineal approach
combined androgen blockade (CAB)
combined hormonal therapy (CHT)
combined kidney and pancreas transplant (CKPT)
combined laparoscopic-vaginal approach
combined pregnancy
combined vaginal-abdominal approach in surgery
combined version
CombiPatch (estradiol/norethindrone) transdermal patch
comedocarcinoma
comedomastitis
Comfort Cath I or II
commissure
  posterior
  vulvar
commode
commodious
common law
common iliac artery
common iliac nodes
communicating hydrocele
communicating hydrocephalus
communicating vessel
community-acquired bacteremia
community dialysis center
Companion 2 blood glucose monitor
comparative mapping
compelling need to urinate
compensatory renal hypertrophy
competence, bladder outlet

competence of ureterovesical junction
competitive inhibition of DHT-AR
  complex by antiandrogens
complaint
  chief
  primary
complement (C)
complementary DNA (cDNA)
complementary RNA
complementary sequence
complementation
complementation test
complement component (C56-9)
complement or platelet activation
complement proteins
complete abortion
complete and pushing
complete androgen blockade (CAB)
complete androgen insensitivity
  syndrome (CAIS)
complete birth
complete bladder emptying
complete blood count (CBC)
complete breech
complete breech presentation
complete hemostasis
complete hysterectomy
complete linkage
completely mixed flow
completely penetrant
complete mastectomy
complete omentectomy
complete penectomy
complete placenta previa
complete spontaneous abortion
complete uterine prolapse
complete vaginectomy
complex
  castration
  IgA antigen
  juxtaglomerular
  LBW (limb-body wall)
  membrane-attack
complex *(cont.)*
  nipple-areola
  pulmonary-renal
  tuberous sclerosis
  UMCD (nephronophthisis-uremic
    medullary cystic)
complexation rate constant
complex cystic ovary
complex endometrial hyperplasia
complex glycoproteins
complex intracavitary radium implants
complex PSA
complex renal cyst
compliance
  bladder
  detrusor
  dietary
  low bladder
Compliance Pak treatment for STDs
compliant pre-stress prosthetic bone
  implant device
composite membrane
complications
  antepartum
  intrapartum
  hemodialysis
  peritoneal dialysis
  postoperative
  postpartum
  puerperal
Composite Cultured Skin
Composix mesh
compound heterozygote
compound pregnancy
compound presentation
Comprecin (enoxacin)
comprehensive health enhancement
  support system (CHESS) for breast
  cancer patients
compression of cord
compressor urethrae
compressor venae dorsalis penis
compressus, fetus

compromise
  circulatory
  renal
  respiratory
  umbilical cord
  ureteral vascular
compromised renal function
compromised tumescence
compromised ventilatory support
compulsive sexual behavior
compulsive water drinking
computed tomographic mammography
computed tomography (CT)
computed tomography laser
computed tomography laser mammography (CTLM)
computed tomography, single photon emission (SPECT)
computer-aided ^{192}IR afterloading dosage
computerized axial tomography (CAT)
computerized peristaltic pump
computerized treatment planning
concealed hemorrhage
concealed penis
Conceive Fertility Planner
Conceive Ovulation Predictor
concentrated carbohydrate feeding
concentrated urine
concentrated urine specimen
concentrate, electrolyte
concentrating defect
concentration factor
concentration, gonadotropin
concentration gradient
concentration of contrast media
concentration of dye
concentration polarization
concentric fibroma
concentric mastopexy
conception rate
conception, retained products of
Conceptrol contraceptive cream
Conceptus fallopian tube catheter
Conceptus Robust guide wire
Conceptus Soft Seal cervical catheter
Conceptus Soft Torque uterine catheter
Conceptus VS (variable softness) catheter
Concise Performance Plus hCG-Combo pregnancy test
Concise Performance Plus pregnancy test
concomitant bleeding
concretion, prostatic
concurrent chemotherapy and radiation therapy
condition, fibrocystic (of the breast)
condom
  lambskin
  latex
  Silastic
  The Female Condom
condoms and foam
conductivity of fluid
conduit
  Bricker ileal
  colon
  ileal
  incontinent ileal
  intestinal urinary
  ureteroileal
  urinary
conduit reservoir
condyloma (pl. condylomata)
  anal
  genital
  penile
  perianal
  vaginal
  venereal
condyloma acuminatum (pl. condylomata acuminata)
condyloma lata
Condylox (podofilox) gel
cone biopsy
cone biopsy of cervix
cone catheter tip

cone dystrophy
cone of tissue
cone-shaped expansion plug
cone-tip catheter
cone, weighted
confinement, estimated date of (EDC)
conformation sensitive gel electrophoresis (CSGE)
confirmatory checks of coagulation
confirmatory needle biopsy
Confirm 1-Step pregnancy test
conformational therapy
congenital absence of abdominal muscles
congenital absence of kidney
congenital absence of vagina
congenital adrenal hyperplasia (CAH)
congenital anemia
congenital anomaly (pl. anomalies)
congenital aplasia of vagina and uterus
congenital bronchiectasis
congenital cervical stenosis
congenital complement component deficiency immune reaction
congenital cytomegalic inclusion disease
congenital cytomegalovirus infection
congenital debility
congenital diaphragm
congenital diaphragmatic hernia
congenital dilation of collecting tubules
congenital dislocation of knee (CDK)
congenital dysplastic angiectasia
congenital endometrial hyperplasia
congenital epulis of newborn
congenital facial dysplasia syndrome
congenital fecalith
congenital goiter
congenital heart defects
congenital heart problems
congenital hemidysplasia with ichthyosis erythroderma and limb defects (CHILD) syndrome
congenital hemihypertrophy
congenital hepatic fibrosis
congenital herpes simplex
congenital hydrocele
congenital hydrocele of tunica vaginalis
congenital hydrocephalus
congenital hydronephrosis
congenital hydroureter
congenital hypoplasia of kidney
congenital hypoplastic anemia
congenital hypothyroidism
congenital ichthyosiform erythroderma (CIE)
  bullous
  nonbullous
congenital ichthyosis
congenital immune deficiency syndrome
congenital immune derangement
congenital keratoconus
congenital listeriosis
congenital liver cirrhosis
congenitally defective gonads
congenital malaria
congenital malformation incompatible with life
congenital malformation of major organs
congenital megalourethra
congenital mesoblastic nephroma
congenital mesodermal dysmorphodystrophy
congenital multiple arthrogryposis
congenital muscular dystrophy (CMD)
congenital myodystrophy
congenital myotonic dystrophy
congenital nephrosis
congenital nephrotic syndrome, Finnish-type
congenital neurogenic bladder
congenital neutropenia
congenital nevus
congenital obstruction of bile duct
congenital obstruction of lacrimal duct
congenital oculofacial paralysis
congenital pelvic enterocele

congenital phimosis
congenital pneumonia in the newborn
congenital polycystic disease
congenital renal anomaly
congenital renal cyst
congenital renal hyperplasia
congenital rubella
congenital rubella pneumonitis
congenital sacral agenesis
congenital sensory neuropathy
  with anhidrosis
congenital stricture of urethra
congenital syphilis
congenital thymic aplasia
congenital toxoplasmosis
congenital tuberculosis
congenital tubular impairment
congenital ureteral stricture
congenital ureteropelvic obstruction
congenital urethral stricture
congenital vaginal aplasia
congenital vaginal enterocele
congenital vesicoureteral reflux
congenital word blindness
congested kidney
congestion
  pelvic
  pelvic vein
  splanchnic
  vascular
congestion-fibrosis syndrome
congestion of prostate
congestion of superficial veins of
  prostatic urethra
congestive cardiac failure with uremia
congestive prostatitis
conical mass
conization
  cautery
  cervical
  cold knife
  laser
conization by electrosurgery
conization by laser
conization by scalpel
conization of cervix
conjoined asymmetric twins
conjoined equal twins
conjoined symmetric twins
conjoined tendon deficiency
conjoined twins
conjoined unequal twins
conjoint tendon
conjugate
  obstetric, of pelvic inlet
  obstetric, of pelvic outlet
conjugated estrogens
conjugation
conjunctivitis, neonatal
conjunctivourethrosynovial syndrome
Conn syndrome
conotruncal anomaly face syndrome
  (CTAF)
Conradi disease
Conradi-Hünermann syndrome
consanguineous mating
consanguinity
consensual sexual relations
consensus sequence
consent to adoption revocable
conserved sequence
consort
constant infusion principle
constant proteinuria
constipation interfering with dialysis
  catheter drainage
constituent, host
constitutional cause
constitutive heterochromatin (C)
  chromosome staining method
constriction of ureter
constriction, postglomerular arteriolar
construction of ileal conduit
construction of intestinal ureter
consultant
consultation, nephrology
consumption coagulopathy
contact dermatitis

contact hysteroscope
contact, sexual
contact spotting
contaminated urine sample
contamination
contents of axilla
contents of scrotum
contested paternity
ContiCath catheter
Contigen Bard collagen implant
Contigen collagen implant
Contigen glutaraldehyde cross-linked collagen injection
contiguous gene syndrome
continence mechanism
continence ring (see *urinary incontinence device*)
continent ileostomy
continent supravesical bowel urinary diversion
continent urinary diversion (see *pouch*; *reservoir; urinary incontinence treatment*)
continuous ambulatory peritoneal dialysis (CAPD)
continuous arteriovenous hemodialysis (CAVHD)
continuous arteriovenous hemofiltration (CAVH)
continuous bladder irrigation
continuous catheter drainage
continuous cycler peritoneal dialysis (CCPD)
continuous cyclic peritoneal dialysis (CCPD)
continuous descending pressure (CDP)
continuous diffusion dialysis
continuous drainage
continuous hemofiltration
continuous membrane column
continuous peritoneal dialysis
continuous positive airway pressure (CPAP)
continuous pulsatile hypothermic perfusion
continuous renal replacement therapy (CRRT)
continuous venovenous hemodiafiltration (CVVHDF)
continuous venovenous hemodialysis (CVVHD)
contour
  bladder wall
  breast
contoured tilting compression mammography
Contour Profile silicone breast implant
contraception (see *contraceptive device, contraceptive method, oral contraceptive*)
contraception use
contraceptive device (see also *contraceptive methods*)
  arching-type diaphragm
  barrier
  coil-spring diaphragm
  Conceptrol
  condom
  combination oral
  Copper 7 IUD
  Cu-Safe 300 IUD
  Dalkon shield IUD
  Delfen foam
  Depo-Provera long-term injection
  desogestrel
  diaphragm
  emergency hormonal
  Emko foam
  Empirynol Plus gel
  flat-spring diaphragm
  foam
  Gynol II
  Implanon
  IUD (intrauterine device)
  jelly
  Kormex II
  Lippes loop IUD
  Norplant long-term injectable
  NuvaRing (etonogestrel/ethinyl estradiol)

contraceptive device *(cont.)*
  oral contraceptive (OC)
  Ortho-Cream
  Ortho-Gynol
  Preceptin
  Protectaid contraceptive sponge with F-5 Gel
  Savvy contraceptive vaginal gel
  spermicidal
  STOP (selective tubal occlusion procedure)
  subdermal implant
  Surete gel
  TCu380A IUD
  vaginal contraceptive film (VCF)
  vaginal cream
  vaginal foam
  vaginal sponge
  vaginal suppository
contraceptive cream
contraceptive jelly
contraceptively sterile
contraceptive methods
  abstinence
  calendar rhythm
  cervical cap
  coitus interruptus
  condoms
  diaphragm
  foam
  implantable contraceptives
  injectable contraceptives
  intrauterine device (IUD)
  jelly
  morning-after pill
  oral contraceptive (OC)
  periodic abstinence
  rhythm
  spermicide
  subdermal implant
  withdrawal
contracted bladder
contracted kidney
contracted pelvis
contraction (C)
  bladder
  Braxton Hicks
  duration of
  frequency of
  hourglass
  hypertonic uterine
  impaired voiding
  incoordinate uterine
  inlet
  intense uterine
  irregular uterine
  outlet
  painless uterine
  palpable
  poor
  prolonged uterine
  quality of
  reflex detrusor
  rhythmic uterine
  tetanic
  uterine
contraction ring
contraction stress test (CST)
contracture
  capsular
  cervical
  cervix
  vesical outlet
  wound
contraindications for hemodialysis
contraindications for peritoneal dialysis
contralateral kidney
contrast
  bladder
  extravasated
  extravasation of
  iodinated
contrast-enhanced CT scan
contrast-enhanced scan
contrast enhancement
contrast epididymogram
contrast extravasation

contrast medium (pl. media) (see *imaging agents*)
contrast reaction
contrast reaction with anaphylaxis
contrast vasogram
control, birth (see *contraceptive devices; contraceptive methods; oral contraceptives*)
control gene
controlled bladder filling
controlled cooling
controller, Actis VFC (venous flow controller) for erectile dysfunction
convection-based removal of uremic solutes
convection-based therapy
convective transport
convective transport of nitrogenous solutes
convective transport of solute
conventional abdominal hysterectomy
conventional access
conventional cytogen
conversion of androgens to estrogens
conversion of nitrate to nitrite
conversion to laparotomy
convertible slip knot
convexion-based removal of uremic solutes
convoluted tubular cells
convoluted tubule
ConXn (recombinant human relaxin)
Cook continence ring
Cook-Cope loop suprapubic catheter
Cook cystotomy catheter
Cook hysteroscopic catheter
Cook insemination cup
Cook introducer
Cook silicone balloon HSG (hysterosalpingography) catheter
Cook sperm filter
Cook Stratasis urethral sling
Cook tissue morcellator
Cooley anemia
cooling slush
Coombs test
Cooper hernia
Cooper ligaments of breast
Cooper Surgical cystoscope
Cooper syndrome
COP (coefficient of parentage)
Copeland fetal scalp electrode
Cope nephrostomy tube
coping reactions to chronic dialysis
copious amounts of saline
copious irrigation
copious urination
copper IUD
copper metabolism disease
coproporphyria
  hereditary
  fecal
copulation
copulines
cord (see also *umbilical cord*)
  bandolier
  bruising of
  double nuchal
  entanglement of
  fibromuscular
  genital
  gonadal
  hematoma of
  hydrocele of spermatic
  knot in
  nuchal
  presentation of
  prolapse of
  prolapse of umbilical
  prolapsed
  prolapsed umbilical
  short
  short umbilical
  spermatic
  testicular
  testis
  three-vessel
  thrombosed

cord *(cont.)*
  torsion of umbilical
  two-vessel
  umbilical
  vascular lesion of
  velamentous insertion of umbilical
  vitelline
cord accident
cord around the neck
cord around the neck x 2
cordate pelvis
cord blood
cord blood banking
cord blood gases (CBG)
cord blood pH
cord blood sampling, percutaneous umbilical (PUBS)
cord clamp
cord compression
cord doubly-clamped and cut
Cordguard II
cord hydrocele
cordiform uterus
cordlike mass
cordocentesis
cord of umbilical artery
Cordonnier ureteroileal loop
cord prolapse
cord serially clamped and cut
cord tightly around neck
cord wrapped around neck
Core aspiration/injection needle
core biopsy needle
Core cannula system
Core CO_2 insufflation needle
Core trocar system
Cori disease
corkscrew maneuver
corneal dystrophy
Cornelia de Lange syndrome (CdLS)
corner fracture
cornification
cornified
cornify
cornu (pl. cornua)
cornual obstruction
cornu of bladder
cornu of uterus
cornual pregnancy
Corometrics maternal/fetal monitor
coronal Dentin dysplasia
coronal epispadias
coronal hypospadias
coronal plane
coronal sulcus
corona of glans
corona of glans penis
corpora cavernosa-corpus spongiosum shunt
corpora lutea cyst
corporal rupture
corporeal body
corporeal cesarean section
corporotomy
corpus
corpus albicans
corpus callosum abnormalities
corpus callosum agenesis
corpus cavernosum (pl. corpora cavernosum)
  atrophy of
  embolism of
  fibrosis of
  hematoma of
  hypertrophy of
  thrombosis of
corpus cavernosum abscess
corpus cavernosum cellulitis
corpus cavernosum clitoridis dextrum
corpus cavernosum clitoridis sinistrum
corpus cavernosum of clitoris
corpus cavernosum penile electromyography
corpus cavernosum penis
corpus cavernosum spongiosum shunt
corpus cavernosum urethrae virilis

corpuscle
  genital
  malpighian
  renal
corpus luteal cyst
corpus luteum
corpus luteum cyst
corpus luteum dysfunction
corpus luteum hematoma
corpus luteum hemorrhage
corpus of cervix
corpus spongiosum
corpus spongiosum penis
corpus uteri, polyp of
correction of placenta previa, spontaneous
corregation of tissue
correlation, mammographic-histopathologic
corresponding allele
corresponding phenotype
Corson probe
cortex (pl. cortices)
  fetal adrenal
  ovarian
  patchy atrophy of renal
  pubic symphysis
  renal
  suprarenal
cortical cyst
cortical interstitium
corticalis defornaris
cortical necrosis
cortical renal cyst
cortical scarring of kidney
cortical scintigraphy
corticomedullary junction
corticosteroid premedication
corticosteroids
corticostriatal-spinal degeneration (CJD)
cortisol deficiency
cor triatriatum
corynebacterium (pl. corynebacteria)
co-segregation
Cosman coagulator
cosmid
Costello protocol for laser ablation of prostate
Costello syndrome
costovertebral angle (CVA)
costovertebral angle tenderness
cot death
cot, finger
cottage cheese-like discharge
co-trimoxazole
co-twin, fetal hemorrhage into
cotyledon (pl. cotyledons)
  fetal
  maternal
  retained
cotyledonary placenta
coudé catheter
Coumadin (warfarin sodium)
coumarin
coumarin pulsed-dye laser
Councill catheter
counseling
  genetic
  marital
counter-current flow
counter-current flow mechanism
counterregulatory hormones
counterregulatory mechanism
coupled transport
coupling
course of labor
course, postpartum
Couvelaire uterus
coverage, prophylactic
covert asymptomatic candiduria
covert embryopathy
covert renal bacteruria
cow's kidney
cow's milk anemia
cow's milk-based infant formula
cow's milk hypocalcemia
Cowper gland abscess

cowperitis
coxsackievirus
Cox-Uphoff International (CUI) tissue expander
CP (cerebral palsy)
CPAP (continuous positive airway pressure)
CPD (cephalopelvic disproportion)
CPD (continuous peritoneal dialysis)
cpDNA (chloroplast DNA)
CPK (creatine phosphokinase)
CPP (chronic pelvic pain)
CPS (carbamyl phosphate synthetase) deficiency
CR, CRL (crown-rump length)
crablike lesion on mammogram
crabs
crack baby
cracked nipple
cradle cap
Craft aspiration needle
Cragg hemodialysis thrombolytic brush
cramping, suprapubic
cramplike pains
cramps, uterine
crampy abdominal pain
cranial bones, overlapping of
cranial bosses
cranial bossing
cranial fontanelle
cranial meningoencephalocele
craniectomy, endoscopic strip
CranioCap for infants
craniocaudal view of breast
craniocarpotarsal dysplasia
craniocele
craniofacial dysostosis
craniofrontonasal dysplasia
craniometaphyseal dysplasia or dystrophy
craniorachischisis
craniosynostosis-radial aplasia syndrome
craniosynostosis
  choanal atresia-radiohumeral synostosis
  midfacial hypoplasia and foot anomalies
  primary
craniorachischisis
cranium bifidum (pl. bifida)
Cranley Maternal-Fetal Attachment Scale
"crash" cesarean section
cream
  cervical
  contraceptive
  spermicidal
  vaginal
creamy discharge
creamy vulvitis
crease
  inframammary
  palmar
  plantar
  simian
creatine kinase (CK)
creatine phosphokinase (CPK)
creatinine
  serum
  urinary
creatinine clearance
  endogenous
  24-hour
creatinine level
creation of pseudovagina for transsexual surgery
Credé maneuver of uterus
Cre-loxP system
cremasteric reflex
crescent formation
crescentic glomerulonephritis
crescent mastopexy
crescents, epithelial
crest
  iliac
  interureteric

crest *(cont.)*
 pubic
 sacral
 urethral
cretinism
Creutzfeldt-Jakob disease
CRF (chronic renal failure)
crib
 closed
 open
crib death
cribriform hymen
cri du chat (cat's cry) syndrome
CRIES neonatal postoperative pain assessment tool
Crigler-Najjar syndrome
criminal abortion
Crinone bioadhesive progesterone gel
crisis
 Dietl twisted kidney
 sickle cell
criteria
 Amsel
 gestational dating
 renal replacement therapy
 Spiegelberg
 Studdiford
Crit-Line
CRL (crown-rump length)
cRNA
Crohn disease
Cronin breast breast implant
Cronkhite-Canada disease
cross birth
crossbreeding
cross-clamp
cross-clamping
crossed ectopic kidney
crossed ectopic renal unit
crossed renal ectopia
crossed testicular ectopia
cross flow
crossing
crossing over
crossmatch
"cross-the-heart" augmentation mammoplasty
croup
Crouzon disease
crowned
crown-heel length (CH, CHL)
crowning
crown of fetal head
crown-rump length (CR, CRL)
CRRT (continuous renal replacement therapy)
cruciate incision
crude urine
cruenta, lochia
crus (pl. crura)
crushing of ureter, accidental
crush kidney
crus of clitoris
crus of diaphragm
crus of penis
cryoablation
 Endocare renal
 endometrial
 transperineal prostatic
cryoablation for prostate cancer
cryoablation reduction of menstruation (CARMEN) procedure
cryobank
CRYOCare cryosurgical system
CRYOCare endometrial cryoablation system
CRYOCare laser treatment for prostate carcinoma
cryocauterization
cryoconization of cervix
cryogenic surgery
cryoglobulinemia, mixed
CRYOguide ultrasound system
Cryomedics colposcope
cryoprecipitate infusion
cryopreservation
cryopreservation of fetal tissues
cryopreservation of spermatozoa

CRYOprobe
cryoprostatectomy
cryosurgery of the cervix
cryosurgery, targeted
cryosurgical unit
cryotherapy, FemRx Soprano
cryotherapy of prostate
CryoVein SG vascular graft
cryptic chromosome translocation/
  rearrangement
cryptococcosis
Cryptococcus neoformans
cryptomenorrhea
cryptophthalmus-syndactyly syndrome
cryptorchid testes
cryptorchidism
cryptorchism
crystallographic analysis
crystalloid fluid
crystalluria
crystals
  oxalate
  phosphate
  urate
Crystal Vision smoke evacuation unit
cry, uterine
CSA (colony survival assay)
CsA (cyclosporin A)
CSD (chronic spasmodic dysphonia)
C-section (cesarean section)
CSF (cerebrospinal fluid)
CSF (colony-stimulating factor)
CS-5 cryosurgical system
CSGE (conformation sensitive gel
  electrophoresis)
CST (contraction stress test)
CT (*Chlamydia trachomatis*) assay
CT (computed tomography)
  renal helical CT (RHCT)
  ultrafast
  ultrafast CT electron beam
    tomography
CTAF (conotruncal anomaly faces)
  syndrome
CTCb (Cytoxan, thiotepa, carboplatin)
  chemotherapy protocol
CTD (clitoral therapy device)
CT dialyzer
CT-guided brachytherapy
CT laser mammography (CTLM)
CT pelvimetry
CT scan
CT-2584 mesylate
C3b receptors
C3 deposition
C3 nephritic factor
C3 proactivator
C3 proactivator convertase
CTLM (CT laser mammography)
CTNS gene
cube pessary
Cuda laparoscope
cuff
  bladder
  transected vaginal
  vaginal
CUI (Cox-Uphoff International)
CUI gel breast prosthesis
CUI saline breast prosthesis
CUI tissue expander
cul-de-sac
  anterior
  Douglas
  free fluid in the
  posterior
  retrouterine
  uterine
cul-de-sac hernia
cul-de-sac of Douglas, endometriosis of
cul-de-sac of uterus
cul-de-sac smear
culdocentesis
culdolaparoscopy
culdoplasty (culdeplasty)
  Halban
  high McCall
  Mayo
  McCall modified posterior

culdoplasty *(cont.)*
  McCall posterior
  Moschcowitz
culdoscope
culdoscopy
culdotomy
Cullen sign
culpoperineorrhaphy
culpopexy, transvaginal sacrospinous
Culp pyeloplasty
cultivar
culture
  bacterial
  blood
  cerebrospinal fluid (CSF)
  cervical
  endometrial
  failed
  fluid
  gonorrhea
  herpes
  in situ
  lower-tract localization
  McCoy cell
  quantitative urine
  short-term lymphocyte
  sputum
  Thayer-Martin cell
  urine
  vaginal
  viral
culture and sensitivity (C&S)
culture failure
culture medium, Thayer-Martin
cumulus mass
cunnilingus
Cunningham clamp for male urinary incontinence
CUOG (Canadian Urology Oncology Group)
cup
  Bird
  Bird OP
  CMI/Mityvac cup

cup *(cont.)*
  CMI/O'Neil
  Cook insemination
  insemination
  Malmstrom
  Mityvac
  Murless
  Tender Touch Ultra
cuprammonia process
cuprophane
cup-shaped placenta with raised edges
curative intervention
curdy discharge
curet (also curette)
  Accurette endometrial
  banjo
  Bumm uterine
  EndoCurette endometrial suction
  endometrial aspiration biopsy
  endometrial biopsy suction
  Explora endometrial
  Greene uterine
  GynoSampler endometrial
  Hofmeister biopsy
  Kevorkian-Younge
  large sharp
  Masterson endometrial sampling
  Novak endometrial suction biopsy
  optical aspirating (OAC)
  Pipelle endometrial
  Randall endometrial suction biopsy
  rigid suction
  SelectCells endometrial
  serrated
  sharp and blunt
  Sims uterine
  suction
  Thomas uterine
  uterine
  Vacurette suction
curettage
  aspiration
  blunt
  endocervical (ECC)

curettage *(cont.)*
  endometrial (EMC)
  fractional
  sharp
  suction
curette (see *curet*)
curettement
curettings, endometrial
curlicue ureter
curly hair osteosclerosis
Curosurf (poractant alfa)
currant jelly stools
Curretab (medroxyprogesterone)
Curth-Maklin-type ichthyosis
Curtis–Fitz-Hugh syndrome
Curtis Marmorata telangiectatica congenita
curve
  contraction
  Friedman
  labor
  renal flow
  renogram
  washout
curved needle driver
curved ribbon retractor
curved unipolar scissors
curvilinear incision
CUSA (Cavitron ultrasonic aspirator)
Cu-Safe 300 IUD
CUSALap
Cusco "Swiss pattern" vaginal speculum
Cusco vaginal speculum
Cushieri two-hand maneuver
Cushing disease
Cushing forceps
Cushing syndrome
custody dispute
custom breast implant
Cutalon nylon polyamide surgical suture
cutaneous hemorrhage
cutaneous intubated nephrostomy
cutaneous intubated ureterostomy
cutaneous loop ureterostomy
cutaneous metastatic breast cancer (or carcinoma) (CMBC)
cutaneous nephrostomy tube
cutaneous photosensitivity
cutaneous stoma
cutaneous ureteroileostomy
cutaneous ureterostomy
cutaneous vesicostomy
cutis laxa
cutis marmorata
cutter
  BiLAP bipolar cutting and coagulating probe
  bipolar cutting loop
  Bissinger detachable bipolar coagulation forceps
  Bovie
  Endopath ETS-FLEX endoscopic articulating linear
  Endopath EZ45 endoscopic linear
  Endopath EZ-RF linear
  LaparoSonic coagulating
  Modulap coagulation
cut, clamp, and tie technique
cutting Bovie
CVA (cerebrovascular accident)
CVA (costovertebral angle)
CVAT (CVA tenderness)
CVB (chorionic villi biopsy)
CVC (central venous catheter)
CVP (central venous pressure) line
CVS (chorionic villus sampling)
CVS pregnancy test
CVVHD (continuous venovenous hemodialysis)
cyanosis
  circumoral
  dusky
  peripheral
cyanotic attacks
cyanotic heart disease
cyanotic infant

cyanotic kidney
cyanuria
cycle
  anovulatory
  gonadotrophic
  irregular menstrual
  menstrual
  menstrual-ovarian
  normal menstrual
  ovulatory
  physiologic
Cycle Check ovulation prediction kit
Cyclessa (desogestrel/ethinyl estradiol) oral contraceptive pill
cyclic adenosine monophosphate (cAMP)
cyclic endometrial shedding
cyclic estrogen-progestin regimen
cyclic vomiting syndrome (CVS)
Cyclofem (now Lunelle) injectable contraceptive
cyclophosphamide rescue
cyclopia
Cyclo-Provera (now Lunelle) injectable contraceptive
Cyclops procedure
cyclosporin A (CsA)
cyclosporine
CycloTech cyclosporine delivery system
Cycrin (medroxyprogesterone)
cyesis
CYFRA 21-1 tumor marker for breast carcinoma
CYFRA 21-1 tumor marker for gynecology neoplasm
cylinduria
CyPat
cypridophobia
cyproterone
cyst
  acoustic
  acquired
  adenocarcinoma
  adnexal

cyst *(cont.)*
  amniotic
  aspiration of ovarian
  Bartholin
  Bartholin duct
  benign
  benign hemorrhagic corpus luteum
  Blessig
  blue dome
  blue dome breast
  breast
  calcified outline of
  chocolate
  complex renal
  congenital renal
  corpus luteum
  cortical
  cortical renal
  Dandy-Walker
  dermoid
  drainage of
  dysontogenetic
  endometrial
  epithelial
  fluid-filled
  follicular
  functional ovarian
  Gartner
  germinal epithelial
  glomerular
  hemorrhagic ovarian
  hydatid
  hydatid of Morgagni
  kidney
  luteal
  lutein
  lymphatic
  mammary
  medullary
  mucinous
  müllerian
  multilocular
  multiloculated
  nabothian

cyst *(cont.)*
neoplastic ovarian
non-neoplastic ovarian
omphalomesenteric
ovarian
ovarian dermoid
ovarian follicular
parapelvic
paratubal
parovarian
perimesonephric
peripelvic
prostatic
pyelogenic
renal
ruptured ovarian
ruptured renal
sebaceous
simple renal
solitary
spermatic
testicular
theca lutein
unilocular
urachal
urethral
urinary
utricular
vulvar
Cystadane (betaine anhydrous)
cystadenocarcinoma
mucinous
ovarian
papillary serous
cystadenofibroma, papillary
cystadenoma
ovarian
serous
Cystagon (cysteamine bitartrate)
cystathionine alpha-betasynthase deficiency
cysteamine bitartrate
cystectomy
Bartholin
partial

cystectomy *(cont.)*
radical
salvage
total
vulvovaginal
cystectomy with urinary diversion
Cystex (methenamine)
cystica
cystitis
pyeloureteritis
ureteritis
cystic adenomatoid malformation
cystic appearance
cystic breast
cystic cancer
cystic degeneration
cystic disease of breast
cystic fibrosis (CF)
cystic goiter
cystic hygroma
cystic hyperplasia of breast
cystic kidney
cystic mass
cystic mastitis
cystic mastopathy
cystic mole
cystic neoplasm
cystic ovary
cystic renal dysplasia
cystic renal lesion
cystic sac
cystic structure
cystic teratoma
cystic tumor
cystic wall
cystine, benzine-ring crystals
cystine stone
cystinosis, neuropathic
cystinuria
cystis urinaria
Cystistat (sterile sodium hyaluronate solution)
cystitis
acute
acute hemorrhagic

cystitis *(cont.)*
  allergic
  bacterial
  bullous
  chronic interstitial
  diphtheritic
  emphysematous
  eosinophilic
  follicular
  fungal
  gonococcal
  hemorrhagic
  honeymoon
  Hunner interstitial
  incrusted
  interstitial (IC)
  irradiation
  monilial
  radiation
  subacute
  submucous
  trichomonal
  tuberculous
  vesicular
  viral
cystitis glandularis
cystocarcinoma
Cystocath
cystocele
cystocele bulging below the bladder neck
cystocele with rectocele
cystocele with urinary incontinence
cystochromoscopy
cystocolic anastomosis
cystocolpoproctography
cystocyst
cystoenterocele
cystoenterostomy
cystoepiplocele
cyst of broad ligament
cyst of vulva
cystogram, cystography
  antegrade
  delayed

cystogram *(cont.)*
  double-voiding
  excretory
  postdrainage
  postoperative
  postvoiding
  radionuclide (RNC)
  retrograde
  straining
  stress
  triple voiding
  voiding
cystolith
cystolithiasis
cystolithic
cystolithotomy
cystoma
  endometrial
  simple
cystometer
cystometrics
cystometrogram (CMG)
cystometrography
cystometry, LuMax
cystomorphous
cystomyxoma
cystopanendoscopy
cystopexy
cystophotography
cystoplasty, augmentation
cystoplegia
cystoproctogram, dynamic
cystoprostatectomy
  nerve-sparing radical
  radical
cystopyelitis
cystopyelonephritis
cystorrhaphy
cystorrhea
cystosarcoma
cystosarcoma phyllodes
cystoscope
  ACMI
  ACN flexible
  Brown-Buerger

cystoscope *(cont.)*
  Cabot
  Cooper Surgical
  Dyonics
  Elder Helio
  infant
  InjecTx
  InjecTx customized
  Jarit
  Morganstern continuous-flow operating
  MR-915 podiatric
  MR-Series
  Olympus A2010
  Olympus CHF-P10
  Olympus CYF-3 OES cystofiberscope
  pediatric
  rigid
  Solos
  Storz
  suprapubic
  transurethral
  Visicath
  Wappler
  Wolf
cystoscopically
cystoscopic basket extraction
cystoscopic urography
cystoscopy
  follow-up
  periurethral
  transurethral
cystoscopy table
cystoscopy through artificial stoma
cystospasm
cysto table (cystoscopy table)
cystostomy, suprapubic
cystostomy tube
cysto table (cystoscopy table)
cystotome
cystotomy, suprapubic
cystoureteritis
cystoureterogram
cystoureterography
cystoureteroscope, operative
cystourethritis
cystourethrocele
cystourethrogram, cystourethrography
  micturating
  Pollack bead chain
  retrograde
  voiding (VCUG)
cystourethroplasty
cystourethroscope
cystourethroscopy
Cytadren (aminoglutethimide)
cytochrome C oxidase (COX) deficiency
CytoGam (cytomegalovirus immune globulin)
cytogenetic abnormality
  fetal
  parental
cytogenetic cell lines
cytogenetic map
cytogeneticist
cytogenetics
cytogenic analysis
cytogenic reproduction
cytologic diagnosis
cytology
cytology brush, Detect
cytomegalovirus
cytometric urinalysis
cytoplasm
cytoplasmic organelles
cytosine
cytosine bases
Cytolex (pexiganan)
cytologic smear
cytology
  abnormal
  urinary sediment
  urine
cytolytic therapy
cytomegalovirus (CMV), congenital
cytomegalovirus titers

cytometry, Urocyte diagnostic
cytopathic effect
cytoplasmic ANCA (c-ANCA, cANCA)
cytosine (C)
cytosolic androgen receptors
CytoTAb purified monoclonal antibody
cytotoxic drugs
cytotoxic immune reaction
cytotrophoblast cell
cytotrophoblast, extravillous
cytotrophoblastic elements
Cytovene (oral ganciclovir)
Cytovene-IV (ganciclovir sodium for injection)
Cytoxan (cyclophosphamide)
CY2010

D, d

DA (developmental age)
dacliximab (also daclizumab)
daclizumab (also dacliximab)
Dacomed snap gauge to test impotence
Dacron patch
Dacron suture
Dacron velour bolster
dacryocystitis, neonatal
dactinomycin
DAF (DNA amplification
  fingerprinting)
Dafilon suture
Dagrofil suture
Dahedi 25 insulin pump
daidzein (soy protein)
daily metabolic load of fixed hydrogen
  ions
daily urine output
DA (direct agglutination) latex test for
  pregnancy
Dale Foley catheter
Dale Foley catheter holder
Dalgan (dezocine)
Dalkon shield intrauterine device (IUD)
Dalrymple sign
daltonism
damage
  papillary
  renal papillary
  renal vascular
damaged fallopian tube
DAMD (directed amplification of
  minisatellite region DNA)
Damkohler number
dam, rubber
danazol
dancing eye syndrome
D&C (dilation and curettage)
  diagnostic
  fractional
  suction
D&E (dilation and evacuation)
D&X (partial birth abortion)
Dandy-Walker cyst
Dandy-Walker malformation
Dandy-Walker malformation-joint
  contractures-cleft palate
Dandy-Walker syndrome
Danforth sign
Danubian endemic familial nephropathy
darbepoetin alfa
Dardik clamp

Darier disease
darifenacin
dark-field microscopy
dark urine
dartos fascia
darwinian fitness
data, morphologic
dates
  embryologic
  heavy for
  large for
  light for
  obstetric
  small for
dating, endometrial
daughter cell
daughter, DES (diethylstilbestrol)
DaunoXome (liposomal daunorubicin)
Davol
Davydov vagina construction
dawn phenomenon
day
  first postpartum
  first postoperative
Dayto Himbine (yohimbine)
DBest pregnancy test
DCC tumor suppressor gene
D-chiro-inositol
DCIS (ductal carcinoma in situ)
DDAVP (desmopressin, 1-deamino-8-D-arginine vasopressin)
DDD (dense-deposit disease)
dead birth
dead cells
dead-end flow
dead fetus syndrome
deafness-myopia-cataract-saddle nose, Marshall-type
deafness, sensorineural, with imperforate anus and hypoplastic thumbs syndrome
dead space
death
  cot
  crib

death *(cont.)*
  early fetal
  fetal
  genetic
  infant
  intermediate fetal
  intrauterine fetal
  late fetal
  late neonatal
  maternal
  neonatal
  perinatal
Deaver retractor
DeBakey pickups
DeBarsy syndrome
debility, congenital
debrancher enzyme deficiency (DBD)
debridement
debris
  amorphous
  cellular
debulking of tumor
debulking tumor by ultrasonic aspirator
Decadron (dexamethasone)
decapeptide analogue, synthetic
decapsulation of kidney
deceleration in labor
deceleration of fetal heart rate
decelerations
  early
  fetal heart rate
  late
  variable
  variable fetal heart rate
decels (decelerations)
decidua
  ectopic
  infected
  menstrual
  retained
decidua basalis
decidua capsularis
decidual cast
decidual endometritis
decidual reaction

decidua menstrualis
decidua parietalis
decidua polyposa
decidua spongiosa
deciduate placenta
deciduation
deciduitis
deciduoid reaction
deciduoma, Loeb
decision, gender assignment
decompensation
  acute circulatory
  acute metabolic
  cardiac
  circulatory
  end-stage fetal cardiac
  metabolic
  respiratory
decompression, bladder
decortication of kidney
decreased concentrations of circulating estrogen
decreased fetal movement
decreased renal perfusion
decreased testicular volume
decreased tubular resorption of normal filtered proteins
decreased urinary output
decreased variability of contractions
decreased venous flow in pregnancy
decrease in force and strength of urination
decrease in renal blood flow
decrease in renal concentration capacity
decrease, split renal function
dedicated breast biopsy system
deep artery of clitoris
deep artery of penis
deep diverticulum
deep dorsal vein of clitoris
deep dorsal vein of penis
deep dyspareunia
deep fascia of penis
deep pelvic node dissection
deep perineal pouch
deep photocoagulation
deep retention sutures
deep tendon reflexes (DTRs)
deep transverse arrest
deep vein phlebothrombosis
deep veins of clitoris
deep veins of penis
deep vein thrombophlebitis (DVT)
deep vein thrombosis (DVT)
defatting of panniculus
defect
  atrial septal (also atrioseptal)
  coagulation
  concentrating
  endocardial cushing
  filling
  hernia
  intrinsic renal concentration
  neural tube (NTD)
  polypoid filling
  renal concentrating
  renal tubular
  scrotal
  skin
  tubular
  ureteral filling
  vasopressin-resistant renal concentrating
  ventricular septal
defect in continuity of ureteral muscle
defective gonadal development
defeminization
deferens, vas
deferent canal
deferent duct
deferral of childbearing
defervesce, defervesced
defervescence of fever
defervescing
defibrination syndrome
deficiency
  ADH
  $alpha_1$-antitrypsin

deficiency *(cont.)*
- Arnold-Chiari
- biotinidase
- clotting
- cortisol
- glucagon
- gonadotropin
- intrinsic sphincter
- isolated gonadotropin hormone
- isolated pituitary hormone
- isolated thyroid stimulating hormone
- lipoprotein lipase
- placental sulfatase
- polyglandular
- prolactin
- 17-alpha-hydroxylase
- 3-beta-hydroxysteroid dehydrogenase
- thyroid
- urethral sphincter

deficiencies in sperm quantity
deficiens, ejaculatio
deficient conjoint tendon
deficit, endocrine
Definity ultrasound contrast agent
defloration pyelitis
Deflux
defocused (laser) beam
deformity (pl. deformities) (see also *syndrome)*
- Arnold-Chiari
- bell-clapper
- caliceal
- cockscomb
- Dandy-Walker
- fetal
- lobster-claw
- pelvic
- Sprengel
- tubular breast

degassed, demineralized water
degeneration
- breast
- carneous
- cystic

degeneration *(cont.)*
- fibroid
- infantile neuronal
- Kleeblattschadel
- lobster claw
- Madelung
- split-hand
- Sprengel
- testicular
- uterine myoma

degenerative chorea
degloving of penis
degradation, pigmentary retinal
dehiscence, wound
dehydrate, dehydrated
dehydration fever in newborn
dehydration, neonatal
dehydroepiandrosterone sulfate (DHEAS)
dehydroepiandrosterone (DHEA) test
DEI (diffraction-enhanced imaging) of breast
deionization water purification system
Dejerine palsy
Dejerine-Sottas disease
Delange syndrome
Delaprem (hexoprenaline sulfate)
delayed breast implant insertion
delayed cystography
delayed development
delayed ejaculation
delayed films
delayed implantation of prosthesis
delayed menarche
delayed menses
delayed neuromuscular maturation of lower urinary tract
delayed passage of meconium
delayed puberty
delayed pulmonary toxicity syndrome (DPTS)
delayed virilized adrenal hyperplasia
DeLee-Hillis stethoscope
DeLee maneuver (or rotation) of fetal head

DeLee obstetrical forceps
DeLee pelvimeter
DeLee suction
Delestrogen (estradiol)
deletion (del)
  chromosomal
  gene
  interstitial
  nucleotide
  point
  tandem (tan)
  terminal (ter)
deletion syndrome (see also *syndrome*)
  1p21-22
  1p22-p36.2
  1p36
  1p36.3
  1q
  1q41
  2q
  2q37.1
  4p
  4p15
  4q21-q25
  4q32-q34
  5p
  5q
  6p
  6p24
  7p
  7q21.3
  7q21-q22
  8p
  8p23.1-8pter
  10p
  10qter
  11q
  13p
  13q
  13q14
  13q23-q25
  13q32
  13q33-34
  14p16.3
deletion syndrome *(cont.)*
  14q31-q32.3
  14q32.3
  18p
  18q-
  18q23
  21q
  22q
  22q11
  22q11.2
  22q13.3
  Xp21
  Xp22.1-Xp22.3
  Xq22.3
Delfen foam
delivery (also see *presentation*)
  assisted breech
  assisted cephalic
  assisted vaginal
  breech
  cephalic
  cesarean section
  en caul
  failed forceps
  forceps
  full-term
  high forceps
  low forceps
  manual assisted
  Mauriceau method
  Mauriceau-Smellie-Veit maneuver
  McRoberts maneuver
  midforceps
  missed
  outlet forceps
  perimortem
  postmortem
  precipitate
  premature
  preterm
  Smellie method
  Smellie-Veit maneuver
  spontaneous cephalic
  spontaneous vaginal

delivery *(cont.)*
- vacuum
- vacuum-assisted
- vacuum extraction
- vaginal
- vaginal breech
- vertex

delivery by ventouse
delivery instruments, vectis
delivery room
Delta OD450 test (in amniocentesis)
Delta 32 digital stereotactic system
Delta 32 TACT three-dimensional breast imaging system
Deltec long-term dual-lumen hemodialysis catheter
deltopectoral fascia
Demadex (torsemide)
deme
dementia, dialysis
dementia paralytica
Demerol (meperidine)
demineralization of fetal spine
demise
- embryonic
- fetal

de Morsier syndrome
Demser (metyrosine)
Demulen oral contraceptive
denature
denaturing gradient
denaturing gradient gel electrophoresis (DGGE)
denaturing high performance liquid chromatography (DHPLC)
denervation, ovarian
Denis Browne pouch
Denonvilliers fascia
de novo
de novo duplication
de novo mutation
de novo post-transplant glomerulonephritis
de novo robertsonian translocation
de novo tandem duplication (see *duplication syndrome*)
dense adhesions
dense breast tissue
dense deposit disease (DDD)
dense film
dense (nonporous) membrane
densitometry, dual photon
density
- calcific
- nuclear
- ovoid-shaped calcific

dental embryonic groove
dentate line
denticular hymen
dentin dysplasia
dentinogenesis imperfecta type 3
dento-oculo-osseous dysplasia
denuded area
Denys-Drash syndrome
DeOrio intrauterine insemination catheter
deoxy-D-glucose
deoxyribonucleic acid (DNA)
deoxyribonucleotide
deoxyspergualin
department, Labor and Delivery (L&D)
dependent drainage
dependent edema
Depend pads for incontinence
depGynogen (estradiol cypionate)
depleted of penetrants
depletion, carbohydrate
Depo-Estradiol Cypionate (estradiol)
DepoGen (estradiol)
Depo-Provera (medroxyprogesterone)
deposit
- epimembranous
- mesangial

deposition
- immune complex
- mesangial IgG

deposition of antigenic stimulation
deposition of suspended or dissolved
  substances on external membrane
  surfaces
Depo-Testadiol (estradiol)
Depotestogen (estradiol)
depressed cell-mediated immunity
depressed skull fracture
depression
  cerebral
  endogenous
  exogenous
  fetal heart rate
  postmenopausal
  postpartum
  premenopausal
  prolonged fetal
depression of fetus, prolonged
depression of interactive behavior in
  newborns
deprivation
  estrogen
  oxygen
depuration, adequacy of
de Quervain thyroiditis
deranged electrolyte balance
derangement
  metabolic
  renal failure
  tubular function
Dercum disease
derivative chromosome
Dermabond topical skin adhesive
Dermagraft-TC
DermaLase laser system
dermal bridge of penile shaft
dermal layer
Dermalon suture
dermatitis
  contact
  diaper
  exfoliative
  scrotal
  seborrheic
dermatitis gangrenosa infantum
dermatitis herpetiformis
dermatitis of pregnancy, papular
dermatoglyphics
dermatomyositis
dermatosclerosis
Derma-Trans roll-on system
dermis
dermoid cyst
dermoid epithelium
dermoid plug
dermopathy, infiltrative
DeRoyal surgical cannula
DeRoyal surgical trocar
DES (diethylstilbestrol)
DES daughter
DES exposure
DES in utero, exposure to
DeSanctis-Cacchione syndrome
descended testicles
descended testis
descensus testis
descensus uteri
descensus, uterine
descent
  arrest of
  fetal
desferoxamine mesylate
desiccating tissue
desired pore structure
desire for permanent sterilization
desire for permanent surgical sterility
desire, sexual
deslorelin
desmopressin
Desogen (ethinyl estradiol, desogestrel)
desogestrel and ethinyl estradiol
desogestrel/ethinyl estradiol oral contraceptive pill
DeSouza exercises to encourage
  position change of fetus
desquamated cells
desquamation, germinal cell
desquamation of vaginal cells

desquamative inflammatory vaginitis
destruction, endoscopic
destruction of fetus
destruction of prostate gland by freezing
destruens, chorioadenoma
desultory labor
detachment of placenta
detectable pores
Detect cytology brush
determination, intrauterine pressure
DeToni-Fanconi syndrome
detorsion of testicle
detorsion of testis
Detrol, Detrol LA (tolterodine tartrate)
detrusor compliance
detrusor contraction, impaired
detrusor hypotonia
detrusor instability
detrusor muscle
  bladder
  involuntary contraction of
  spasticity of
detrusor pressure
detrusor spasticity
detrusor-sphincter dyssynergia
detrusor-sphincter incoordination with urinary incontinence
detrusor stability
detrusorrhaphy
detubularizing
detumescence
deuteranopia
deuteranomaly
developing fetus
development
  cognitive
  defective gonadal
  follicular
  life-span
  psychomotor
  psychosexual
  rapid premature sexual
  Tanner staging of
  zygote
developmental age (DA)
developmental anatomy
developmental anomaly
developmental cyst of ovary
developmental disability
developmental hip dysplasia
developmental milestones
developmental pediatrician
deviation, standard
device (see also *contraceptive device*)
  Acurette endometrial sampling
  Acutrainer electronic bladder retraining
  amniohook
  Arrequi laparoscopic knot pusher ligator
  Autocath 100 bladder-control
  AVA 3Xi advanced venous access
  AxyaWeld Bone Anchor System
  Bard Biopty gun
  BD Sensability breast self-examination aid
  BiliBottoms phototherapy
  Bili mask
  bipolar urological loop
  BladderManager ultrasound
  bladder neck spreader
  Bovie 1250 electrosurgical
  Bovie 2100 electrosurgical
  breast bolster
  BreastCheck
  BreastExam
  breast lesion localizing grid
  Calcutript lithotripter
  Capio CL transvaginal suture-capturing
  CaverMap surgical aid
  cavernotome
  C-bloc continuous nerve block
  CellCept
  ChromaVision digital analyzer
  clitoral therapy (CTD)
  CloseSure wound closure
  Clot Buster Amplatz thrombectomy

device *(cont.)*
CMI/Mityvac cup
CMI/O'Neil cup
colpomicroscope
Conceive Fertility Planner
contraceptive
Crystal Vision smoke evacuation unit
CTD (clitoral therapy)
cystotome
Dacomed snap gauge
Dalkon shield intrauterine
Disetronic Insulin Pen
Diva laparoscopic morcellator
Dopplex
Dornier compact lithotriptor
Dynamic Optical Breast Imaging System (DOBI)
Ellik kidney stone basket
Ellik kidney stone elevator
Ellik kidney stone evacuator
endocoagulator
Endo Stitch endoscopic suture
Eros-CTD (clitoral therapy)
Estring (estradiol-loaded silicone vaginal ring)
Evershears
Explora endometrial sampling
ExpressView blood sugar monitoring
ExtendEVAC smoke evacuation pencil
Extractor three-lumen retrieval balloon
eXtract specimen bag
FemSoft insert urinary incontinence
First Warning breast cancer screening
Fletcher applicator
Fletcher-Suit applicator
Forma water-jacketed incubator
Freeman cookie cutter areola marker

device *(cont.)*
Fria pelvic muscle training
Futura resectoscope sheath
GelPort abdominal access
Gene Gin cloning
GE Senographe 20001 digital mammography system
Gynecare Verascope Hysteroscopy System
HandPort hand-assist
Hartley balloon inflation
Hasson trocar
Hemasure r/LS red blood cell filtration system
Hemocor HPH high performance hemoconcentrator
Humatro-Pen growth hormone delivery
HUMI uterine manipulator/injector
ImageChecker M1000 computer aid
ImageChecker mammography detection
In Charge Diabetes Control System
inflation pencil
InnoSense urinary incontinence
Innovo insulin delivery
InPath (for cervical cancer screening)
inSync miniform menstrual
InterStim implantable continence-control therapy
InterStim neurostimulation
InterStim urinary neurostimulation
intrauterine (IUD)
Karl Storz Calcutript
Karl Storz N_2O Endoflator
laparoscopic biopsy
LaserSonics SurgiBlade colposcopic Lasette finger stick
LightSheer SC diode laser hair removal
Lilly Pen for insulin
Lymphedema Alert bracelet

device *(cont.)*
lyodura loop
Macroplastique implantable urinary continence
Majoli uterine manipulator/injector
Makler insemination
Mammex TR computer-aided mammography system
Mammotome handheld breast biopsy
Marsupial adjustable belt with attachable pouch
Masterson endometrial sampling
Medi-Jector Choice needle-free insulin injection
Medworks urinary incontinence surgical
Microlet Vaculance finger stick
Microsulis microwave endometrial ablation system
Millin bladder neck spreader
Miniguard urinary incontinence
Mobetron electron accelerator
Multispatula cervical sampling
Neocontrol incontinence control
NeoCure Cryoablation System
Nibbler
Nibblit laparoscopic
Oasis thrombectomy system
Opal R.F. tissue ablation
Origin Tacker laparoscopic tacking
OR1 electronic endoscopy system
OvuStick
OxyHood
Palpagraph breast mapping
Palpagraph breast tissue examination
PAPNET cervical smear screening
P.D. Access
PelvX pelvic support
percutaneous Stoller afferent nerve stimulation system (PerQ SANS)
PerQ SANS urge incontinence
pHEM-ALERT vaginosis screening

device *(cont.)*
Philips ultrasound machines endovaginal transducer
Photon radiosurgery system
Pipelle endometrial sampling
Plastibell
Pneumo Sleeve laparoscopic airlock
Pneumo Sleeve laparoscopic assist
portable blood irradiator
Prostatron
Prostatron mobile microwave
Prostatron 2.5
prosthetic
Protect-a-Pass suture passer
Raz double-prong ligature carrier
R.F. tissue ablation
RigiScan penile tumescence
Sadowsky hook wire breast
Sahara Clinical Bone Sonometer
SANS (Stoller afferent nerve stimulation) urinary incontinence
Scopette genital prolapse
Sea-Band acupressure wristband
SelectCells
Sensability breast examination sheet
SoftScan laser mammography system
stapling
STAR (specialized tissue aspirating resectoscope)
StatLock dialysis catheter securement
stereotactic vacuum-assisted biopsy (SVAB)
STOP (selective tubal occlusion procedure) nonsurgical permanent contraception
SurgiScope robotic surgery
Suspend sling implant
TCI-31 Lifelong Ovulation Tester
The Female Condom
The Whittlestone Physiological Breastmilker
transcutaneous access (TQa) flow

device *(cont.)*
TUOD (transurethral occlusive)
ureteral stimulator
Uroloop surgical
UroVive sphincter deficiency system
vacuum erection (VED)
vectis
venous access
VersaPoint hysteroscopic fibroid removal
Vesica percutaneous bladder neck stabilization kit
Vocare Bladder System
Wallace pipette
Wallach Endocell endometrial cell sampler
Wedge electrosurgical resection
Zelsmyr Cytobrush
ZUMI uterine manipulator
Dewan suprapubic urodynamic catheter
Dewey obstetrical forceps
dexamethasone
DEXA (dual-energy x-ray absorptiometry) scan for bone density determination
Dexon sutures
dextran 1
dextran 10
dextran 40
dextran 70
dextran 75
dextrocardia, bronchiectasis, and sinusitis
dextrocardia with situs inversus
dextrorotation
Dextrostix
dezocine
D5W
DGGE (denaturing gradient gel electrophoresis)
DGS (diabetic glomerulosclerosis)
DGS (DiGeorge syndrome)
DHE (dehydroepiandrosterone)
DHE (dihematoporphyrin ether)
DHEA-S sulfate (dehydroepiandrosterone sulfate) test
DHPG (dihydroxypropoxymethylguanine)
DHPLC (denaturing high performance liquid chromatography)
DHT (dihydrotestosterone)
DiaBeta (glyburide)
diabetes (see also *diabetes mellitus*)
adult onset (type 2)
brittle
bronze
calcinuric
familial nephrogenic
galactose
gestational
insulin-dependent
insulin-resistant associated with acanthosis nigricans
juvenile onset (type 1)
lipoatrophic
maternal
maturity onset, of the young (MODY)
non-insulin-dependent
post-transplant diabetes mellitus
Priscilla White classification of
type 1
type 2
uncontrolled maternal
diabetes associated with other endocrine diseases
diabetes attributed to pancreatic disease
diabetes induced by beta-cell toxins
diabetes insipidus
acquired
central
complete form
idiopathic
nephrogenic
partial form
primary
secondary
vasopressin-sensitive

diabetes insipidus, diabetes mellitus, optic atrophy, and deafness syndrome
diabetes mellitus (see also *diabetes*)
  brittle
  adult onset (AODM)
  gestational (GDM)
  insulin-dependent (IDDM)
  juvenile (JDM)
  juvenile onset (JODM)
  ketosis-prone
  ketosis-resistant
  maturity onset (MODM)
  neonatal
  stable
  type 1 (insulin-dependent)
  type 2 (non-insulin-dependent)
diabetes mellitus syndrome in newborn
diabetic acidosis
diabetic fetopathy
diabetic glomerulopathy
diabetic glomerulosclerosis (DGS)
diabetic hyperglycemia
diabetic hyperosmolar nonketotic coma
diabetic ketoacidosis
diabetic kidney disease
diabetic nephropathy (DN)
DiabetiSweet Sugar Substitute
diabetologist
DiabGel hydrogel dressing
DiabKlenz wound cleanser
DiaCan fistula needle
diaceturia
Diacyte DNA ploidy analysis
diagnosis (pl. diagnoses)
  antenatal (of fetal disorder)
  clinical
  cytologic
  differential
  final
  frozen section
  genetic
  histologic
  neonatal

diagnosis *(cont.)*
  pathologic
  preimplantation genetic diagnosis
  preliminary
  prenatal
  prenatal genetic
diagnosis by exclusion
diagnostic biomarker
diagnostic D&C (dilation and curettage)
diagnostic hysteroscope
diagnostic hysteroscopy
diagnostic laparoscopy
diagnostic/operative hysteroscope
diagnostic system
diagonal conjugate
diakinesis
Dialock hemodialysis access system
Dialock system
Dialog dialysis system
Dialose, Dialose Plus (docusate sodium)
dialysate
  bicarbonate-based
  leakage of
  peritoneal
dialysate bags, collapsible polyvinyl chloride
dialysate contaminant
dialysate delivery system
dialysate drainage system
dialysate exchange
dialysate infusion
dialysate infusion method, "flush-before-fill"
dialysate leak
dialysate port
dialyser
dialysis (see also *dialyzer*; *hemodialysis*; *peritoneal dialysis*)
  Aksys PHD hemodialysis system
  automated-cycler intermittent peritoneal
  automated peritoneal (APD)

dialysis *(cont.)*
 continuous ambulatory peritoneal (CAPD)
 continuous cyclical peritoneal (CCPD)
 continuous peritoneal (CPD)
 Dialock hemodialysis access system
 Dialog
 equilibrium peritoneal (EPD)
 extracorporeal
 hemodialysis
 Home Choice automated PD (peritoneal dialysis) system
 HomeChoice Pro with PD Link
 immediate
 intermittent peritoneal (IPD)
 kidney
 LifeSite hemodialysis system
 maintenance
 manual intermittent peritoneal
 nocturnal automated-cycler intermittent peritoneal
 partner-assisted
 peritoneal (PD)
 personal hemodialysis system (PHD)
 postoperative
 RenaClear dialyzer cleaning system
 self-care
 short-time
 urgent
dialysis access
dialysis amyloidosis
dialysis-associated cystic disease
dialysis catheter
 Deltec long-term dual-lumen hemodialysis
 double-cuff
 Flexxicon Blue
 Hemo-Cath
 Hurwitz
 Meostar hemodialysis
 Niagra temporary
 Oreopoulos-Zellerman peritoneal
 polyurethane pail-handle coil-tipped peritoneal

dialysis catheter *(cont.)*
 porous polyethylene
 Quinton
 Quinton Mahurkar dual-lumen hemodialysis
 S.E.T. hemodialysis
 single-cuff
 soft silicone rubber
 SPI-Argent II peritoneal
 surgically implanted hemodialysis
 Tenckhoff peritoneal
 Tesio hemodialysis
 Uldall subclavian hemodialysis
 Vas-Cath Opti-flow long-term dual-lumen hemodialysis
 Vas-Cath Soft-Cell permanent dual-lumen hemodialysis
dialysis catheter securement device
dialysis center
dialysis coordinator
dialysis delivery system
 Drake-Willock automatic
 HomeChoice Pro with PD Link
dialysis dementia
dialysis fistula needle
dialysis machine (see *dialysis, dialyzer, hemodialyzer, hemodialysis*)
dialysis monitor, OLC (On Line Clearance)
Dialysis Outcome Quality Initiative (DOQI)
dialysis regimen
dialysis-related amyloid deposits
dialysis-related ascites
dialysis-related carpal tunnel syndrome
dialysis service
dialysis solution pumped through ultrafiltrate chamber
dialysis shunt
dialysis unit
dialytic loss of water soluble vitamins
dialytic therapy
Dialyvite, Dialyvite 800
dialyzed blood

dialyzer (see also *dialysis*)
- Biospal
- capillary flow
- Clirans
- CT (computed tomographic)
- Filtryzer
- Gambro Lundia
- high flux
- hollow fiber capillary
- Hospal Biospal
- large-surface
- parallel flow
- parallel plate
- Terumo Clirans
- Toray Filtryzer
- twin-coil

diameter
- biparietal (BPD)
- fetal biparietal
- fetal chest
- gestational sac (GS)
- intertuberous
- obstetric conjugate

diamnionic twins
diamniotic twins
Diamond-Blackfan anemia
diamond-shaped wedge of fibromuscular tissue
diamond tip electrode
Dianon prostate profile and diagraph
Diapact CRRT system
diaper dermatitis
diaper rash
diaphanography
diaphanoscope
diaphanous
diaphonography
diaphoresis
diaphragm
- arching-type
- coil-spring
- congenital
- contraceptive
- flat-spring
- urogenital

diaphragmatic hernia
diaphyseal aclasis
diaplacental
DIAPPERS (delirium; infection; atrophic urethritis; vaginitis; pharmaceuticals; psychological; excess urine output; restricted mobility; stool impaction)
diarrhea, *Clostridium difficile*-associated (CDAC)
DiaScreen urine chemistry test strip
Diasensor 1000 blood glucose monitor
diastasis of symphysis pubis
Diastat vascular access graft for dialysis
diathesis, bleeding
diastrophic dysplasia
diatrizoate meglumine imaging agent
Dibenzyline (phenoxybenzamine)
DIC (disseminated intravascular coagulation)
dicarboxylic aciduria
DICC (dynamic infusion cavernosometry and cavernosography)
dicentric chromosome
dichogamy
dichorionic-diamniotic (di-di)
dichorionic twins
dichromasy
diclofenac
di-di (dichorionic-diamniotic)
didelphia, uterine
didelphic uterus
didelphys
dideoxynucleoside
Didronel (etidronate)
didymus
diecious
diembryony
diencephalic syndrome
dienestrol (estrogen)
diet
- fluid-restricted
- high biologic value protein content
- low-fat
- low-sodium

diet *(cont.)*
  Portagen
  protein-restricted
diet ad lib
dietary amenorrhea
dietary ketoacidosis
dietary management in renal failure
dietary supplement
  Amin-Aid
  Ensure
  Glucerna
  Nepro
  Trinovin
dietetic albuminuria
diethylenetriaminepentaacetic acid (DTPA)
diethylstilbestrol (DES)
diethylstilbestrol diphosphate
diethylstilbestrol exposure in utero
Dietl twisted kidney crisis
differential diagnosis
differential renal function test
differential temperature sensor (DTS) breast screening
  BreastAlert
differential ureteral catheterization test
differentiation
difficult childbirth
difficulty in achieving erection
difficulty in attaining orgasm
difficulty in maintaining erection
difficulty voiding
diffraction-enhanced imaging (DEI) of breast
diffuse breast involvement
diffuse cystic mastopathy
diffused hydrocele
diffuse glomerulonephritis
diffuse goiter
diffuse inspiratory crepitant rales
diffuse intravascular coagulation (DIC)
diffusely swollen prostate
diffuse membranous lupus nephritis
diffuse mesangial sclerosis
diffuse nephritis
diffuse proliferative glomerulonephritis
diffusion across a semipermeable membrane
diffusion of glomerular filtrate
diffusion of HCO_3
diffusive solute transport
Diflucan (fluconazole)
DiGeorge anomaly
DiGeorge syndrome (DGS)
digestive glycosuria
Digiscope
digital Add-On Bucky
digitalization, prophylactic
digital mammography
digital pelvic examination
digital rectal examination
digital subtraction angiogram
digital subtraction angiography
digital subtraction imaging technique
digito-otopalatal syndrome
digoxin induction
dihematoporphyrin ether (DHE)
dihybrid cross
dihydropyrimidine dehydrogenase
dihydrotestosterone (DHT), transdermal
dihydroxypropoxymethylguanine (DHPG)
Dilamezinsert (DMI) penile prosthesis dilator
Dilamezinsert (DMI) penile prosthesis inserter
Dilantin (phenytoin sodium)
Dilapan hygroscopic cervical dilator
Dilapan synthetic laminaria for cervical dilation
dilated caliceal system
dilated calix
dilated loops of ureter
dilated, tight fingertip (TFD)
dilated ureter
dilatation (see *dilation*)

dilation (also dilatation)
appreciable
arrested
caliceal
cervical
distal ureteral
transvaginal uterine cervical dilation with fluoroscopic guidance
urethral
tubular
ureteral
ureteric
urethral
ventral
dilation and curettage (D&C), suction
dilation and effacement of cervix
dilation and evacuation (D&E)
dilation and extraction
dilation and suction
dilation/arterialization of forearm veins
dilation of caliceal system
dilation of calices
dilation of foreskin
dilation of ureter
dilator
Bakes common duct
cervical
Dilamezinsert (DMI) penile prosthesis
Dilapan hygroscopic cervical
Garrett
Goodell uterine
graduated
Hanks uterine
Hegar cervical
Key-Med
Kollmann urethral
laminaria cervical
osmotic
Pharmaseal cervical
Pratt uterine
Walther urethral
dildo (pl. dildos)
dilute oxytocin drip
dilute urine excretion
dilute urine sample
dilution technique for access flow measurement
dilution, ultrasound velocity
DiMattina laparoscopic catheter
dimercaptosuccinic acid (DMSA)
dimerizing
dimethyl sulfoxide (DMSO)
diminished fetal perfusion
diminished libido
diminished renal reserve
diminished sensorium
diminished uterine blood flow
DIMOAD syndrome (diabetes inspidus, diabetes mellitus, optic atrophy, and deafness)
dimorphism, sexual
dimpling of skin
dinitrophenylhydrazine screening test for maple sugar urine disease
dinoprost tromethamine
dinoprostone
dinucleotide/trinucleotide/tetranucleotide repeats
dioecious (also diecious)
Diovan HCT (valsartan and hydrochlorothiazide)
diovular twins
dipalmitoyl phosphatidylcholine (DPPC) test
diphosphonate
diphtheria
diphtheria-tetanus (DT) toxoid
diphtheritic cystitis
diploid
diploid sperm
diplotene
diplotene stage of meiotic prophase
dipslide
dipstick urinalysis
dipstick, urine

dipyridamole
directable coaxial catheter
direct agglutination (DA) latex test for pregnancy
direct complement-activated immune reaction
direct Coombs test
direct diuretic
directed amplification of minisatellite region DNA (DAMD)
directed biopsy
direct DNA analysis
direct endothelial cell injury
direct IBT (immunobead test)
Directigen latex agglutination test
direction
  clockwise
  counterclockwise
direct maternal death
direct replacement of embryos (DREM) technique
direct tissue destruction
direct-vision internal urethrotomy (DVIU)
direct-vision urethrotome
direct visual control of biopsy
direct visualization
disability (pl. disabilities), developmental
disassortative mating
discharge
  bloody
  brown
  candidal
  cheesy
  clear
  cottage cheese
  creamy
  curdy
  fishy
  foul
  foul-smelling
  foul-smelling vaginal
  frothy

discharge *(cont.)*
  green
  KOH-positive
  mucopurulent
  mucosanguineous
  odorous
  preputial
  subpreputial
  thick
  thin
  urethral
  vaginal
  watery
  white
  white and cheesy
  yellow
discharge from the nipple
discission
discoidal placenta, uterine surface
discoid lupus erythematosus
discoid placenta
discontinuity of vas deferens
discoplacenta
Discrene breast implant
discrete mass
discriminatory zone of beta hCG
disease (see also *disorder*; *syndrome*)
  ABO hemolytic
  acquired cystic
  acute intermittent porphyria (AIP)
  acute pelvic inflammatory
  acute proliferative glomerulonephritis
  Addison
  Addison-Schilder
  ADH deficiency
  ADPKD (autosomal dominant polycystic kidney)
  adrenal
  adult immune thrombocytopenic purpura (TCP)
  adult onset medullary cystic
  adult polycystic kidney
  Aicardi-Goutieres syndrome

disease *(cont.)*
- Alexander
- allergic tubulointerstitial renal
- Alport post-transplant anti-GBM
- Alström
- Alzheimer
- amyloid
- Andersen
- anti-GBM
- anti-TBM
- atheroembolic renal
- atherosclerotic renovascular
- autoimmune
- autosomal dominant polycystic kidney (ADPKD)
- autosomal recessive polycystic kidney
- azorean
- Barlow
- Bartter syndrome
- Basedow
- Batten
- Batten-Spielmayer-Vogt
- Behçet
- Berger
- Berger nephritic
- biotinidase
- Bourneville
- Bowen
- breast fibrocystic
- Bright
- broad beta
- bronze
- Bronze-Schilder
- Byler
- calculus
- Camurati-Englemann
- Canavan
- Caroli
- celiac
- central core
- Charcot-Marie-Tooth
- Charnin-Dorfman
- chlamydia pelvic inflammatory

disease *(cont.)*
- cholesterol ester storage
- Christensen-Krabbe
- chronic alcoholic liver
- chronic lung
- Coats
- congenital cytomegalic inclusion
- congenital polycystic
- congestive cardiac failure with uremia
- Conradi
- Cori
- Creutzfeldt-Jakob
- Crohn
- Cronkhite-Canada
- Crouzon
- Cushing
- cyanotic heart
- cystic kidney
- Darier
- Dejerine-Sottas
- dense deposit (DDD)
- Dercum
- diabetes mellitus
- diabetic kidney
- dialysis-associated cystic
- diffuse proliferative glomerulonephritis
- distal tubal
- Durhing
- end-organ
- end-stage kidney
- end-stage renal (ESRD)
- Erdheim Chester
- ESRD (end-stage renal)
- extramammary Paget
- Fabry
- Fahr
- Fairbanks
- familial juvenile nephronophthisis
- familial nephrogenic diabetes
- Farber
- fetal liver
- fibrocystic

disease *(cont.)*
fibrocystic breast
Flatan-Schilder
Folling
foot process
Forbes
Forbes-Albright
Fournier
Friedreich
fulminant
functional bowel
fungal
gastroesophageal reflux (GERD)
Gaucher
Gaucher-Schlagenhauffer
gestational trophoblastic (GTD)
giant cell
Gilbert
glomerular
glycogen storage
Goodpasture syndrome
graft versus host (GVHD)
granulomatous
Graves
GTD (gestational trophoblastic)
Günter (Guenter)
Hailey-Hailey
Hallervorden-Spatz
Hartnup
hemolytic (of newborn)
hemorrhagic (of newborn)
Henoch-Schönlein purpura
hereditary
heredofamilial
Hirschsprung
Huntington
hyaline membrane (of newborn)
hypersensitivity angiitis
hypertensive renal
I cell
idiopathic immune complex glomerulonephritis
idiopathic membranous glomerular
immune complex

disease *(cont.)*
immune renal (IRD)
immune tubular interstitial
immunologically mediated
inclusion cell
infantile phytanic acid storage
infantile celiac
infantile Refsum
infectious
infectious hepatitis
interstitial
intramembranous dense deposit
intrauterine cytomegalic inclusion
intrinsic genitourinary
intrinsic renal
intrinsic urinary system
iron storage
irreversible
juvenile nephronophthisis
Kimmelstiel-Wilson
kinky hair
Kugelberg-Welander
legionnaires
Leigh
Lesch-Nyhan
Lindau
lipid storage
Little
Lobstein
Lou Gehrig
lymphoma
Machado-Joseph
maple syrup urine
Marie-Sainton
McArdle
measles
medullary cystic
mesangial
metastatic
metastatic trophoblastic (MTD)
microcystic, of renal medulla
micrometastatic
microvillus inclusion
Miege

disease *(cont.)*
- Milroy
- minimal change
- mixed connective tissue (MCTD)
- mixed cryoglobulinemia
- Mondor
- Morvan
- motor neuron
- moyamoya
- MSUD (maple sugar urine)
- multiple myeloma
- multisystem
- mumps
- muscle core
- mycotic penile
- myoclonic
- myoencephalopathy ragged red fiber
- myoneurogenic
- nephronophthisis-uremic medullary cystic (UMCD)
- neurocutaneous
- neuromuscular
- neutral lipid storage
- Niemann-Pick
- nil
- Norrie
- oasthouse urine
- occult renal
- oculocraniosomatic neuromuscular
- Ormond
- overt urologic
- Paget
- parasitic
- parasitic urinary tract
- parenchymatous renal
- Parry
- pauci-immune rapidly progressive glomerulonephritis
- Pelizaeus-Merzbacher
- pelvic inflammatory (PID)
- persistent trophoblastic (PTD)
- Peyronie
- phenylketonuria (PKU)
- Pick

disease *(cont.)*
- Plummer
- polyarteritis nodosa
- polycystic kidney
- polycystic liver
- polycystic ovary
- Pompe
- primary renal
- pseudo-Hurler
- pulmonary-renal syndrome
- ragged red fiber
- Recklinghausen
- Reclus
- Refsum
- remittent
- renal
- renal bone
- renal limited
- renal parenchymal
- renal vein thrombosis
- renovascular
- right-sided bacterial endocarditis
- rubella
- Sandhoff
- Santavouri
- sarcoidosis
- Schimmelbusch
- scleroderma
- sclerosing
- secondary membranous
- Seitelberger
- sexually transmitted (STD)
- sickle cell
- silicon nephropathy
- Simmonds
- Sinding-Larsen-Johansson
- slowly progressive glomerular
- Spielmeyer-Sjögren
- Steinert
- systemic inflammatory
- systemic lupus erythematosus (SLE)
- Tangier
- Tauri
- Tay-Sachs

disease *(cont.)*
 Thomsen
 Thomsen-Becker
 Tis
 trophoblastic
 tubo-ovarian inflammatory disease
 tubulointerstitial
 UMCD uremic medullary cystic)
 urethral stricture
 venereal
 von Gierke
 von Willebrand
 Waldmann
 Wegener granulomatosis
 Werdnig-Hoffman
 West
 Wilson
 Wohlfart-Kugelberg-Welander
 Wolman
 Woody Guthrie
 Ziehen-Oppenheim
disease-causing mutation
disease-free interval
disease-free survival
Disetronic Insulin Pen
disjoined pyeloplasty
disk kidney
disk, Molnar
dislodged calculus
dislodgment of ureteral stone
dismembered pyeloplasty
disomy
disorder
 amino acid metabolic
 anterior lobe
 arrest
 autoimmune
 autosomal dominant genetic
 autosomal recessive
 coagulation
 female sexual arousal (FSAD)
 genetic
 gestational carbohydrate intolerance (GCI)

disorder *(cont.)*
 hereditary
 hyperprolactinemic
 intersex
 late luteal phase dysphoric (LLPDD)
 mendelian
 multifactorial
 myoneurogenic
 neural tube
 polygenic/multifactorial
 polyglandular
 postpartum mood
 protraction
 premenstrual dysphoric (PMDD)
 rare benign X-linked
 sexual
 X-linked recessive
disperse placenta
displacement of ovary and fallopian tube
displacement of kidney
disposable cervical dilator
disposable douche
disposable uterine sound
disproportion
 cephalopelvic (CPD)
 fetal
 fetal-pelvic
 fetopelvic
disruption in contour
disruption of corporeal body
disruption of perineal wound
dissecting scissors
dissection
 bladder flap
 blunt
 deep pelvic node
 en bloc axillary node
 en bloc pelvic lymph node
 finger
 groin
 meticulous
 mucosal

dissection *(cont.)*
  paravesical blunt
  scissor
  sharp
dissection of ureter, inadvertent
dissector
  Agris-Dingman submammary
  Kitner (also Kittner)
  Maryland
  Spacemaker balloon
  ultrasonic
  water-jet
disseminated candidiasis
disseminated coccidioidomycosis
disseminated cutaneous gangrene
disseminated infection
disseminated intravascular coagulation (DIC) in newborn
disseminated intravascular coagulopathy
dissolved NaCl
dissolved polymer
distal acorn tip
distal arthrogryposis type 2A
distal convoluted tubule
distal end of ureter was fishmouthed
distal fallopian tube
distillation column
distillation process
distal muscular dystrophy (DMD)
distal nephron
distal orifice
distal part of prostatic urethra
distal renal tubular acidosis
distal right ureter
distal RTA
distal splenorenal shunt (DSRS)
distal stump of artery
distal tubal disease
distal ureteral dilation
distal urethral stenosis
distended bladder
distended kidney
distended urinary bladder
distended vagina
distention
  abdominal
  bladder
  pelvicaliceal
  ureteral
  uterine
  vesical
distinctive sequences of DNA
distortion of bladder position
distortion of calices
distress
  fetal
  iatrogenic fetal
  maternal
distribution of body fat
  android
  gynecoid
disturbance
  fluid-electrolyte
  metabolic
disturbance of acid-base metabolism
  mixed
  simple
disturbance of enchondral ossification
Ditropan, Ditropan XL (oxybutynin chloride)
diuresis
  osmotic
  postobstructive
diuretic
  cardiac
  direct
  high ceiling
  indirect
  loop
  mercurial
  osmotic
  potassium sparing
  saline
  thiazide
diuretic medication
diuretic phase of acute tubular necrosis
diuretic renal imaging
diuretic renal scan

diuretic therapy, potassium sparing
diurnal enuresis
diurnal rhythm
Diva laparoscopic morcellator
diversionary bladder drainage
diversion, urinary
diverticular prostatitis
diverticulectomy
  open
  urethral
diverticulum (pl. diverticula)
  acquired
  bladder
  caliceal or calyceal
  colonic
  deep
  fallopian tube
  false
  left-sided bladder
  Meckel
  metanephric
  pseudodiverticulum
  urethral
  vesical
  wide-mouthed mucosal
diving goiter
division of sacrouterine ligaments
division of zygote
division, ureteral
dizygotic twins
DMD (Duchenne muscular dystrophy)
D-Modem and insulin pump therapy
DMSA (dimercaptosuccinic acid)
DMSO (dimethyl sulfoxide)
DN (diabetic nephropathy)
DNA (dioxyribonucleic acid)
DNA amplification fingerprinting (DAF)
DNA banking
DNA-based testing
DNA clone
DNA fingerprinting
DNA genetic determination
DNA heteroduplexes
DNA hybridization
DNA ploidy analysis
DNA polymerase
DNA probe
DNA repair genes
DNA repair pathway
DNA replication
DNA sequencing
DNA typing
DOBI (Dynamic Optical Breast Imaging) system
docetaxel
documentation by serial ultrasound examinations
Döderlein (Doederlein)
Döderlein bacillus
Döderlein laparoscopic hysterectomy
Döhle body (Doehle)
dolens, phlegmasia alba
dolichopellic pelvis
DoLi S extracorporeal shock wave lithotriptor
Dolphin hysteroscopic fluid management system
Dolsed (methenamine)
domain
domelike portion of uterus
dome of bladder
dome of prostate
dome of urinary bladder
dome of uterus
domestic violence
dominance variance
dominant allele
dominant gene
dominant inheritance
dominant negative mutation
dominant breast mass
dominant follicles in ovary
dominant mass
dominant X-linked inheritance pattern
Dominion aspiration needle
Donahue syndrome
donate a zygote

donation of genetic material
Donnan exclusion
donor
  bilateral
  cadaver
  cadaveric
  egg
  IVF egg
  kidney
  living
  living-related
  organ
  renal transplant
  semen
  third-party
  unilateral
donor egg cycle
donor egg/gestational carrier surrogacy
donor insemination
donor kidney
donor oocyte
donor source for neophalloplasty
donor-specific transfusion (DST)
donor sperm
donor twin transfusion
Donovan bodies
donut mastopexy
donut of prostatic tissue
DOOR (deafness, onychodystrophy, osteodystrophy, and mental retardation) syndrome
dopamine
Doppler Perfusion Index
Doppler study, penile
Doppler ultrasonic blood flow detector
Doppler ultrasonic fetal heart monitor
Doppler ultrasonography
Doppler ultrasound
Doppler waveform analysis
Dopplex device
Doptone monitoring of fetal heart tones
DOQI (Dialysis Outcome Quality Initiative)
doral slit of prepuce
Dormia stone basket
Dornier compact lithotriptor
Dorner HM3 lithotripsy machine
Dornier lithotriptor (also lithotripter)
Dorros brachial internal mammary guiding catheter
dorsal artery of clitoris
dorsal artery of penis
dorsal hood
dorsal hood of foreskin
dorsal hood of penis
dorsal hood of prepuce
dorsalis pedis pulse
dorsal lithotomy position
dorsal nerve of clitoris
dorsal nerve of penis
dorsal onlay graft urethroplasty
dorsal penile nerve block (DPNB)
dorsal recumbent obstetric position
dorsal supine position
dorsal vein complex
dorsum of penis
dosage analysis
dose-dense therapy
dose-limiting toxicity
dospirenone/ethinyl estradiol oral contraceptive
Dostinex (cabergoline)
double-armed suture
double-blind clinical trial
double breast coil
double-bubble ultrasound appearance of fetus
double-cuff dialysis catheter
double-footling breech
double helix
double heterozygote
double-J indwelling catheter
double-J stent placement
double-J ureteral catheter
double-J ureteral stent
double kidney
double-loop stoma
double-lumen breast implant

double-lumen catheter
double-lumen venous umbilical catheter
double minute chromosomes
double-mouthed uterus
double nuchal cord
double penis
double-pigtail ureteral catheter
double skin mastopexy
double-stranded DNA
double-toothed tenaculum (also double tooth tenaculum)
double uterus
double uterus with double cervix and double vagina
double vagina
double-voided a.m. urine specimen
double-voided specimen
double-voided urine specimen
double-voiding cystography
double-walled incubator
doubling time
doubly ligated and divided
doubly refractile fat bodies
douche
  baking soda
  baking soda and vinegar
  Betadine
  disposable
  Massengill
  Novofem disposable
  povidine-iodine
  Summer's Eve
  Tanafem
  therapeutic
  Vagi-Guard
  vaginal
  vinegar
  yogurt
douche bag
douching
doughnut kidney
doughnut pessary
Douglas
  abscess of pouch of
  cul-de-sac of
  pouch of
Douglas cul-de-sac
douglasectomy
Douglas rectouterine pouch
doula
Dow Corning breast implant
down-regulation, pituitary
downsizing
downstaging
downstream side of the membrane
Down syndrome
doxazosin mesylate
doxercalciferol
Doxil (doxorubicin)
doxorubicin
doxycycline
Doyen vaginal retractor blade
Doyle operation for paracervical uterine denervation
DPC4 tumor suppressor gene
DPI (Doppler Perfusion Index)
DPNB (dorsal penile nerve block)
DPPC (dipalmitoyl phosphatidylcholine) test
DPTS (delayed pulmonary toxicity syndrome)
drain
  Blake
  flat Silastic suction
  Hemovac
  Jackson-Pratt
  Penrose
  Ring-McLean sump
  silicone Penrose
  silicone Pezzer
  suction
  sump
drainage
  catheter
  closed wound suction
  continuous

drainage *(cont.)*
  continuous catheter
  dependent
  feculent
  gravity
  intermittent
  intraoperative bladder
  nephrostomy
  percutaneous nephrostomy
  postoperative
  preliminary
  tidal
  transvaginal ultrasound-guided
  wound
drainage films
drainage of bulbourethral gland
drainage of ovarian cyst
drain and replenish in tidal fashion
DR antigen
Drake-Willock automatic dialysis
  delivery system
drape
  adhesive plastic
  fenestrated drape
  Ioban
  Ioban Vi-Drape
  sterile
  sterile paper
draping, gowning, and gloving
Drash syndrome
DREM (direct replacement of embryos)
  technique
dressing
  ABD pad
  Acticoat
  Adaptic
  Band-Aid
  breast support
  bulky
  Coban
  collodion
  compression
  Dermabond topical skin adhesive

dressing *(cont.)*
  DiabGel hydrogel
  Elastoplast
  Flexinet
  fluff
  4 x 4 (four-by-four)
  Interceed TC7
  Iodoflex
  Iodoform gauze
  Iodosorb
  Jobst breast support
  Koch-Mason
  Op-Site
  perineal compression
  Peri-Strips Dry
  pressure
  PSD Gel
  Repliderm
  Steri-Strips
  sterile
  Tegaderm
  Telfa
  3M Clean Seals
  tie-over
  transparent polyurethane
  Vaseline gauze
  Xeroform
dribbling incontinence
dribbling, terminal
drip incontinence
droloxifene
dromedary kidney
drooping lily sign in urography
droplets
  free fat
  tubular protein
dropped bladder
drug delivery system, AERx pulmonary
drug-induced acute renal failure (ARF)
drug-induced hypoglycemia
drug-induced nephrotoxicity
drug-induced teratology
drug-induced virilization

drug intoxication, acute
drug metabolites in renal failure
  a-methyldopamine
  acetylated metabolites
  adriamycinol
  chlorophenoxyisobutyric acid
  daunorubicinol
  desacetylcephalothin
  desacetylrifampin
  digoxigenin-bis-digitoxoside
  digoxigenin-mono-digitoxoside
  digoxin
  hydroxyhexamide
  N-acetyl analog
  N-acetylprocainamide
  normeperidine
  norpropoxyphene
  oxazepam
  oxypurinol
  phenobarbitone
  6-mercaptopurine
  2-hydroxychlorpropamide
drug overdose with dialyzable toxin
drug reaction
drug therapy infertility
drug toxicity
drug withdrawal syndrome in newborn
drugs (see *medications)*
  antestrogen or antiestrogen
  anticholinergic
  antischistosomal
  beta-adrenergic blocking
  cytotoxic
  immunosuppressive
  oxytocic
  sympathomimetic
  synergistic
Drummond syndrome
DRx quantitative hCG patient monitor
DRYalysate
dry heaves
dry labor
dry-phase separation membrane
  formation
dry weight
dry-wet phase separation membrane
  formation
DSRS (distal splenorenal shunt)
DST (donor-specific transfusion)
DT (diphtheria-tetanus) vaccine
DTaP (diphtheria-tetanus-pertussis)
  vaccine
D10W (dextrose in 10% water)
DTPA (diethylenetriaminepentaacetic
  acid) renography
DTP (diphtheria-tetanus-pertussis)
  vaccine
DTRs (deep tendon reflexes)
DTS (differential temperature sensor)
  breast screening device, BreastAlert
dual-check valve
dual-energy x-ray absorptiometry
  (DEXA) scan
dual-lumen catheter color-coded for
  inflow and outflow
dual-photon densitometry
Duane syndrome
DUB (dysfunctional uterine bleeding)
Dubecq-Princeteau angulating needle
  holder
Dubin and Amelar classification of
  varicocele
Dubin-Johnson syndrome
Dubowitz-Ballard maturity rating
Dubowitz exam
Dubowitz scale for infant maturity
Dubowitz syndrome
Duchenne muscular dystrophy (DMD)
Duchenne palsy
Ducrey bacillus
duct
  amniotic
  Bartholin
  breast
  bulbourethral gland
  collecting
  deferent
  ejaculatory

duct *(cont.)*
excretory
galactophorous
Gartner
gasserian
genital
Guérin
Haller aberrant
lactiferous
Leydig
mammary
mesonephric
metanephric
milk
Müller (Mueller)
müllerian
occlusion of breast
obstruction of efferent
omphalomesenteric
ovarian
paramesonephric
paraurethral
primordial
pronephric
prostatic
renal
Schüller
secretory
seminal
Skene
spermatic
stenosis of breast
subvesical
testicular
umbilical
urogenital
vitelline
vitellointestinal (VID)
wolffian
ductal carcinoma in situ (DCIS)
ductal carcinoma of prostate
ductal ectasia
ductal ectasia of breast
ductal hyperplasia
ductal hyperplasia in subareolar region of breast
ductal proliferation
ductal transitional cell carcinoma of prostate
duct ectasia
duct hyperplasia
ductogram, mammary
ductule, prostatic
ductus arteriosus
patent (PDA)
persistent
persistent patency of
reversed
ductus arteriosus patency
ductus deferens
ampulla of
artery to
scrotal part of
ductus venosus patency
due date
Duet vascular sealing device
Duhrssen incision of cervix
Duke pouch for continent urinary diversion
Dukes classification of colon carcinoma (*not* Duke's)
Dulcolax (bisacodyl) suppositories
Dumontpallier pessary
Duncan placenta
Duncan presentation
Duo-Cyp (estradiol)
duodenal atresia or stenosis
Duo-Flow dual-lumen catheter
Du Pen epidural catheter
Duplay uterine tenaculum forceps
duplex kidney
duplex, placenta
duplex uterus
duplicated marker
duplication, bilaterality of ureteral
duplication mutations (see *duplication syndrome*)
duplication of left kidney

duplication of right kidney
duplication syndrome (see also *syndrome*)
  4q21-q28
  4q23-q27
  5q
  6q23
  6p
  7
  7p11.2-p13
  7p15.1-p21.3
  7p21.1-p14.2
  8p
  8p12-p23
  9
  10p11.2-p12.2
  10q
  12
  12p11.2-p13.3
  14q12-q13
  15q11-q13
  15q11.2-q14
  17
  17p11.2
  18
  19
  21
  22q11-q12
  FLT3 gene
  MLL gene
  P gene
  Xq23
  Xq27-28
Dupuytren contracture
Dupuytren hydrocele
Duraphase inflatable penile prosthesis
Durasphere bladder bulking agent
duration of contractions
duration of periods
DUR flexible ureteropyeloscope
Dura-II positional penile prosthesis
Durhing disease
Duricef (cefadroxil)
dusky cyanosis
Dutch pessary
Duvoid (bethanechol)
DVIU (direct-vision internal urethrotomy)
DVT (deep vein thrombosis; deep venous thrombosis)
dwarf
  achondroplastic
  asexual
  geleophysic
  hypophysial
  Lévi-Lorain
  micromelic
  normal
  phacomelic
  physiologic
  pituitary
  polydystrophic
  renal
  rhizomelic
  sexual
  Silver-Russell
  thanatophoric
dwarfism
dwarf pelvis
dwell time of dialysate
dwell volume
dye extravasation
dye (also see *contrast*)
  aniline
  Berwick
  indigo carmine
  Lymphazurin
  methylene blue
  radioactive
Dyggve-Melchior-Claussen syndrome
Dynaflex penile prosthesis
dynamic cystoproctogram
dynamic infusion cavernosography
dynamic infusion cavernosometry
dynamic infusion cavernosometry and cavernosography (DICC)

dynamic membrane formation
Dynamic Optical Breast Imaging
(DOBI) system
Dynepro (gene-activated erythropoietin)
Dyonics cystoscope
dysautonomia, familial
dysbetalipoproteinemia
dyschondroplasia with hemangiomas
dyschondrosteosis
dyscoordinate labor
dyscrasia (pl. dyscrasias)
hematologic
plasma cell
dysencephalia splanchnocystica
dysfunction
allograft
bladder
bowel and bladder
corpus luteum
endocrine
erectile
female sexual (FSD)
hypertonic uterine
hypothalamic
hypotonic uterine
male sexual (MSD)
medication-induced allograft
mitochondrial
pituitary
placental
psychosexual
renal
renal tubular
sexual
sphincter
tubular
venous leak
vesical
dysfunctional kidney
dysfunctional labor
dysfunctional uterine bleeding (DUB)
dysfunctional uterine hemorrhage
dysfunction of hypothalamus
dysgenesis
gonadal
müllerian
ovarian
seminiferous tubule
testicular
XO gonadal
XY gonadal
dysgenic
dysgerminoma
dyskeratosis congenita
dyslexia
dyslipidemia
dysmaturity
dysmenorrhea
acquired
essential
functional
mechanical
membranous
obstructive
ovarian
primary
psychogenic
secondary
spastic
tubal
ureteric
uterine
vaginal
dysmenorrheal membrane
dysmorphic RBCs (red blood cells)
dysmorphism
dysmorphogenesis
dysmorphology
dysmucorrhea
dysmyelogenic leukodystrophy-megalo-
barencephaly
dysontogenesis
dysontogenetic cyst
dyspareunia
collision
deep

dyspareunia *(cont.)*
  introital
  psychogenic
  secondary
dysphonia, chronic spasmodic
dysphoria, late luteal phase
dysplasia
  arthro-onychodysplasia
  benign mammary
  bronchopulmonary
  cervical
  cystic renal
  developmental hip
  epiphysealis hemimelica
  epiphysialis punctata
  fibromuscular
  fibrous
  intraepithelial cervical
  mammary
  microcystic
  minimal cervical
  obstructive renal
  onycho-osteodysplasia
  osteodenta
  osteo-onychodysplasia
  renal
  renal-retinal
  residual
  septo-optic
  sheetlike retroareolar
  skeletal
  tubular
dysplasia gigantism syndrome, X-linked
dysplasia of nails and hypodontia
dysplasia of cervix
dysplastic cystic malformation of kidney
dysplastic kidney
dysplastic nevus syndrome
dysponderal amenorrhea
dysproteinemia
dysspermatogenic sterility
dyssynergia
  bladder
  detrusor-sphincter
  esophageal
  sphincter
  uterine
dysthyroidal infantilism
dystocia
  arrest of active phase
  arrest of descent
  fetal
  maternal
  placental
  shoulder
  uterine
dystocia-dystrophia syndrome
dystonia, torsion
dystrophic epidermolysis bullosa
dystrophy
  adiposogenital
  asphyxiating thoracic
  Jeune thoracic
  Landouzy-Dejerine
  muscular
  myotonic
  vulvar
dysuria
dysuric
DYT-1 dystonia
DYT-1 gene

E, e

early amniocentesis
Eagle Barrett syndrome
early constraint defects
early decelerations
early embryonic cells
early fetal death
early intervention program
early labor
early latent syphilis
early menarche
early neonatal death
early onset preeclampsia
early syphilis
ear oximeter
ear, patella, short stature syndrome
Eastern Cooperative Oncology Group (ECOG) performance status
Eaton-Lambert syndrome
EBO (estimated blood loss)
EBRT (external beam radiation treatment/therapy)
Ebstein anomaly
E-cadherin expression test for classification of breast carcinoma
E-Cath tunneled epidural catheter
ECC (endocervical curettage)
Eccentric "Y" retractor
ecchymosis, fetal
ECD (endocardial cushion defect)
ECF (extracellular fluid)
Echinococcus infestation
echo (echocardiogram)
echocardiogram, echocardiography
  endometrial
  fetal
  in utero
  renal sinus
Echo-Coat ultrasound biopsy needle
echo-Doppler duplex flow meter
EchoEye ultrasound imaging system
echography, transvaginal
echolucency, posterior nuchal
echolucent fluid of gestational sac
EchoSeed (iodine-125) brachytherapy seed
Echosight Jansen-Anderson intrauterine catheter
Echosight Patton coaxial catheter
Echotip amniocentesis needle
Echotip Baker amniocentesis needle
Echotip culdocentesis needle
Echotip Dominion aspiration needle
Echotip Foothills needle
Echotip Kato-Asch coaxial needle
Echotip LANCET needle
Echotip Mannuti sampling needle

Echotip Norfolk aspiration needle
Echotip percutaneous entry needle
Echotip Pivet-Cook double lumen needle
echovirus
Eckbom syndrome
eclampsia
eclampsia with convulsions
ECLS (extracorporeal life support)
ECM (extracellular material)
ECM (extracellular matrix)
ECMO (extracorporeal membrane oxygenation)
ECOG (Eastern Cooperative Oncology Group)
ECOG performance status
E. coli (Escherichia coli)
E. coli H157:H7
Econolith lithotripter
ectasia
  duct
  ductal
  mammary
  mammary duct
  mammary ductal
  renal tubular
  tubular
  ureteral
ectatic ureter
ectocervical smear
ectocervix
ectoderm
ectodermal dysplasia
ectopia
  crossed kidney
  crossed renal
  crossed testicular
  renal
  renal cross-fused
  testis
  ureteral
ectopia cloacae
ectopia cordis
ectopia vesicae
ectopic adrenocorticotropic hormone deficiency
ectopic decidua
ectopic kidney
ectopic pregnancy
  aborted
  hemorrhage in
  persistent
  ruptured
  tubal ring in
ectopic pregnancy locations
  abdominal
  ampullar tube
  cervical
  cornual (interstitial)
  eccentric
  extrauterine
  fallopian tube
  heterotopic
  infundibular tubal
  intraligamentous
  intramural
  isthmic tubal
  interstitial
  ovarian
  peritoneal
ectopic test
ectopic testis
ectopic ureter
ectopic ureterocele
ectopic urethral orifices
ectoplacental
ectrodactilia
ectrodactyly-electrodermal dysplasia-clefting syndrome
ectropion, cervicitis with
ectropion of cervix
ECV (external cephalic version) maneuver
eczema
EDC (estimated date of confinement)
EDD (estimated date of delivery)

edema
 acute urethral
 bullous
 cerebral
 cervical
 dependent
 generalized
 gestational
 idiopathic
 infantile acute hemorrhagic (of skin)
 interstitial
 local
 massive
 menstrual
 nephrotic
 nonpitting
 nutritional
 pedal
 penile
 pitting
 placental
 preeclamptic
 premenstrual
 presacral
 pretibial
 pulmonary
 renal
 sacral
 trace
 villous
 vulvar
edema neonatorum
edema of pregnancy
edematous fallopian tube
edematous kidney
Eder probe
Edex (alprostadil for injection)
EDMD (Emery-Dreifuss muscular dystrophy)
EDR (extreme drug resistance) score
Edwards-Steptoe method of in vitro fertilization (IVF)
Edwards syndrome
EEA stapler
EEC (ectrodactyly-electrodermal dysplasia-clefting) syndrome
EEDC (ectrodactyly-electrodermal dysplasia-clefting syndrome)
effaced foot process
effacement
 cervical
 foot process
 pelvocaliceal
effacement of cervix
effacement of podocytes
effect
 androgen
 antiestrogenic
 Bohr
 estrogen
 estrogenic
 long-term radiation
 testosterone
effective renal blood flow (ERBF)
effective renal plasma flow (ERPF)
effector system
effemination
efferent ductule of testis
efferent glomerular arteriole
effluent, urine
efflux of urine
effusion
 pericardial
 pleural
 massive
eflornithine
EFM (electronic fetal monitoring)
EFRT (extended-field radiotherapy)
EFW (estimated fetal weight)
EG/BUS (external genitalia/Bartholin glands, urethra, and Skene) glands
EGA (estimated gestational age)
Egan mammography
EGF (epidermal growth factor)
EGFR (epidermal growth factor receptor) test
egg activation
egg cell

egg donor
egg membrane
egg production
egg retrieval
egg transfer
Egnell breast pump
EHK (epidermolytic hyperkeratosis)
EHL (electrohydraulic lithotripsy)
Ehlers-Danlos syndrome
EIC (extensive intraductal component) of breast tumor
EIFT (embryo intrafallopian transfer)
eight-cell embryo
8p deletion syndrome
18 duplication syndrome
8p duplication syndrome
8p12-p23 duplication syndrome
18p deletion syndrome
18p23.1-8pter syndrome
18q- deletion syndrome
18q23 deletion syndrome
Eisenmenger complex
Eisenmenger syndrome
ejaculate (noun, verb)
  split sperm
  whole-sperm
ejaculated semen
ejaculation
  delayed
  premature
  retarded
  retrograde
ejaculatory duct
ejaculatory duct obstruction
elaboration of toxins
elasticity, bladder
elasticity of cervical mucus
elastic vagina
elastic vaginal pessary
Elastoplast dressing
ELBW (extremely low birth weight) infant
Elder Helio cystoscope
ejaculatio deficiens
ejaculatio praecox
ejaculatio retardata
elderly primigravida
elderly primiparous patient
Elecare infant formula
Elecsys total PSA immunoassay
elective abortion
elective bilateral vasectomy
elective cesarean section
elective induction of labor
elective low forceps
elective mutism or selective mutism
elective sterilization
elective termination of pregnancy
elective TURP (transurethral resection of prostate)
elective vasectomy
electrical impedance breast scanning system
electrically mediated separations
electrical stimulation for incontinence
electrical stimulation of bladder
electrical stimulation of sacral nerves
electrical stimulation of spinal cord
electrocardiogram, fetal scalp
electrocautery (also *electrosurgical instruments*)
  bipolar
  Bovie
  Coaguloop resection electrode
  Electroscope disposable scissors
  Evershears
  Fine-Lap bipolar cutting device
  low current
  monopolar
  needlepoint
  needle-tip
  Neoflex bendable knife
  NeoKnife electrosurgical
electrocautery therapy
electrochemical glucose-monitoring test strip
electrocoagulate
electrocoagulation

electrode
  Aspen laparoscopy
  ball tip
  BiLAP bipolar needle
  Bugbee
  Coaguloop resection
  Copeland fetal scalp
  diamond tip
  fetal scalp
  resection
  resectoscope
  RollerLOOP surgical
  scalp
  SingleBAR
  StarBAR resection
  V+Loop cutting
  VaporTrode roller
electrode for incontinence
electrode needle
electrodiagnostic testing
electrodialysis
electroejaculation
electrohydraulic lithotripsy (EHL)
electrohydraulic lithotriptor
electrohydraulic shock wave lithotripsy (ESWL)
electrohysterograph
Electroloop cautery
electrolyte balance
electrolyte concentrate
electrolyte disturbance
electrolyte imbalance
electrolytes, urinary
electromicturition
electromyogram (EMG)
  pelvic floor
  ureteral
  sphincter
  urethral sphincter
electromyography of penile corpus cavernosum muscles
electron accelerator, Mobetron
electron-dense material
electronic fetal monitor (EFM)
electron microscopy
electron transfer flavoprotein (ETF) deficiency
electro-osmosis
electrophoresis
  hemoglobin
  serum protein
electrophoretic pattern of heteroduplexes
electroporation therapy
Electroscope disposable scissors
electrosurgery
electrosurgical instruments (see *electrocautery*)
electrosurgical pencil
electrosurgical plume
electrosurgical probe
electrosurgical unit (ESU)
electrovaporization of prostate tissue
elements, particulate
elephantiasis, genital
elephant pelvis
elevated serum acid phosphatase
elevated serum progesterone
elevated venous pressure in pregnancy
elevation of scrotum
elevation of vesical neck
elevation, uterine
elevator
  Boyle uterine
  Ellik
  Hulka
  Maher
  Ramathibodi uterine
  Somer uterine
  Valtchev
11q deletion syndrome
Eligard (leuprolide acetate)
Elipten (aminoglutethimide)
ELISA (enzyme-linked immunosorbent assay)
Elite nephroscope
Ellence (epirubicin)
Ellik elevator

Ellik evacuator
Ellik kidney stone basket
Ellik kidney stone elevator
Elliott obstetrical forceps
ellipse of skin
elliptical incision
elliptocytosis
Ellis-van Creveld syndrome
Elmiron (pentosan polysulfate sodium)
Elmore radiofrequency tissue morcellator
elongated cervix
elongated mass
elongated urethra
elongation of cervix
emancipated minor
embedded ovarian follicles
embolectomy
embolic episode
embolism
  air
  amnionic fluid
  amniotic fluid
  corpus cavernosum
  fat
  gas
  massive
  obstetrical air
  obstetrical blood clot
  penile
  peripheral
  puerperal pulmonary
  pulmonary
  pyemic
  renal artery
  septic
embolization
  atheromatous
  fibroid
  selective renal artery
  transcatheter
  tumor
embolization to regional lymph nodes
embolization to retina
embolize
EMBP (estramustine-binding protein)
embrace reflex
embrace, startle
embryo
  eight-cell
  frozen
  Janosik
  micromanipulating and cloning
  presomite
  previllous
  somite
  Spee
  stored
embryo adoption
embryo biopsy
embryoblast
embryocardia
embryo culture
embryofetoscopy, transabdominal (TGEF) thin-gauge (TGEF)
embryo frozen in liquid nitrogen
embryogenesis
embryogenetic
embryogenic
embryogeny
embryography
embryo intrafallopian transfer (EIFT)
embryologic dates
embryologist
embryology
embryomorphous
Embryon GIFT catheter
Embryon HSG (hysterosalpingography/hysterosonography) catheter
embryonal carcinoma
embryonal cell tumor
embryonal rhabdomyosarcoma
embryonal sarcoma
embryonate
embryonic demise
embryonic germ layers
  ectoderm
  endoderm
  mesoderm

embryonic ovary
embryonic pole of blastocyst
embryonic reduction to twins
embryonic sac
embryoniform
embryonization
embryonoid
embryony
embryopathy
embryophore
embryoplastic
embryoscopy
embryotomy
embryotoxicity
embryo transfer (ET)
embryotroph
embryotrophic
embryotrophy
EMC (endometrial curettage)
Emcyt (estramustine phosphate sodium)
emergency hormonal contraception
emergency laparotomy
emerging infectious disease
Emery-Dreifuss muscular dystrophy (EDMD)
emesis
EMG (electromyogram)
eminence, genital
Emit 2000 cyclosporine specific assay
EMIT (enzyme-multiplication immunoassay technique)
Emko foam
EMLA (eutectic mixture of local anesthetic)
EMLA anesthetic disc
Emmet-Gelhorn pessary
Emmet uterine tenaculum hook
emotional amenorrhea
emphysema
  congenital lobar
  interstitial
  neonatal cystic pulmonary
  subcutaneous
emphysematous cystitis
emphysematous pyelonephritis
Empirynol Plus contraceptive gel
emptying, complete bladder
empty sella syndrome
empty sella turcica
empty uterus
empyocele
EMS Swiss lithoclast intracorporeal lithotriptor
E-MVAC (escalated methotrexate, vinblastine, Adriamycin, cisplatin or Cytoxan) chemotherapy protocol
EnAbl thermal ablation system
enalapril
en bloc
en bloc augmentation mammoplasty
en bloc axillary node dissection
en bloc dissection of bladder, reproductive organs, perineum, rectum, and pelvic lymph nodes
en bloc pelvic lymph node dissection
en bloc removal
en bloc resection
en bloc transplantation of small pediatric kidney into adult recipient using interposition technique
encapsulated breast implant
encapsulated mass
encapsulated neoplasm
en caul delivery
encephalitis neonatorum
encephalitis periaxialis diffusa
encephalocele
encephalocystocele
encephalodysplasia
encephalofacial angiomatosis
encephaloid
encephalomyelocele
encephalomyelopathy
encephalopathy
  bilirubin
  neonatal hyperammonemic
  uremic
encephalotrigeminal angiomatosis

enchondromatosis
enchondromatosis with multiple cavernous hemangiomas
encopresis
encroachment of tumor
encrusted pyelitis
encysted calculus
encysted hydrocele
endarteritis obliterans
endarteritis, proliferative
endemic goiter
endemic hematuria
endemic syphilis
endemic tubulointerstitial nephritis of the Balkans
End-Flo laparoscopic irrigating system
endoanal ultrasound
Endo-Babcock surgical grasping device
Endobag laparoscopic specimen retrieval system
endocardial cushion defect (ECD)
endocardial fibroelastosis
endocarditis
Endocare Horizon prostatic stent
ENDOcare nitinol urinary stent
Endocare renal cryoablation
Endo Catch specimen retrieval bag
endocervical aspiration
endocervical biopsy
endocervical brush, Zelsmyr Cytobrush
endocervical canal
endocervical curettage (ECC)
endocervical curettement
endocervical glands
endocervical gonorrhea
endocervical mucosa
endocervical polyp
endocervical sample
endocervical sampling
endocervical smear
endocervical speculum
endocervical tissue obtained by scrapings
endocervicitis
endocervix
Endo Clip laparoscopic clip applier
Endoclosure suture carrier
endocoagulator
endocrine ablation
endocrine deficit
endocrine disorders-epilepsy-mental retardation
endocrine dysfunction
endocrine status
endocrine therapy
endocrinology, reproductive
EndoCurette endometrial suction curette
endocystitis
endoderm
endogenous arteriovenous fistula
endogenous creatinine clearance
endogenous depression
endogenous gonadotropin secretion
endogenous nuclear proteins
endogenous protein catabolism
endogenous pyrogenic cytokines
Endo GIA surgical stapler
Endo Hernia stapler
Endoknot suture needle
Endoloop disposable chromic ligature suture instrument
Endoloop ligature
EndoLumina bougie
EndoLumina II transillumination system
endoluminal ultrasound (EUS)
EndoMate Grab Bag endoscopic specimen retrieval bag
EndoMed LSS laparoscopic system
endometrectomy of bladder
endometria (see *endometrium*)
endometrial ablation
  laser
  Microsulis
  NovaSure
  PEARL
  rollerbar or roller bar electrode

endometrial ablator
endometrial adenocanthoma
endometrial aspiration biopsy curette
endometrial biopsy
endometrial biopsy suction curette
endometrial cancer
endometrial carcinoma
endometrial casts
endometrial cavity
endometrial cell sampler, Wallach
  Endocell
endometrial cryoablation
endometrial culture
endometrial curettage (EMC)
endometrial curettings
endometrial cyst
endometrial cystic hyperplasia
endometrial cystoma of ovary
endometrial dating
endometrial destruction
endometrial echo
endometrial glands
endometrial hyperplasia
endometrial implant
endometrial intraepithelial neoplasia
endometrial laser ablation
endometrial layers
endometrial lining
endometrial malignancy
endometrial necrosis
endometrial neoplasia
endometrial polyp
endometrial resection
endometrial resection and ablation
  (ERA) resectoscope sheath
endometrial scarring
endometrial screening
endometrial smear
endometrial stripe
endometrial stroma
endometrial stromal sarcoma
endometrial tissue
endometrioid carcinoma
endometrioid tumor
endometrioma, perforated
endometriosis
  abdominal
  adhesive
  appendiceal
  bladder
  broad ligament
  burned-out
  cervical
  colonic involvement of
  fallopian tube
  implantation theory of
  intestinal
  intra-abdominal
  lung
  myometrial
  ovarian
  patchy
  peritoneal
  rectal
  rectovaginal nodules of
  sciatic
  stromal
  studding of
  ureteral
  uterine
  vaginal
  vulvar
endometriosis in skin of scar
endometriosis of cul-de-sac of Douglas
endometriosis of rectovaginal septum
  and vagina
endometritis
  bacteriotoxic
  decidual
  exfoliative
  glandular
  hyperplastic
  membranous
  puerperal
  secondary
  superficial
  syncytial
  tuberculous

endometritis dissecans
endometritis related to prolonged
  rupture of membranes
endometrium (pl. endometria)
  atrophic
  benign secretory
  carcinoma of
  hyperechoic
  normal-appearing
  predecidual changes in the
  secretory
  Swiss cheese
  uterine
endometropic
endomyocardial fibrosis
endonuclease
end-organ disease
Endopath ETS-FLEX endoscopic
  articulating linear cutter
Endopath EZ45 endoscopic linear
  cutter
Endopath EZ45 No Knife endoscopic
  linear stapler
Endopath EZ-RF linear cutter
Endopath laparoscopic trocar
Endopath Ultra Veress needle
endopelvic fascia
endophytic ulcer
Endopouch Pro specimen retrieval bag
endopyelotomy
  Acucise
  antegrade
  retrograde ureteroscopic
Endosac specimen collection bag
endosalpingiosis
endosalpingitis
endosalpinx
endoscope
  Accuscope colposcope
  ACMI cystoscope
  ACMI flexible cystoscope
  ACMI hysteroscope
  ACMI nephroscope
  ACMI rotating continuous flow
    resectoscope

endoscope *(cont.)*
  ACMI ureteroscope
  ACMI USA series endoscope
  amnioscope
  AUR-7 flexible ureteroscope
  babyscope
  Baggish hysteroscope
  Baumrucker resectoscope
  binocular fiberoptic colposcope
  Brown-Buerger cystoscope
  Cabot cystoscope
  Cerveillance vaginal/cervical scope
  Circon Cryomedics colposcope
  Circon hysteroscope
  colpohysteroscope
  Cooper Surgical cystoscope
  Cryomedics colposcope
  Cuda laparoscope
  culdoscope
  cystoscope
  cystoureteroscope
  diaphanoscope
  Digiscope
  DUR flexible ureteropyeloscope
  Dyonics cystoscope
  Elder Helio cystoscope
  falloposcope
  fetoscope
  flexible fallopian tube endoscope
  flexible hysteroscope
  flexible video laparoscope (FVL)
  Futura resectoscope
  galactoscope
  Galileo rigid hysteroscope
  Gautier ureteroscope
  Gynecare Verascope hysteroscope
  Gyne-Tech B101-D colposcope
  Hysteroser contact hysteroscopy
    system
  hysterocolposcope
  hysteroscope
  Iglesias fiberoptic resectoscope
  infant cystoscope
  InjecTx cystoscope
  InjecTx customized cystoscope

endoscope *(cont.)*
Jarit cystoscope
Karl Storz flexible ureteropyeloscope
KryMed F0-101 colposcope
lactoscope
laparoscope
Leica colposcope
McCarthy panendoscope
Micro-H hysteroscope
microlaparoscope
MicroSpan minihysteroscope
MiniSite laparoscope
Morganstern continuous-flow operating cystoscope
mother and baby endoscope
nephroscope
Nesbit resectoscope
Olympus A2010 0° 4 mm cystoscope
Olympus CHF-P10 cystoscope
Olympus CYF-3 OES cystofiberscope (fibroscope)
Olympus HYF-XP flexible hysteroscope
OPERA STAR SL hysteroscope
Ovation falloscope
pediatric cystoscope
pelviscope
Pentax ECN-1530 choledochonephroscope
Pixie fiberoptic scope
resectoscope
rigid cystoscope
rigid hysteroscope
Seiler colposcope
Solos cystoscope
StereoEndoscope
Stern-McCarthy resectoscope
Storz cystoscope
Storz cystourethroscope
Storz hysteroscope
Storz resectoscope
suprapubic cystoscope
Surgiview laparoscope

endoscope *(cont.)*
3Dscope laparoscope
transurethral cystoscope
ureterocystoscope
ureteroscope
urethroscope
uteroscope
Valle hysteroscope
VerreScope microlaparoscope
videofetoscope
Visicath cystoscope
Wallach ColpoStar colposcope
Wallach PentaScope colposcope
Wallach TriScope colposcope
Wallach TriScope Quantum colposcope
Wallach Tristar colposcope
Wallach ZoomScope Quantum colposcope
Wappler cystoscope
Wappler cystourethroscope
Welch Allyn coloposcope
Welch Allyn Video Path colposcope
Wolf cystoscope
Wolf ureteroscope
Wolf videoresectoscope
Zeiss colposcope
Zoomscope colposcope

endoscopic-assisted mastopexy
endoscopic-assisted transumbilical augmentation mammoplasty
endoscopic bladder neck suspension
endoscopic cyst aspirator
endoscopic cap
endoscopic curved needle driver
endoscopic cyst aspirator
endoscopic destruction of fallopian tubes
endoscopic fetal surgery
endoscopic grasping forceps, 100°
endoscopic introducer/extractor
endoscopic Kitner (also Kittner)
endoscopic knife, Selikowitz
endoscopic needle bladder neck suspension

endoscopic needle suspension of bladder
endoscopic scissors
endoscopic stone disintegration
endoscopic strip craniectomy
endoscopic suspension of bladder neck
endoscopic suspension of vesical neck
endoscopic transaxillary augmentation mammoplasty
endoscopic ultrasound-guided fine-needle aspiration (EUS-FNA)
endoscopy (pl. endoscopies)
  OR1 electronic
  pelvic
  transabdominal thin-gauge embryofetoscopy (TGEF)
  ureteral
endospeculum (see also *speculum*)
  Gynex
  laser Kogan
endosperm
Endo Stitch endoscopic suture device
endothelial glomerulonephritis
endotheliochorial placenta
endothelium, renal capillary
EndoTIP cannula
endotoxemia
endotoxin
endotracheal intubation
endotracheal tube
endovaginal coil
endovaginal sonography
endovaginal transducer
endovaginal ultrasonography, ultrasound (EVUS)
Endoview endoscopy camera
endproduct
end-stage chronic renal failure
end-stage disease
end-stage fetal cardiac decompensation
end-stage kidney disease
end-stage liver disease
end-stage renal disease (ESRD)
end-stage renal failure (ESRF)
end-tidal carbon dioxide monitor
end-to-end anastomosis
end-to-end renal artery to hypogastric artery anastomosis
end-to-side anastomosis
end-to-side renal vein to iliac vein anastomosis
en face ("ahn fahs")
Enfamil 22 infant formula
Enfamil formula
Enfamil Human Milk Fortifier
Enfamil infant formula
Enfamil Premature Formula
Enfamil Premature Formula with Iron
Enfamil with Iron infant formula
enforced maturity of fetal lungs
engage
engaged head
engagement of fetal head
Engelmann syndrome
Engerix-B
engineering, genetic
English lock
English position
engorged breasts
enhanced sperm survival
enhancement factor
enhancer
enhancing mass
enisoprost
enlarged clitoris
enlarged kidney
enlarged prostate
enlarged thymus
enlarged tongue
enlargement
  fundal
  prostate
  uterine
en masse
enmesh
enmeshed

enoxacin
Enpresse (levonorgestrel/ethinyl estradiol tablets)
ensure hemostasis
Entamoeba histolytica
entanglement of cords
enterically transmitted non-A non-B hepatitis
enterobacteria
Enterobius vermicularis
enterocele
  acquired vaginal
  congenital pelvic
  congenital vaginal
  vaginal
enterocele repair, transvaginal
enterococci
enterocolitis
  necrotizing
  pseudomembranous
enterocystoplasty method of bladder augmentation
enterorenal
enterotomy scissors
enterourethral fistula
enterovaginal fistula
enterovesical fistula
entrapment of Cooper ligament by growing tumor
entrapment of smegma
enucleation
  adenomatous tissue
  extracervical
  transurethral
enuresis
  diurnal
  nocturnal
envelope, axillary
Enview camera
environment
environmental variance
environmental incontinence
enzygotic twins
enzyme
  angiotensin-converting (ACE)
  aromatase
  cathepsin D lysozoma
  dihydropyrimidine dehydrogenase
  intracellular
  matrix metalloproteinase
  proteolytic
  thymidine phosphorylase
enzyme assay
enzyme-linked immunosorbent assay (ELISA)
enzyme-multiplication immunoassay technique (EMIT)
eosinophilic cystitis
eosinophilic fasciitis
eosinophilic infiltration in kidney
eosinophilic prostatitis
eosinophils, urinary
epamniotic cavity
EPD (equilibrium peritoneal dialysis)
epicranial subaponeurotic hemorrhage
epicystitis
epidemic hemorrhagic fever
epidemiologic genetics
epidermal growth factor (EGF)
epidermal growth factor receptor (EGFR) test
epidermal nevus
epidermoid carcinoma
epidermolysis bullosa letalis
epidermolytic hyperkeratosis (EHK)
epididymal appendix
epididymal aspiration catheter
epididymal sperm aspiration (ESA)
epididymectomy
epididymis (pl. epididymides)
  appendix of
  superior ligament of
  torsion of
epididymitis
  bacterial
  nonbacterial
  tuberculous

epididymogram, contrast
epididymo-orchitis
epididymoplasty
epididymostomy
epididymotomy
epididymovasostomy, microsurgical (MSEV)
epidural analgesia
epidural anesthesia
epidural block
epidural catheter
epigenesis
epigenetic
epilepsy, hereditary
epiloia
epimembranous deposit
epimembranous nephritis
epimenorrhagia
epimenorrhea
epiphyseal changes and high myopia
epiphyseal osteochondroma, benign
epiploic
epiploica
epirubicin
episcleral plaque brachytherapy
episioperineorrhaphy
episioplasty
episioproctotomy
episiorrhaphy
episiotomy
  fourth degree
  Matsner median
  mediolateral
  midline
episiotomy extension
episiotomy repair
episode, embolic
episome
epispadias
  balanitic
  coronal
  penile
  penopubic
epistasis
epistatic
epithelial alteration
epithelial cell hyperplasia
epithelial cell proliferation
epithelial cells in urine
epithelial crescents
epithelial cyst
epithelial podocyte
epithelial thickness
epitheliochorial placenta
epithelium
  acetowhite
  coelomic
  columnar
  necrosis of bladder
  ovarian
  squamous
  tubular
  urinary bladder
  vaginal
EPL (extracorporeal piezoelectric lithotriptor)
EPO (erythropoietin)
EPO coordinator
epoetin alfa (EPO)
epoetin beta
Epogen (epoetin alfa)
EPP (erythropoietic porphyria)
EPP (erythropoietic protoporphyria)
Eppendorfer biopsy punch
Eppendorfer-Krause biopsy forceps
Eprex (recombinant human erythropoietin)
Epstein nephrosis
e.p.t. pregnancy test
epulis gravidarum
epulis, pigmented
equation
  Cockcroft-Gault renal function
  Jeliffe
  Rossavik fetal growth
  Schwartz
equilibrate
equilibration

equilibration between maternal blood
 and fetal tissues
equilibrium peritoneal dialysis (EPD)
equilibrium concentration
ER (estrogen receptor)
ER- (estrogen-receptor negative)
ER+ (estrogen-receptor positive)
ERA (endometrial resection and
 ablation) resectoscope sheath
eradicate
eradicated
eradication of stones
Erb palsy
Erb paralysis
erbB-2
ERBF (effective renal blood flow)
erbium:YAG laser system
ErCr:YAG (erbium chromium;
 yttrium-aluminum-garnet) laser
Erdheim Chester disease
ErecAid Classic system
erectile
erectile dysfunction, rigidity in
erectile dysfunction treatment
 Actis venous flow controller (VFC)
 Alibra (alprostadil/prazosin)
 alprostadil
 Alprox-TD (alprostadil)
 aminobenzoate potassium
 Androderm testosterone transdermal
 patch
 Aphrodyne (yohimbine)
 apomorphine
 Aphrodyne (yohimbine)
 Caverject (alprostadil)
 Cialis
 Dayto Himbine (yohimbine)
 Edex (alprostadil)
 ErecAid Classic system
 intracavernous injection test
 Invicorp (phentolamine mesylate)
 minoxidil
 Muse (alprostadil)
 Plaquase (collagenase)
erectile dysfunction *(cont.)*
 prostaglandin E1 (alprostadil)
 ProstaJect ethanol injection system
 RigiScan
 sildenafil citrate
 Topiglan (alprostadil topical gel)
 Uprima (apomorphine)
 vasoactive intestinal polypeptide
 (VIP)
 Vasomax (phentolamine)
 VED (vacuum erection device)
 V.E.T. (Vacuum Erection
 Technologies)
 VFC (venous flow controller)
 Viagra (sildenafil citrate)
 VTU-1 vacuum
 Yocon (yohimbine)
 yohimbine
 Yohimex (yohimbine)
erectile failure
erectile function
erectile impotence
erectile organ
erection
 artificial
 difficulty in achieving
 difficulty in maintaining
 inability to get an
 inability to maintain an
 inability to sustain an
 morning
 painful
 physiologic
erection mechanism
Ergoset (bromocriptine mesylate)
ergotamine
ER-ICA (estrogen-receptor immunochemical assay)
erogenous zones
Eros-CTD (clitoral therapy device)
erosion
 cervical
 phagedenic
erotic

eroticism
erotism, anal
erotogenesis
erotogenic
erotomania
erotopathy
ERPF (effective renal plasma flow)
ERT (estrogen replacement therapy)
  patch
ERxin multicomponent penile injection
erythema
  angry
  vulvar
erythema neonatorum
erythema toxicum neonatorum
erythematosus, systemic lupus
erythematous vulvitis en plaque
erythroblastosis, fetal
erythroblastosis fetalis
erythroblastosis neonatorum
erythrocyte
erythrocyte phosphoglycerate kinase deficiency
erythrocyte sedimentation rate (ESR)
erythrocyturia
erythroid hyperplasia of marrow
erythrokeratodermia heimalis
erythrokeratodermia progressiva symetrica
erythrokeratodermia variabilis
erythropoietic protoporphyria (EPP)
erythropoietin (EPO)
erythropoietin production
erythroplasia of Queyrat
erythropoiesis
erythropoietic stimulation
erythropoietin (epoetin alfa)
erythropoietin, recombinant human
ESA (epididymal sperm aspiration)
escape of amniotic fluid
escape phenomenon
Escherichia coli (*E. coli*) infection
Esclim (estradiol) transdermal system
Escobar syndrome
Escort balloon stone extractor
escutcheon
  female
  male
  normal female
esophageal atresia
esophageal atresia and/or tracheo-esophageal fistula
ESR (erythrocyte sedimentation rate)
ESRD (end-stage renal disease)
ESRF (end-stage renal failure)
ESS (euthyroid sick syndrome)
essential dysmenorrhea
essential hematuria
essential hypertension
essential pentosuria
EST (expressed sequence tag)
Estalis (estrogen/progesterone) transdermal system
Estes operation for sterility
estimated at term
estimated blood loss
estimated date of confinement (EDC)
estimated date of delivery (EDD)
estimated fetal size
estimated fetal weight (EFW)
estimated gestational age (EGA)
Estinyl (ethinyl estradiol)
Estrace
Estraderm (estradiol)
estradiol cypionate and medroxy-progesterone
estradiol
estradiol level
estradiol-loaded silicone ring
estradiol/norethindrone
estradiol/norethindrome patch
estradiol/norgestimate
estradiol transdermal patch
estradiol vaginal cream
Estra-L 40 (estradiol)
estramustine
estramustine-binding protein (EMBP)
estramustine phosphate sodium

Estrasorb (17-beta-estradiol) cream
Estring (estradiol-loaded silicone vaginal ring)
Estrinor oral contraceptive
estriol determinations, serial
estrogen
conjugated
ovarian hormone
tissue-selective
unopposed
estrogen breakthrough bleeding
estrogen conversion, peripheral
estrogen deficiency
estrogen-dependent adenocarcinoma of breast
estrogen deprivation
estrogen effect
estrogenic effect
estrogen-induced change
estrogen-induced prolactinoma
estrogen level
estrogen loss
estrogen-producing neoplasm
estrogen-producing ovarian tumor
estrogen/progesterone replacement therapy (EPRT)
estrogen-progestin
estrogen receptor (ER)
estrogen-receptor analysis
estrogen-receptor immunochemical assay (ER-ICA)
estrogen-receptor negative (ER-) tumor
estrogen-receptor positive (ER+) tumor
estrogen-receptor status
estrogen replacement
estrogen replacement patch, Climara Pro
estrogen replacement therapy (ERT)
estrogen-secreting testicular tumor
estrogen secretion
estrogen withdrawal effect
estrone
Estrone Aqueous (estrogen)
Estrophasic
estropipate
Estrostep (norethindrone)
ESU (electrosurgical unit)
ESWL (extracorporeal shock wave lithotripsy)
ESWT (extracorporeal shock wave therapy)
ET (embryo transfer)
etching of the damaged region
ETF (electron transfer flavoprotein deficiency)
ethchlorvynol
ETH (ethanol) intoxication
ethanol (ETH, ETOH)
Ethibond suture
Ethicon Surgiport 10-11 trocar
Ethicon Teflon paste
ethinyl estradiol
ethinyl estradiol/levonorgestrel
Ethmozine (moricizine)
ethnocephaly
ethoglucid
ethylene glycol
ethylene glycol poisoning
ethynodiol diacetate/ethinyl estradiol oral contraceptive
Ethyol (amifostine)
etidronate disodium
etoglucid
ETOH (ethanol) intoxication
etoposide
etretin
etretinate
ET (endotracheal) tube
ETT (endotracheal tube)
E2 (estradiol)
E2 prostaglandin suppository
EUA (examination under anesthesia)
eucalcemia
euchromatin
eugenics
euglycemia
eukaryote
Eulexin (flutamide)

Eulexin plus LHRH-A protocol
eunuch
eunuchism
eunuchoid gigantism
eunuchoidism
  hypergonadotropic
  hypogonadotropic
euploid
euploidy
Euro-Collins multiorgan perfusion kit
Euro-Collins solution
EUS (endoscopic ultrasonography)
EUS-FNA (endoscopic ultrasound-guided fine-needle aspiration)
euthymic
euthyroid goiter
euthyroid sick syndrome (ESS)
Evacet (doxorubicin [liposomal])
evacuating cannula
evacuation
  dilation and
  uterine
evacuation forceps
evacuation of prostatic chips
evacuation of smoke plume
evacuation pouchography
evacuator
  Ellik
  Toomey
evaluation
  fertility
  genetic
  qualitative
  quantitative
  staging
  urologic
evanescent
evaporation of solvent
event
  antepartum
  intrapartum
  postpartum
everolimus
Evershears electrosurgical instrument
Evershears II bipolar curved scissors
eversion
  cervical
  nipple
  umbilical
  vaginal
everted cervix
everted nipples
everted umbilicus
EVII endoscopic video system
evisceration, pelvic
Evista (raloxifene)
evolution
evolutionarily conserved
EVUS (endovaginal ultrasound)
ExacTech blood glucose monitor
examination
  annual
  bimanual
  bimanual palpation of adnexa
  bimanual palpation of uterus
  bimanual pelvic
  dark-field microscopic
  digital rectal
  external genital
  gynecologic
  pelvic
  pelviscopic
  prostate
  rectal
  rectovaginal
  speculum
  urinary sediment
  vaginal
examination under anesthesia (EUA)
Excel GE electrochemical glucose monitoring test strip
excellent visualization
excess, base
excess crystalloid removed by hemofiltration
excessive bone resorption
excessive extraglandular estrogen production

excessive fetal growth
excessive hair growth
excessive menstruation
excessive secretions
excessive urinary sodium excretion
excessive vomiting
excessive water loss
excess ultrafiltrate
excess vaginal mucosa
exchange, fetal-maternal
exchange transfusion
excision
  LEEP (loop electrosurgical excision procedure)
  suprapubic
  wide
excisional biopsy
excision of adnexa uteri
excision of appendix testis
excision of bladder dome
excision of cervix uteri
excision of cone of tissue
excision of cyst of Morgagni
excision of fallopian tube and ovary
excision of median bar of prostate
excision of spermatocele
excitation, sexual
exciting cause
excoriation
excrescence
excrete
excretion
  dilute urine
  kallicrein
  potassium
  protein
  renal sodium
  urinary calcium
  urinary sodium
excretion of acid urine
excretion of contrast medium
excretion of food pigments
excretion of radionuclide
excretion of urine
excretory cystography
excretory duct
excretory duct of seminal gland
excretory function
excretory intravenous pyelogram
excretory intravenous pyelography
excretory phase
excretory process
excretory urogram
excretory urography
excruciating left flank pain
exencephaly
exenteration
  anterior pelvic
  pelvic
  posterior pelvic
  total pelvic
exenterative surgery for pelvic cancer
exercise-induced amenorrhea
exercise proteinuria
exercise
  biofeedback
  DeSouza
  FemTone pelvic
  Kegel pubococcygeal muscle
  pelvic floor
  pelvic muscle (PME)
exfoliated cells
exfoliative dermatitis
exfoliative endometritis
exhibitionism
exhibitionist
exit site
exit site infection
ExMI (extracorporeal magnetic innervation)
exocervix
exogenous ACTH
exogenous depression
exogenous DNA
exogenous insulin
exogenous obesity

exogenous prosthesis
  bovine carotid xenograft
  expanded polytetrafluoroethylene (PTFE)
exomphalos-macroglossia-gigantism syndrome
exon
exon scanning
exonuclease
exophthalmic goiter
exostoses, multiple
Exosurf Neonatal (colfosceril palmitate)
Expand-a-Band breast binder
expanded basement membrane
expanded polytetrafluoroethylene (PTFE) exogenous prosthesis
expanded polytetrafluoroethylene graft
expander
  four-way vaginal
  Hextend blood plasma volume
expansile mass
expansion, mesangial
expectantly managed
expectant management
explantation of breast implants
Explora endometrial sampling device
exploration
  manual
  pelvic
  retropubic
  surgical
exploration of scrotum
exploratory laparotomy
exploratory pelvic laparotomy
exposure, diethylstilbestrol (DES)
exposure to DES in utero
exposure to excessive heat
exposure to industrial/environmental toxins
expressed gene
expressed phenotype
expressed prostatic secretions
expressed sequence tag (EST)
expression of trinucleotide repeat mutation
ExpressView blood sugar monitor
expulsion from the uterus of embryo or fetus
expulsion of gas from the vagina
expulsion rate for IUDs
expulsive pain
exquisitely tender prostate
exquisitely tender to palpation
exsanguination, fetal
exstrophic
exstrophy
  bladder
  cloacal
extended-field radiotherapy (EFRT)
extended pyelotomy
extended radical mastectomy
extended-survival graft
ExtendEVAC smoke evacuation pencil
extension
  episiotomy
  fourth degree
extensive intraductal component (EIC) of breast tumor
exteriorized stoma
exteriorize the uterus
external anal sphincter
external arteriovenous shunt
external beam radiation treatment (EBRT)
external blow over a full bladder
external cephalic version (ECV) maneuver
external cephalic version of fetus
external chondromatosis syndrome
external fetal monitor
external fetal monitoring
external genital examination
external genital/Bartholin, urethral, and Skene glands (EG/BUS)
external genitalia
external hemorrhage

external hemorrhoid
external iliac artery
external iliac node
external mammary artery
external meatus
external oblique
external oblique aponeurosis
external os
external os of uterus
external phase
external ring
external spermatic fascia
external sphincter
external ureteral ileostomy
external urethral meatus
external urethral orifice
external urethral sphincter
external urethrotomy
external version
extirpation of tissue
extirpation of uterus and adnexa
extirpative surgery
extra-amniotic pregnancy
extracaliceal
extracapillary lesion
extracapillary proliferation
extracapsular extension of prostate cancer
extracellular buffer system
extracellular diplococci
extracellular fluid (ECF)
extracellular fluid volume
extracellular fluid volume depletion
extracellular material (ECM)
extracellular matrix (ECM)
extracellular volume
extracellular volume depletion
extracellular volume expansion
extracervical enucleation
extrachorial pregnancy
extrachromosomal gene
extra chromosomes
extracorporeal circuit
extracorporeal circulation of blood
extracorporeal dialysis
extracorporeal life support (ECLS)
extracorporally tied sutures
extracorporeal magnetic innervation (ExMI)
extracorporeal membrane oxygenation (ECMO)
extracorporeal perfusion
extracorporeal piezoelectric lithotriptor (EPL)
extracorporeal shock wave lithotripsy (ESWL)
extracorporeal shock wave therapy (ESWT)
extracorporeal therapy
extracting solvent
extraction
  breech
  forceps
  Malstrom
  stone
  ureteral stone
  vacuum
extractor
  Bird vacuum
  CMI
  Fasflo mucus extractor
  Glassman stone extractor
  IUD
  Malmstrom vacuum
  Miltex IUD
  Mityvac vacuum
  Murless fetal head
  O'Neil
  vacuum
Extractor three-lumen retrieval balloon
eXtract specimen bag
extraembryonic coelom
extrafascial total abdominal hysterectomy with wide vaginal cuff
extragenital chancre
extragenital organs
extramammary Paget disease
extramembranous pregnancy

Extraneal (7.5% icodextrin) peritoneal
  dialysis solution
extranodal extension of lymph node
  metastases
extraosseous deposit of calcium
extraovarian mass
extraperineal
extraperitoneal abdominal approach
extraperitoneal cesarean section
extraperitoneal excision of one-third
  of ureter
extraperitoneal pelvioscopy
extraperitoneal space
extrapyramidal
extrarenal involvement by tumor
extrarenal pelvis
extrarenal uremia
extratesticular scrotal mass
extratubal
extrauterine gestation
extrauterine IUD (intrauterine device)
extrauterine pregnancy
extravaginal
extravaginal torsion
extravasate
extravasation
  bile
  blood
  contrast
  contrast agent
  dye
  fluid
  radiopaque fluid
  urinary
extravesical opacification
extravesical reimplantation
extravillous cytotrophoblast
extreme drug resistance (EDR) score
extreme immaturity of newborn
extreme lithotomy
extremely low birth weight (ELBW)
  infant
extrinsic compression of inferior vena
  cava
extrinsic compression of renal vein
extrinsic malignant ureteral obstruction
extrinsic ureteral compression
extubation
exuberant keratin formation
exudate
  bloody
  gray
  serosanguineous
  serous
  shaggy grayish
exudative glomerulonephritis
exudative nephritis
exudative stage of proliferative
  glomerulonephritis
ex utero fetal surgery
ex vacuo, hydrocephalus
ex vivo extracorporeal kidney surgery
ex vivo perfusion
ex vivo revascularization of kidney
eye patch
EZ-Screen Profile
E-Z Tac soft tissue reattachment system

F, f

FA (Fanconi anemia)
FAA gene
fabric
  biodegradable
  knitted
  satinlike
fabric polyester catheter cuff
Fabry disease
Fabry syndrome
face presentation
facial-digital-genital syndrome
facial dysplasia-short stature-
  penoscrotal anomalies
facial hemiatrophy
facial nerve palsy
facial palsy
facial paralysis
facial puffiness
facies
  moon
  Potter
facies anterior prostatae
facies inferolateralis prostatae
facies intestinalis uteri
facies lateralis ovarii
facies lateralis testis
facies medialis ovarii
facies medialis testis
facies posterior prostatae
facies posterior renis
facies renalis glandulare suprarenalis
facies renalis lienis
facies renalis splenis
facies urethralis penis
facilitation factor, F
facioauriculovertebral anomaly
faciocardiocutaneous syndrome
faciodigitogenital syndrome
faciofrontonasal dysplasia
faciogenital dysplasia
facioscapulohumeral muscular
  dystrophy
FACOG (Fellow of the American
  College of Obstetricians and
  Gynecologists)
factitial proctitis
factitious hematuria
Factive (gemifloxacin)
factor
  chemotactic (C567)
  coagulation
  colony-stimulating
  C3 nephritic
  epidermal growth (EGF)
  growth
  mammotropic

factor *(cont.)*
  nephritic
  risk
  testis-determining (TDF)
  tumor necrosis
  vascular endothelial growth (VEGF)
factor H deficiency
Fader Tip ureteral stent
factor V Leiden (FVL) mutation
factor IX deficiency
factor XIII deficiency
Fact Plus pregnancy test
Fact Plus Pro pregnancy test
Factrel (gonadorelin)
FAE (fetal alcohol effects)
FAG gene
FAH gene
Fahr disease
failed culture
failed forceps delivery
failed induced abortion
failed nipple valve
failed trial of labor
failed vacuum extraction
failed vaginal breech delivery
failure
  acute renal (ARF)
  chronic end-stage
  chronic renal
  end-stage chronic renal
  fetal heart
  intrauterine cardiac
  intrauterine heart
  intrinsic renal
  obstructive renal
  oligoanuric renal
  oliguric acute renal
  ovarian
  pituitary
  post-traumatic renal
  premature ovarian
  renal
  respiratory
failure of child to mature
failure of lactation
failure of version
failure to descend
failure to experience orgasm
failure to progress in active labor
failure to thrive (FTT)
Fairbank disease
falciform hymen
falciform ligament
falciparum infection
falciparum malaria
Falcon tube
falling of the womb
fallopian canal
fallopian ligament
fallopian neuritis
fallopian pregnancy
fallopian tube
  abscess of
  accessory
  clubbed
  consistency of
  damaged
  displacement of
  endometriosis of
  fill and spill of dye in
  fimbriated end of
  infarction of
  mobility of
  nonfunctioning
  outline of
  position of
  patent
  removal of
  size of
  torsion of
fallopian tube diverticulum
fallopian tube endometriosis
fallopian tube infarction
fallopian tube occlusion
fallopian tube perfusion
fallopian tube pregnancy
fallopian tube prosthesis
falloposcope

falloposcopy
falloscope, Ovation
Fallot, tetralogy of
Falope-Ring band applicator
Falope-Ring band sterilization
false diverticulum of bladder
false hematuria
false hermaphroditism
false labor
false negative
false pains
false passage
false paternity
false pelvis
false positive
false pregnancy
famciclovir
familial adenomatous polyposis (FAP)
familial alphalipoprotein deficiency
familial ataxia
familial breast cancer
familial cancer
familial dysautonomia
familial endocrine adenomatosis
familial factors
familial glycinuria
familial high density lipoprotein
  deficiency
familial hypogonadotropic hypogonadism
familial incomplete male pseudohermaphroditism
familial inheritance pattern of
  endometriosis
familial juvenile nephronophthisis
familial juvenile nephrophthisis
familial lecithin cholesterol acyltrans-
  ferase deficiency
familial lipoprotein lipase deficiency
familial Mediterranean fever
familial multiple endocrine neoplasia
familial nephritic syndrome
familial nephritis
familial nephrogenic diabetes
familial nephrosis
familial pemphigus
familial spastic paraparesis
familial splenic anemia
family-centered obstetric unit
family history
  negative
  positive
family history of breast cancer
family law
family planning
family practitioner
family selection
Famvir (famciclovir)
Fanconi anemia, group C
Fanconi syndrome
Fanconi II
FAP (familial adenomatous polyposis)
Farber disease
Farber lipogranulomatosis
Fareston (toremifene citrate)
FAS (fetal alcohol syndrome)
fascia
  anterior rectus
  autologous rectus abdominis
  Buck
  clavipectoral
  dartos
  deep
  deltopectoral
  Denonvilliers
  endopelvic
  external spermatic
  Gerota
  internal spermatic
  pectoral
  pectoralis
  perirenal
  preperitoneal
  pubocervical
  rectus
  rectus muscle
  renal
  Scarpa
  transversalis

fascia lata harvesting
fascia lata suburethral sling
fascial absorbable suture
fascial layer of perineum
fascial plane
fascial sling
fascia reapproximated
fascia renalis
fasciitis, necrotizing
Fasflo mucus extractor
FASIAR (follicle aspiration, sperm injection, and assisted rupture)
Faslodex (ZD 9238)
fastener
  ROC suture
  ROC XS suture
fasting blood glucose
fasting hyperinsulinemia
fasting hypoglycemia
FastPack PSA test
Fasturtec (rasburicase)
fat
  abdominal
  omental
  pararenal
  perinephric
  periprostatic
  perirenal
  renal
  renal sinus
fatal hemorrhage of kidney
fat embolism
fatigability
fat inclusions
fat injection for incontinence
fat lines, subcutaneous
fat necrosis breast mass
fat necrosis of breast
fat planes
fatty acids, unesterified
fatty apron
fatty cast
fatty droplets
fatty epiploica
fatty kidney
fatty liver of pregnancy
fatty renal capsule
fatty tissue
fatty tumor
Fc fragment of IgG
FCAP (fluorouracil, cyclophosphamide, Adriamycin, Platinol) chemotherapy protocol
FCAP (fluorouracil, Cytoxan, Adriamycin, Platinol) chemotherapy protocol
FDA (U.S. Food and Drug Administration)
FDG (fluorine-18-deoxyglucose)
FDG (facial-digital-genital syndrome)
febrile
febrile amnionitis
febrile episode
febrile seizure
febrile urine
FEC (fluorouracil, epirubicin, cyclophosphamide)
fecal diversion by colostomy
fecal impaction
fecal incontinence
fecalith, congenital
fecal mass
fecal material in vagina
fecal occult blood test
fecal soiling
Fechtner syndrome
feculent drainage
fecund
fecundate
fecundation
fecundity
fecundity selection
Federation Internationale de Gynécologie et Obstétrique (FIGO)
feedback
  inappropriate steroid
  tubuloglomerular
feedback effect

feeding
  bottle
  breast
  concentrated carbohydrate
  gavage
feeding tube
feed pretreatment
feed solutions
feed stream
feed-type solutions
Feissinger-Leroy-Reiter syndrome
Felig insulin pump
fellatio
Fellow of the American College of Obstetricians and Gynecologists (FACOG)
female
  fertile donor
  genetic
  X
female body habitus
female castration
female catheter
female circumcision
Female Condom
female escutcheon
female external genitalia
female factor infertility
female gender assignment
female genital mutilation (FGM)
female gonad
female hermaphroditism
female homosexuality
female hypospadias
female impotence
female incontinence ring
female internal genitalia
female pattern alopecia
female prostate
female pseudohermaphroditism
female reproductive cell
female reproductive history
female reproductive system
female sex hormones
female sexual arousal disorder (FSAD)
female sexual dysfunction (FSD)
female sterility
female-to-male transsexual
female urethra
Femara (letrozole) tablets
FemHRT 1/5 (norethindrone and ethinyl estradiol)
feminine secondary sex characteristics
feminization, testicular
feminizing testes syndrome
femoral catheter
femoral dysgenesis, bilateral
femoral-facial syndrome
femoral hypoplasia
femoral pulse
femoral vein
FemPatch transdermal estrogen replacement system
Femprox (alprostadil)
FemRx Soprano cryotherapy
FemSoft Insert urinary incontinence device
Femstat One (butoconazole nitrate)
Femstat 3 (butoconazole nitrate 2%) vaginal cream
femtomole (fmole)
femtomoles per milligram (fmoles/mg)
FemTone pelvic exercises
fenestrated drape
fenestrated hymen
fenestration, laparoscopic
fenretinide
fentanyl
Ferguson scissors
Fer-In-Sol
ferning
fernlike appearance of cervical and uterine mucus on slide
fern-negative Nitrazine test
fern-positive Nitrazine test
fern test
Ferrimin 150
ferritin

Ferrlecit (sodium ferric gluconate complex)
ferrous sulfate
fertile donor female
fertility
  general
  secondary
fertility drugs (see also *medications*)
  Antagon (ganirelix)
  A.P.L. (chorionic gonadotropin)
  Chorex-5 (chorionic gonadotropin)
  Chorex-10 (chorionic gonadotropin)
  chorionic gonadotropin
  Choron-10 (chorionic gonadotropin)
  Clomid (clomiphene citrate)
  clomiphene citrate
  Factrel (gonadorelin)
  Fertinex (urofollitropin)
  Follistim
  follitropin alfa
  follitropin beta
  ganirelix
  gonadorelin
  Gonal-F (follitropin alfa)
  Gonic (chorionic gonadotropin)
  Humegon (menotropins)
  injected
  Lutrepulse (gonadorelin)
  menotropins
  oral
  Pergonal (menotropins)
  Pregnyl (chorionic gonadotropin)
  Profasi (chorionic gonadotropin)
  Puregon (follitropin beta)
  Repronex (menotropins)
  Serophene (clomiphene citrate)
  urofollitropin
fertility device, Oves conception cap
fertility evaluation
fertility monitor, PSC Fertility Monitor
fertilizable life span
fertilization, in vitro (IVF)
fertilization membrane
fertilized ovum
fertilized ovum outside uterine cavity
Fertil MARQ male fertility test
Fertinex (urofollitropin)
fetal abnormality (pl. abnormalities)
fetal acid-base balance
fetal acidemia
fetal acidosis
fetal adrenal cortex
fetal age
fetal alcohol effects (FAE)
fetal alcohol syndrome (FAS)
fetal anemia
fetal anomaly (pl. anomalies)
fetal anoxia
fetal anoxic injury
fetal ascites
fetal asphyxia
fetal aspiration pneumonitis
fetal aspiration syndrome
fetal biophysical profile
fetal biopsy
fetal biparietal diameter
fetal blood loss
fetal blood sampling
fetal bradycardia
fetal capillaries
fetal caput
fetal cardiac anomalies
fetal cardiac motion
fetal chest diameter
fetal chromosome abnormality
fetal chromosome analysis
fetal circulation
fetal congenital hyperplasia
fetal cord blood
fetal cotyledon
fetal cystic hygroma
fetal cytogenetic abnormality
fetal death
  early
  intrauterine
  late
  middle
fetal death rate

fetal deformity
fetal demise
fetal descent
fetal disproportion
fetal distress
fetal ductus arteriosus
fetal dystocia
fetal ecchymosis
fetal echocardiography
fetal echocardiography in utero
fetal endoscopic surgery (fetendo)
fetal erythroblastosis
fetal exsanguination
fetal face syndrome
fetal fibronectin (fFN) test
fetal gallbladder
fetal gigantism
fetal goiter
fetal growth restriction (FGR)
fetal growth retardation
fetal habitus
fetal head
  manual rotation of
  transverse arrest of
fetal head molding
fetal head presenting
fetal head rotation
fetal heart
fetal heart acceleration
fetal heart failure
fetal heart rate (FHR)
  acceleration of
  deceleration of
fetal heart rate decelerations
fetal heart rate depression
fetal heart rate monitoring, electronic
fetal heart tones (FHT)
fetal heart tracing
fetal hemorrhage into co-twin
fetal hemorrhage into mother's
  circulation
fetal hepatitis
fetal hydantoin syndrome
fetal hydrops
fetal hypermetabolism
fetal hyperthyroidism
fetal hypokinesia syndrome
fetal hypothyroidism
fetal hypoxia
fetal imaging in utero
fetal inclusion
fetal intolerance to labor
fetal intracranial bleeding
fetalis
  chondrodystrophia
  erythroblastosis
  hydrops
  ichthyosis
  maternal hydrops
  maternal parvovirus
fetalism
fetal karyotype
fetal kernicterus
fetal lie
fetal limb reduction
fetal liver disease
fetal lobe
fetal lobulation
fetal loss from amniocentesis
fetal lung maturity
fetal maceration
fetal macrosomia
fetal magnetic resonance imaging
fetal malformation
fetal malnutrition
fetal malpresentation
fetal manipulation
fetal-maternal exchange
fetal-maternal hemorrhage
fetal-maternal incompatibility
fetal maturity
fetal meconium
fetal membrane
fetal midface
fetal monitor
  actocardiotocograph
  Corometrics maternal/
  Doppler

fetal monitor *(cont.)*
 electronic (EFM)
 external
 internal
 OxiFirst
 Propaq Encore
 scalp
fetal monitoring
fetal mortality
fetal motion or movement
fetal movement
fetal myelomeningocele
fetal neuron allotransplantation
fetal number
fetal ovary
fetal ovoid
fetal oxygenation
fetal-pelvic disproportion
fetal-pelvic index
fetal perfusion, diminished
fetal petechia
fetal placenta
fetal pole
fetal position
fetal presentation
fetal presenting part
fetal pulmonary maturation
fetal reconstructive surgery
fetal reduction
fetal regressor
fetal reticularis
fetal sac
fetal sacral teratoma
fetal scalp blood sampling for pH
fetal scalp EKG
fetal scalp electrode
fetal scalp monitor
fetal sequelae, serious
fetal skin sampling
fetal small parts
fetal sonography
fetal souffle
fetal spine, demineralization of
fetal squamous cells
fetal stimulation
fetal surgery for spina bifida
fetal tachycardia
fetal tissue implant
fetal transfusion
fetal trimethadione syndrome
fetal tumor
fetal ultrasonography
fetal ultrasound
fetal umbilical artery
fetal umbilical vein injection under sonographic guidance
fetal urine
fetal uterus
fetal valproate syndrome
fetal ventral mesencephalic tissue transplantation
fetal vernix
fetal viability
fetal warfarin syndrome
fetal wastage
fetal well-being
fetation
FETENDO (or fetendo) (fetal endoscopic surgery)
Feth-R-Kath epidural catheter
feticide
fetish
fetishism
fetofetal transfusion
fetoglobulins
fetography
fetology
fetomaternal hemorrhage
fetomaternal incompatibility
fetomaternal transfusion
fetometry
fetopathy, diabetic
fetopelvic disproportion
fetoplacental anasarca
fetoplacental transfusion
fetoproteins
fetoscope
fetoscopic approach

fetoscopic sleeve
fetoscopic technique
fetoscopy
fetouterine cell
Fettouh bladder suspension
Fettouh bladder suspension needle
fetus (pl. fetuses)
  amorphous
  appendage of
  calcified
  external cephalic version of
  growth-retarded
  habitus of
  harlequin
  hydrocephalic
  impacted
  intra-amniotic infection in
  intrauterine
  intrauterine sepsis of
  large for dates
  large for gestational age (LGA)
  macerated
  malpositioned
  malposition of
  malpresentation of
  maturity of
  mummified
  nonviable
  paper-doll
  papyraceous
  parasitic
  presentation of
  previable
  retained dead
  retention of dead
  SGA (small for gestational age)
  sireniform
  small parts of
  small for dates
  small for gestational age (SGA)
  stunted
  tissue of
  umbilical artery in
  viable
fetus acardiacus
fetus amorphus
fetus compressus
fetus in fetu
fetus papyraceus
fetus sanguinolentis
fever
  dehydration
  epidemic hemorrhagic
  intermittent
  low grade
  Mediterranean
  puerperal
  transitory
  urethral
  urinary
fever and chills
fever and malaise
fever, chills, and night sweats
feverish urine
fever of undetermined origin (FUO)
fever of unknown origin (FUO)
fever spike
FGM (female genital mutilation)
FGR (fetal growth restriction)
FGS (focal glomerulosclerosis)
FG syndrome
FHR (fetal heart rate)
FHT (fetal heart tones)
fiberoptic hysteroscope, rigid
fiberoptic instrument
fiberoptic needle scope
fibers of bladder neck
fibril, amyloid
fibrillary glomerulonephritis
fibrillary glomerulopathy
fibrin calculus
fibrin clots in catheter
fibrin deposition
fibrinoid degeneration of astrocytes
fibrinolytic agents
fibrinolytic therapy
  intraluminal
  systemic

fibrinopeptides
fibrinous polyp
fibrin sheath
fibroadenoma
  breast
  prostatic
fibroadenomatous nodule
fibroadenosis of breast
fibroblast growth factor
fibroblast metaphases
fibroblastoma, perineuronal
fibroblasts
fibrocystic breast
fibrocystic breast disease
fibrocystic breast syndrome
fibrocystic residuals
fibrodysplasia
fibrodysplasia ossificans progressiva (FOP)
fibrofatty tissue
fibroglandular tissue
fibroid (pl. fibroids)
  anterior
  benign
  broad ligament
  calcified uterine
  cervical
  degenerated
  interstitial
  intramural
  necrotic
  pedunculated submucosal
  pedunculated submucous
  pedunculated subserous
  pedunculated uterine
  submucous
  subserosal
  subserous
  uterine
fibroid adenoma
fibroidectomy
fibroid embolization
fibroid removal device, VersaPoint hysteroscopic
fibroid tumor categorization
fibroid tumors
fibroid uterus
fibroleiomyoma
fibrolipoma
fibrolipomatous nephritis
fibroma
  concentric
  ovarian
  prostatic
fibroma of prostate
fibroma-thecoma tumor of ovary
fibromatosis
  congenital generalized
  penile
fibromectomy
fibromuscular cord
fibromuscular dysplasia
fibromuscular hyperplasia
fibromuscular prostate
fibromuscular tissue between vagina and anus
fibromyalgia syndrome
fibromyoma (pl. fibromyomata), submucous
fibromyoma of ovary
fibronectin, fetal
fibroplasia, retrolental
fibrosclerosis of breast
fibrosis (pl. fibroses)
  bilharzial
  corpus cavernosum
  idiopathic retroperitoneal
  panmural
  penile
  perineal
  periureteral
  periureteric
  renal
  retroperitoneal
fibrotic kidney
fibrous ankylosis of multiple joints
fibrous capsule of kidney
fibrous core of villus

fibrous goiter
fibrous material
fibrous nephritis
fibrous renal capsule
fibrous tissue of penis
fibrous tumor
field, tangential breast
15-methylprostaglandin F2a
15q11-q13 duplication syndrome
15q11.2-q14 duplication syndrome
fifth digit syndrome
fifth venereal disease
FIGO (Federation Internationale de Gynécologie et Obstétrique) stages 0–IV
FIGO staging for adenocarcinoma of the endometrium
FIGO staging of fimbriae
FIGO staging of gynecologic malignancy
figure-of-8 sutures
filamentous pseudohyphae
filarial funiculitis
filariasis
filial generation
filiforms and followers
Filippi syndrome
fill and spill of dye (in fallopian tubes)
fill, capillary
filling
  controlled bladder
  incomplete
  retrograde
  ureteral
filling defect
  air-bubble
  radiolucent
  ureteral
films
  delayed
  drainage
  lateral
  oblique
  postevacuation
films *(cont.)*
  postvoid
  postvoiding
filmy adhesion
filtering membrane
Filshie female sterilization clip
filter
  Cook sperm
  membrane
  red-free
  sperm
filtered molecules
filtered proteins
filter residue
filtrate, glomerular
filtration, glomerular
filtration procedure
filtration rate, glomerular
Filtryzer dialyzer
fimbria (pl. fimbriae)
  FIGO staging of
  occlusion of
  ovarian
fimbriae of uterine tubes
fimbriae ovarica
fimbrial
fimbriated
fimbriated end of fallopian tube
fimbriated end of oviduct
fimbriated end of tube
fimbriectomy
fimbriocele
fimbrioplasty
final diagnosis
finasteride
findings, mammographic
Findley folding pessary
Fine-Lap bipolar cutting device
Fine-Lap bipolar forceps
Fine-Lap grasping forceps
Fine-Lap probe
fine-needle aspiration
fine-needle aspiration biopsy
fingerbreadth (pl. fingerbreadths)

finger cot
finger dissection
fingerlike amino-acid loop
fingerlike projections
finger stick device
fingertip measurement
fingertip dilation
Finney Flexi-Rod penile prosthesis
Finochietto retractor
Firlit-Sugar intermittent catheter
firm mass
firm neoplasm
firm uterus
first a.m. urine specimen
first and second branchial arch
  syndrome
first degree enterocele
first degree laceration
first degree perineal laceration
first degree prolapse of uterus
first degree relative
first degree uterine prolapse
first morning specimen
first morning voided urine specimen
first morning urine
first postpartum day
First Response ovulation prediction kit
first sigmoid branch
first stage labor
first stage of labor
first trimester
first trimester abortion
first trimester bleeding
first trimester placenta
First Warning breast cancer screening
  device
fishhooking of ureters
fish mouth
FISH (fluorescent in situ hibridization)
  technique in bone marrow transplantation
fish odor syndrome
fishy discharge
fission track analysis of urine
fissure in ano
fissure of nipple
fistula (pl. fistulas or fistulae)
  arteriovenous (AV, AVF)
  AV, AVF (arteriovenous)
  bladder
  bladder to skin
  bladder to uterus
  bladder to vagina
  brachiosubclavian bridge graft
    (BSBGF)
  Brescia-Cimino
  bridge-graft (BGF)
  cervical
  cervicosigmoid
  cervicovaginal
  cervicovesical
  colovaginal
  colovesical
  endogenous arteriovenous
  enterourethral
  enterovaginal
  enterovesical
  genitourinary
  intestinoureteral
  intestinouterine
  intestinovaginal
  intestinovesical
  kidney arteriovenous
  lacteal
  lower ureter and vagina
  mammary
  mammillary (also mamillary)
  perineovaginal
  rectolabial
  rectourethral
  rectovaginal
  rectovesical
  rectovesicovaginal
  rectovestibular
  rectovulval
  rectovulvar
  saphenous vein
  sigmoidovaginal

fistula *(cont.)*
- sigmoidovesical
- spermatic
- umbilical
- ureteral
- ureter and skin
- ureterocervical
- ureterocutaneous
- ureterovaginal
- urethra and penile skin
- urethra and vagina
- urethral
- urethrocutaneous
- urethroperineal
- urethroperineovesical
- urethrorectal
- urethroscrotal
- urethrovaginal
- urethrovesical
- urethrovesicovaginal
- urinary
- urinary tract
- urogenital
- uterine
- uteroperitoneal
- uterorectal
- uteroureteric
- uterovaginal
- uterovesical
- uterus to abdominal wall
- vaginal
- vaginoperineal
- vaginovesical
- vesical
- vesicocervicovaginal
- vesicocolic
- vesicocutaneous
- vesicoenteric
- vesicointestinal
- vesicoperineal
- vesicorectal
- vesicosigmoidovaginal
- vesicoureterovaginal
- vesicouterine

fistula *(cont.)*
- vesicovaginal
- vesicovaginorectal
- vitelline

fistula formation of vaginal wall
fistula in ano
fistula knife
fistula of cul-de-sac of Douglas
fistula of prostate
fistulation
fistulatome
fistula tract study
fistulectomy
- cervicosigmoid
- scrotal
- transurethral
- vulvar

fistulectomy of bladder
fistulization
fistuloenterostomy
fistulotomy
fistulous passage from the urinary bladder
fistulous tract
fitness
fits in newborn
Fitz-Hugh–Curtis perihepatitis syndrome
5-alpha reductase deficiency
5-aminolevulinic acid
5′-DFUR
5-fluorouracil (5-FU)
5 oxoprolinuria
5p deletion syndrome
5q deletion syndrome
5q duplication syndrome
fixation of breast mass to chest wall
fixation of breast mass to overlying skin
fixation, Salute tissue
fixed allele
fixed axillary lymph nodes
fixed drug eruption
fixed hydrogen ions
fixed mass

flaccid bladder
flaccid infant
flaccid paralysis of bladder
flagellated organism
flagellation
flagellum (pl. flagella)
Flagyl (metronidazole)
Flagyl ER (metronidazole)
flank incision
flanking marker
flanking microsatellite analysis
flanking region
flank pain
flank position
flap
  bladder
  gluteal free
  lateral transverse thigh
  latissimus dorsi
  latissimus dorsi island
  latissimus dorsi myocutaneous
  maple leaf flap
  Martius
  Martius labial fat pad
  McGraw gracilis myocutaneous
  meatal-based skin
  muscle
  myocutaneous
  myouterine
  Orandi
  perineal artery fasciocutaneous
  Rubens
  "saddle bags"
  subcutaneous tissue
  Tanagho anterior bladder
  TRAM (transverse rectus abdominis myocutaneous)
  tummy tuck
  vaginal
  vascularized myocutaneous
  vascularized omental
  Young-Dees-Leadbetter posterior bladder
flare reaction
flaring, alar
flaring of ala nasi
flash (pl. flashes), hot
flashlamp-pulsed dye laser
flashlamp-pulsed Nd:YAG laser
FlashPoint optical localizer
flash pulmonary edema with anuria
Flatan-Schilder disease
flat Silastic suction drain
flat-spring diaphragm
flatus vaginalis
flavin-containing mono-oxygenase (FMO) 2
flea-bitten kidney
fleecy mass
Fleet Enema
fleshy mole
Fletcher applicator
Fletcher cervix-holding forceps
Fletcher-Suit applicator
Fletcher-Suit-Delclos (FSD) mini-colpostat tandem and ovoids system
fleur de lis breast reconstruction pattern
flexible fallopian tube endoscope
flexible filiform catheter tip
flexible hysteroscope
flexible retrograde ureterorenoscopy
flexible-shaft biopsy forceps
flexible-shaft foreign body forceps
flexible-tip guidewire
flexible ureteropyeloscope
flexible ureteroscope
flexible video laparoscope (FVL)
Flexinet dressing
FlexStrand cable
Flexxicon dialysis catheter
FLIC (Functional Living Index-Cancer)
Floating-Harbor syndrome
floating head
floating kidney
Flomax (tamsulosin)
flooding

floor
  bladder
  pelvic
  rigid pelvic
floppy baby
floppy infant syndrome
flora
  mixed genital
  normal
  urethral
  vaginal
Florida pouch
Flo-Stat fluid management system
Flo-Stat monitoring system
flow
  access blood
  effective renal blood (ERBF)
  effective renal plasma (ERPF)
  heaviness of menstrual
  heavy
  heavy menstrual
  intra-access blood
  menstrual
  Qb-blood
  reduced urine
  urine
flow cytometry
flow karyotyping
flow pattern
Floxin (ofloxacin)
FLT3 gene
fluasterone
fluconazole
fluctuant abscess
fluctuant bubo
fluctuant lesion
fluctuant mass
flucytosine
fluff dressing
fluid
  amnionic
  amniotic
  ascitic

fluid *(cont.)*
  crystalloid
  echolucent
  high viscosity
  intravenous
  isotonic replacement
  lactated Ringer
  meconium-stained
  meconium-stained amniotic
  parenteral
  peritoneal
  prostatic
  serosanguineous
  testicular interstitial fluid (TIF)
  third spacing of
  urethral
fluid and electrolyte depletion
fluid challenges to stabilize blood pressure
fluid-electrolyte disturbance
fluid-filled cyst
fluid-filled mass
fluid-filled mass in uterus
fluid-filled sac
fluid extravasation
fluid in cul-de-sac
fluid leakage
fluid management system
  Flo-Stat
  Maestro
fluid mass
fluid overload
fluid overload hyperosmolality
fluid-restricted diet
fluid retention
fluid retention due to stasis
fluoexitine
fluorescein
fluorescein-labeled specific antibodies
fluorescein uptake
fluorescence
fluorescence chromosome staining method

fluorescence technique
fluorescence using quinacrine (QFQ) chromosome staining method
fluorescent in situ hibridization (FISH) technique
fluorescent treponemal antibody absorption (FTA-ABS) test
fluorinated topical steroids
fluorine-18-deoxyglucose (FDG)
fluoroscopic control
fluoroscopy
fluorouracil cream
fluoxetine
"flush-before-fill" dialysate infusion method
flushes, hot
flushing port
flutamide
flux, Ji
FMO (flavin-containing mono-oxygenase) 2
FMO (flavin-containing mono-oxygenase), adult liver form
fmoles/mg (femtomoles per milligram)
FNM (fluorouracil, Novantrone, methotrexate) chemotherapy protocol
foam and condoms
foam contraceptive
foam stability test for fetal pulmonary maturity
focal areas of uptake
focal dermal hypoplasia
focal embolic glomerulonephritis
focal glomerulonephritis
focal glomerulosclerosis (FGS)
focal mass
focal mesangial lupus nephritis
focal nephritis
focal sclerosing glomerulopathy
focal segmental glomerulonephritis (FSGN)
focal segmental glomerulosclerosis (FSGS)
focal spermatogenesis
focal squamous metaplasia
focal tenderness
focal tubulointerstitial atrophy
focal vulvitis
focused extracorporeal ultrasound
focused-heat tumor ablation
focus (pl. foci) of metastasis
Foerster capsulotomy knife
Foerster sponge forceps
folate deficiency
fold
  amnionic
  amniotic
  genital
  interureteric
  labiocrural
  labioscrotal
  mammary
  medial umbilical
  peritoneal
  rectouterine
  rectovesical
  sacrogenital
  sacrouterine
  sacrovaginal
  sacrovesical
  transverse vesical
  ureteric
  uterovesical
folds of uterine tubes
Folex PFS (methotrexate)
Foley catheter
Foley catheter introducer
Foley Cordostat
Foley, Release-NF (nitrofurazone Foley)
Foley three-way catheter
Foley ureteral catheter
Foley Y-plasty pyeloplasty
folic acid
follicle
  anovular ovarian
  atretic ovarian
  dominant

follicle *(cont.)*
- graafian
- growing ovarian
- luteinized unruptured
- lymphoid
- mature ovarian
- nabothian
- ovarian
- polyovular ovarian
- presumptive preovulatory
- primary
- primary ovarian
- primordial
- secondary
- vesicular ovarian

follicle aspiration, sperm injection, and assisted rupture (FASIAR)
follicle development
follicle production
follicle stimulation
follicle-stimulating hormone (FSH)
follicular antrum
follicular atresia
follicular cyst
follicular cyst of ovary
follicular cystitis
follicular development
follicular goiter
follicular growth
follicular maturation study
follicular ovarian cyst
follicular phase of menstrual cycle
follicular salpingitis
follicular stigma
follicular urethritis
follicular vulvitis
follicularis, salpingitis
folliculitis
Folling disease
Follistim (follitropin beta)
follitropin alfa
follitropin beta
follow-up clinic
follow-up cystoscopy
fomepizole
F1 (first filial generation)
Fong syndrome
fontanelle (also fontanel)
- anterior
- anterolateral
- bregmatic
- Casser
- closed
- cranial
- frontal
- Gerdy
- mastoid
- occipital
- open
- posterior
- quadrangular
- sagittal
- sphenoidal
- triangular
- wide open

food, regurgitation of
foot drop
Foothills needle
footling breech presentation
footling presentation
footling presentation of fetus
foot presentation
foot process disease
foot process effacement
foot process fusion
foot process of podocytes
foot process, effaced
foot process, fused
foot, prolapsed fetal
FOP (fibrodysplasia ossificans progressiva)
foramen of Luschka
foramen of Magendie
Forbes-Albright disease
Forbes-Albright syndrome
Forbes disease
force (v.)
force fluids

force of urinary stream
force of urination
forceps
- Adson
- Allis
- atraumatic
- Babcock
- baby Tischler cervical biopsy
- Barrett placenta
- Barton obstetrical
- bayonette
- BiCOAG 3-mm bipolar
- Bierer ovum
- biopsy
- bipolar
- bipolar Adson
- bipolar coaptation
- bipolar Cushing
- bipolar Gerald bayonette
- bipolar grasping
- bipolar Hardy bayonette
- bipolar Jansen bayonette
- bipolar jeweler
- bipolar Malis
- bipolar McPherson
- bipolar Semkin
- bipolar Tenzel
- Bissinger detachable bipolar coagulation
- Bozeman uterine dressing
- bullet-tip
- Burke cervical biopsy punch
- Chamberlen
- Cheron dressing
- Cushing
- DeLee obstetrical
- Dewey obstetrical
- Duplay uterine tenaculum
- elective low
- Elliott obstetrical
- endoscopic grasping
- Eppendorfer-Krause
- evacuation
- Fine-Lap bipolar

forceps *(cont.)*
- Fine-Lap grasping
- Fletcher cervix-holding
- flexible-shaft biopsy
- flexible-shaft, foreign body
- Foerster sponge
- Garland hysterectomy
- Gaylor uterine biopsy
- Gerald
- grasping
- Hale obstetrical
- Hardy
- Heaney
- Heaney-Ballentine hysterectomy
- Heaney hysterectomy
- Hildebrandt uterine hemostatic
- Iowa membrane
- Jacobson hemostatic
- Jansen
- jeweler
- Kelly placenta
- Kelly tissue
- Kelly vulsellum
- kidney stone
- Kielland obstetrical
- Kjelland (see *Kielland*)
- Kleppinger
- Kleppinger bipolar
- Lahey
- laser Adson
- laser Allis
- laser Bozeman
- laser Campion
- laser Clemetson
- laser Potts-Smith
- Laufe divergent obstetrical
- Laufe-Piper obstetrical
- Laufe uterine polyp
- Levret
- Llorente dissecting
- Long hysterectomy
- low
- Luikart obstetrical
- Luikart-Simpson

forceps *(cont.)*
Malis
Mayo-Russian tissue
McLane-Tucker-Kielland obstetrical
McLane-Tucker-Luikart obstetrical
McLane-Tucker obstetrical
McPherson
Mengert
MOLLY bipolar
Moolgaoker
Moore ovum
needle nose
Nelson tissue
Neville-Barnes
nonfenestrated
obstetrical
outlet
Pean hysterectomy
Pearl packing
Phaneuf uterine artery
Piper obstetrical
placental
polyp
Powell
Pozzi uterine tenaculum
Randall kidney stone
Randall stone
Re-New
rigid biopsy
ring
Rochester-Pean
Russian tissue
Schroeder-Braun uterine tenaculum
Schubert uterine biopsy
Schweizer uterine
Seitzinger tripolar cutting
Semkin
Simpson
Singley
Sopher
Sovereign bipolar
SpectraScience biopsy
SpectraScience reusable biopsy
spike tooth

forceps *(cont.)*
sponge
spoon
stone-grasping
stone-holding basket
Take-apart
TeleMed reusable biopsy
Tenzel
Therma Jaw hot urologic
Thoms-Allis vulsellum
Thomas-Gaylor uterine biopsy
Tischler cervical biopsy punch
Townsend mini-bite cervical biopsy punch
trial
Tucker-McLane
Tuttle
uterine dressing
vacuum
Wertheim-Cullen
Wertheim vaginal
Willett
Yeoman uterine biopsy
Z-Clamp hysterectomy

forceps delivery
elective
indicated

forceps extraction
forces, Starling
forcible rape
forearm veins
foreign antigen of graft
foreign body, intraluminal
foreign body salpingitis
foreign body vaginitis
foreplay
forepleasure
foreskin of penis (also *prepuce*)
adherent
frenulum of
hooded
nonretractable
penile
redundant

foreskin of penis *(cont.)*
  retractable
  tight
  ventral apron
  ventral penile
forewaters
Formad kidney
Forma in vitro incubator
formation
  bezoar
  gas
  giant cell
  glomeruloid
  hernia
  secondary stricture
  subsequent hernia
formation of open ileal bladder
Forma water-jacketed incubator
form of ultrafiltration
formula (see *infant formula*)
  Cockcroft-Gault formula/equation
    for renal function
  half-strength
  Jeliffe
  quarter-strength
  Schwartz
  three-quarter strength
fornication
fornices (sing. fornix)
fornix (pl. fornices)
  anterior
  anterior vaginal
  lateral
  posterior vaginal
  vaginal
fornix of vagina
fornix vaginae
foroblique lens
FortaGen surgical mesh
FortaPerm surgical sling
Fortel ovulation prediction kit
45,XO syndrome
45,X syndrome
46,XX normal female
46,XY normal male
47,XXY syndrome
47,XY syndrome
47,XYY syndrome
48,XXXX syndrome
48,XXXY syndrome
48,XXYY syndrome
49,XXXXX syndrome
49,XXXYY syndrome
Forvade (cidofovir gel)
Fosamax (alendronate)
Foscan (temoporfin, mTHPC) mediated photodynamic therapy
foscarnet
fosfomycin tromethamine
fossa (pl. fossae)
  adipose (of breast)
  antecubital
  axillary
  intrauterine
  ipsilateral iliac
  obturator
  ovarian
  pararectal
  paravesical
  prostatic
  renal
  supravesical
fossa navicularis
foul discharge
fouling
foul-smelling discharge
foul-smelling vaginal discharge
founder effect
Fountain syndrome
4 x 4 (four-by-four) dressing
fourchette
  anterior
  posterior
  tear of
4-hour glucose tolerance test
4p deletion syndrome
4p15 deletion syndrome
4q21-q25 deletion syndrome

4q21-q28 duplication syndrome
4q23-q27 duplication syndrome
4q32-q34 deletion syndrome
four-quadrant approximation
four-quadrant cervical biopsy
Fournier disease
Fournier gangrene of scrotum
Fournier, syphiloma of
14F dialysis catheter
14p16.3 deletion syndrome
14q12-q13 duplication syndrome
14q31-q32.3 deletion syndrome
14q32.3 deletion syndrome
fourth degree episiotomy
fourth degree extension of episiotomy
fourth degree laceration
fourth degree perineal laceration
four-way vaginal expander
Fowler-Stephens orchiopexy
fractional amount
fractional curettage
fractional dilation and curettage (D&C)
fractionation of calculus
fractionation of stone
fracture
  corner
  depressed skull
  kidney
  intrauterine (of fetus)
  linear
fragile X chromosome
fragile X syndrome
fragmentation of calculus
fragmentation of renal stone
Fraley syndrome
frameshift mutation
Franchetti-Klein syndrome
Francois dyscephalic syndrome
Frank and McIndoe vagina construction
Frankenhäuser ganglion
frank breech
frank breech presentation
Frank vaginal construction
Franseen biopsy needle
Fraser syndrome
fraternal twins
fraught with difficulty
FRAX (fragile X syndrome)
FRED (fog reduction elimination device) anti-fog solution
free air in abdomen
free air in pelvis
free air in scrotum
free alpha subunit of hCG
free beta subunit of hCG
free blood
free border of ovary
free fascial graft
free fat droplets
free flap breast reconstruction
free flap procedures
free-floating testis
free fluid in cul-de-sac
free fluid in pouch of Douglas
freely movable mass
Freeman cookie cutter areola marker
Freeman-Sheldon syndrome
free nipple graft
free nipple transposition technique reduction mammoplasty
free PSA (prostate-specific antigen)
free serum PSA
free thyroxine (T_4) index test
free tie
free tissue transfer
free/total PSA index
free trisomy 21
free water intake
Freeway Graves speculum
French
frenular band
frenulectomy
frenuloplasty
frenulum (pl. frenula)
frenulum of clitoris
frenulum of labia minora
frenulum of prepuce

frenulum of pudendal lips
frequency
  intermittent urinary
  menstrual
  urinary
frequency of contractions
frequency of sexual activity
frequency of urination
frequent urination
Fresenius hemodialyzer
fresh eggs
fresh embryos
freshly voided urine
fresh sperm
Fresh Start breast support
Freund total abdominal hysterectomy
friable lesion
friable mass
friable mucosa
friable tissue
Fria pelvic muscle training device
Friberg test
Friedman curves
Friedreich ataxia
Friedreich disease
Friedreich tabes
frigidity
frog-leg position
frog-leg posture
frond-like appearance
frontal fontanelle
frontoanterior position
frontofacionasal dysplasia or dysostosis
frontonasal dysplasia
frontoposterior position
frontotransverse position
frost, uremic
frothy discharge
frothy urine
frottage
frozen cycle
frozen embryo cycles
frozen pelvis
frozen section
frozen section diagnosis
frozen sperm
frozen sperm specimen
fructosamine
fructosemia
fructose intolerance, hereditary
fructose-1-phosphate aldolase deficiency
fructosuria
Fryns syndrome
FSAD (female sexual arousal disorder)
FSD (female sexual dysfunction)
FSD (Fletcher-Suit-Delclos) system
F-series insemination catheter
FSGN (focal segmental glomerulonephritis)
FSGS (focal segmental glomerulosclerosis)
FSH (follicle-stimulating hormone)
FTA-ABS (fluorescent treponemal antibody absorption) test
FTI (free thyroxine index)
FTT (failure to thrive)
F2 (second filial generation)
fucosidosis
Fukuhara syndrome
fulgurate, fulguration
fulguration of bladder tumor
fulguration of ulcerative lesion
full-bladder technique
full-bladder ultrasound technique
full breech presentation
full-field digital mammography system
full mastopexy
fullness, breast
full systemic anticoagulation
full term
full-term delivery
full-term infant
fulminant disease
fulminant immune-complex RPGN
fulminant renal failure

fulminating hyperpyrexia
function
  abnormal tubular
  erectile
  excretory
  inadequate ovarian
  ovarian
  renal
  renal tubular
  residual renal
  split
functional anatomic mapping
functional androgen excess
functional anovulation
functional bladder capacity
functional bowel disease
functional dysmenorrhea
functional estrogen receptor
functional gene tests
functional hematuria
Functional Living Index-Cancer (FLIC)
functional murmur
functional nephrosis
functional ovarian cyst
functional prepubertal castration
functional tubular impairment
functional ureteral obstruction
functional urethral length
functional uterine hemorrhage
functional vagina, surgical creation of
functioning allograft
functioning neoplasm
fundal enlargement
fundal growth
fundal height
fundal indentation
fundal placenta
fundal pressure
fundectomy
fundoplication, Nissen
fundus (pl. fundi)
  bladder
  globular
  incompetence of pelvic
  normal
  regular in outline
  urinary bladder
  uterine
  vaginal
fundus irregular in outline
fundus 10 weeks' gestational size
fundus uteri
fungal component
fungal cystitis
fungal disease
fungal infection
fungal urinary tract infection
fungating lesion
funguria
fungus
  imperfect
  perfect
  umbilical
funiculitis, filarial
funiculus umbilicalis
funipuncture
funisitis
funnel-shaped pelvis
FUO (fever of unknown origin)
FUO (fever of undetermined origin)
Furadantin (nitrofurantoin)
furosemide
furrow, genital
furuncle of vulva
fused foot process
fused kidney
fusiform ureter
fusion, foot process
Futura resectoscope sheath
FVL (Factor V-Leiden)
FVL (flexible video laparoscope)
FVS (fetal varicella syndrome)

G, g

G (gravida)
GABHS (group A beta-hemolytic streptococcus)
gag reflex
Gail breast cancer model
galactocele
galactogram, mammary
galactography
galactometer
galactophagous
galactophore
galactophoritis
galactophorous
galactopoietic hormone
galactorrhea
galactorrhea-amenorrhea syndrome
galactoscope
galactose diabetes
galactosemia
galactose-1-phosphate uridyl transferase deficiency
galactosialidosis
galactosylceramidosis
Galant reflex
Galileo rigid hysteroscope
gallbladder contractility, impaired
gallbladder, fetal
galling
gallium
gallium nitrate
gallium nitrate infusion
gallium, radioactive
gallium-67 citrate, gallium citrate Ga 67 (^{67}GA) contrast medium
Galloway-Mowat syndrome
gallstone
Galtonian-Fisher genetics
galtonian genetics
Gambro hemodialyzer
Gambro Lundia dialyzer
Gambro Lundia Minor artificial kidney
Gambro Polyflex hemodialyzer
gamete
gamete intrafallopian transfer (GIFT)
gamete intrafallopian tube transfer (GIFTT)
gamete micromanipulation
gametic selection
gametogenesis
gamogenesis
gamophobia
ganciclovir
ganciclovir sodium for injection
ganciclovir triphosphate
ganglia pelvica
ganglia pelvina

ganglion (pl. ganglia)
  aorticorenal
  celiac
  cervical
  Frankenhäuser
  hypogastric
  hypoglossal
  Lee
  olfactory
  sacral sensory nerve
gangliosides
gangliosidosis type 1-GM1
gangrene
  disseminated cutaneous
  Fournier
  ischemic penile
  penile
  scrotal
Gantrisin (sulfisoxazole)
gantry
Garamycin (gentamicin sulfate)
Garceau tapered tip
Gardnerella test
Gardnerella vaginalis
Gardner syndrome
gargantuan mastitis
gargoylism
Gariel pessary
Garland hysterectomy forceps
Garrett dilator
Garrigue weighted vaginal speculum
Gartner cyst
Gartner duct
gas (pl. gases)
gas and vapor permeation systems
gas embolism
gas formation
gas-forming bacteria
gas insufflation
Gaskin shoulder dystocia maneuver
gasless laparoscopy
gas phase
gasserian duct
Gastaldo maneuver
gastric neobladder procedure
gastric tissue patch, vascularized
gastrinoma
gastrocystoplasty
gastroesophageal reflux disease (GERD)
gastrointestinal hemorrhage
gastroschisis
gastrula
gastrulation
gas, vapor, and pervaporation separations
gatifloxacin
Gaucher disease (GD)
Gaucher-Schlagenhauffer disease
Gauss sign
Gautier ureteroscope
gavage feeding
gay (homosexual) sex
Gaylor biopsy punch
Gaylor uterine biopsy forceps
Gazayerli endoscopic retractor
Gazelle balloon dilation catheter
GBA (genetic bit analysis)
G-banding technique of chromosome staining
GBM (glomerular basement membrane)
GC (gonorrhea)
GC (gonorrhea culture)
GCBM (glomerular capillary basement membrane)
GCI (gestational carbohydrate intolerance)
GCPS (Greig cephalopolysyndactyly syndrome)
GD (Gaucher disease)
GDM (gestational diabetes mellitus)
Gehrung pessary
geitonogamy
gel (see also *medications*)
  Crinone bioadhesive progesterone
  Hylagel Uro viscoelastic
  Savvy contraceptive vaginal
  SEPA/testosterone

gel *(cont.)*
Sepragel bioresorbable
Surete contraceptive
testosterone
Topiglan (SEPA/alprostadil)
Tostrex (testosterone gel)
gelatin agglutination test (GAT)
gelatin-sealed sling material
gel-filled breast implant
gel fouling layer
Gelhorn biopsy punch
Gelhorn pessary
GelPort abdominal access device
gemcitabine
gemellary pregnancy
gemellipara
gemfibrozil
gemifloxacin
Gencept oral contraceptive
gender assigned as female
gender assigned as male
gender assignment
gender assignment decision
gender differences
gender dysphoria
gender dysphoric
gender identity
gender identity disorder
gender role behavior
gene (see also *chromosome; deletion syndrome; duplication syndrome; monosomy; pentasomy; tetrasomy; trisomy*)
allelic
AMMECR1
autosomal
AVPR2
beta
beta-globin
BRCA1 (breast cancer 1)
BRCA2 (breast cancer 2)
BTK
C
Cdc2L1-2

gene *(cont.)*
codominant
COL2A1
COL4A5
control
CTNS
DCC tumor suppressor
DNA repair
dominant
DPC4 tumor suppressor
DYT-1
extrachromosomal
FAA
FAC
FACL4
FAG
FAH
FLT3
H
histocompatibility
hitchhiker
HLA-G
holandric
homeotic
housekeeping
human homeobox
IFN-alpha 2
immune response
jumping
K-ras
lethal
LIS1 (lissencephaly-1)
mimic
mitochondrial
MLL
MMP21-22
modifier
MTS1 tumor suppressor
mutant
oncosuppressor
operator
p53 adenoviral
p53 tumor suppressor
pleiotropic

gene *(cont.)*
  polyphrenic
  PTEN
  PTK
  regulator
  repressor
  Rb tumor suppressor
  RhoC
  RhoC GTPase
  sickle
  SOS
  split
  structural
  transfer
  transforming
  UBE3A
  V
  VHL tumor suppressor
  WT1 (Wilms tumor 1)
  X-linked
  Y-linked
  Z
gene activation, NFkB-dependent
gene alteration
gene amplification
gene conversion
gene deletion
gene dose
Genee-Wiedemann syndrome
gene expression
gene expressivity
gene family
gene flow
Gene Gin cloning device
gene interaction
gene library
gene map
gene mapping
gene markers
gene mutation
Genentech biosynthetic human growth hormone
gene penetrance
gene pool
gene product
gene promoter methylation
general anesthesia
general endotracheal anesthesia
general fertility
generalized congenital osteosclerosis
generalized edema
generalized glycogenesis
generalized nephrographic (GNG) phase imaging
generation
  asexual
  filial
  nonsexual
  parental
  sexual
  skipped
  spontaneous
  virgin
generation rate for urea
generator, Medstone STS shock wave generator
gene replication
Genestone 190 lithotripter
gene targeting
gene testing
gene therapy
gene transfer
gene therapy in utero
gene therapy program
genetic (see *genetics*)
genetically engineered transgenic animals
genetically linked to the child
genetically passed disease
genetically related
genetic amplification
genetic analysis
  transabdominal sampling of the chorionic villi
  transcervical sampling of the chorionic villi
genetic bit analysis (GBA)
genetic blood testing

genetic cell lines
genetic code (ATGC)
genetic counseling
genetic death
genetic diagnosis, preimplantation
genetic disorder (see *syndrome*)
genetic distance
genetic diversity
genetic drift
genetic engineering
genetic evaluation
genetic father
genetic female
genetic fine structure
genetic hemochromatosis
genetic heterogeneity
genetic heterogenicity
genetic human male
genetic interference
geneticist
genetic link
genetic linkage maps
genetic male
genetic map
genetic marker
genetic material
genetic maternity
genetic mother
genetic predisposition
genetic relatedness
genetics
  behavioral
  biochemical
  classical
  clinical
  epidemiologic
  galtonian
  Galtonian-Fisher
  human
  mathematical
  medical
  mendelian
  microbial
  modern

genetics *(cont.)*
  molecular
  multilocal
  population
  reverse
  somatic cell
  statistical
  transplantation
genetic screening
genetic stock
genetic testing
genetic trait
  autosomal dominant
  autosomal recessive
genetic variance
Gengraf (cyclosporine)
genistein
genital and urethral reconstructive
  surgery for gender conversion
genital bleeding
genital candidiasis
genital carcinoma
genital condyloma
genital cord
genital corpuscle
genital duct
genital elephantiasis
genital eminence
genital fistula
genital fold
genital furrow
genital gland
genital groove
genital herpes infection
  primary
  recurrent
genital herpes simplex
genitalia
  ambiguous
  ambiguous external
  external
  female external
  female internal
  herpes

genitalia *(cont.)*
  indifferent
  male external
  male internal
  normal female
  normal male
  self-stimulation of
genitality
genital lesion
genital ligament
genital organs
genital phase
genital prolapse
genital ridge
genital swelling
genital system
genital tract
  lower
  upper
genital tract cells
genital tract infection
genital tract tumor
genital tubercle
genital ulcer
genital warts
genitocrural
genitofemoral nerve
genitoinguinal ligament
genitourinary (GU)
genitourinary apparatus
genitourinary fistula
genitourinary infection
genitourinary symptoms
genitourinary system
genitourinary tract
genitourinary tuberculosis
Genline Miller-Dieker syndrome
genome
genome maps
Genome Project, Human
genomic DNA
genomic in situ hybridization (GISH)
genomic library
genoplasm
Genora oral contraceptive
genotype
genotype/phenotype correlation
genotyping
Gen-Probe amplified CT assay
gentamicin
gentamicin solution
gentle suction
genuine stress incontinence (GSI)
genus
Geocillin (carbenicillin)
GER (gastroesophageal reflux)
Gerald forceps
Gerber Baby Formula with Iron
Gerber Soy Formula
GERD (gastroesophageal reflux disease)
Gerdy fontanelle
Geref (sermorelin)
geriatric hypogonadism
geriatrics
germ (germination)
germ cell maturation
germ cell ovarian neoplasm
germinal aplasia
germinal cell aplasia
germinal cell desquamation
germinal epithelial cyst
germinal failure
germinal mosaicism
germination tube
germination tube test
germinoma
germ line
germ line mosaicism
germ line mutation
germline RET proto-oncogene point mutations
germplasm
germ tube
germ tube test
geroderma osteodysplastica
gerontology
Gerota fascia

Gesco umbilical catheter
GE Senographe 20001 (and 2000D)
  digital mammography system
gestating female
gestating male
gestation
  anembryonic
  extrauterine
  intrauterine
  multiple
  tubal
  twin
  uterine
gestational age
gestational age assessment
gestational carbohydrate intolerance
  (GCI) disorder
gestational carrier
gestational dating criteria
gestational diabetes
gestational diabetes mellitus (GDM)
gestational edema
gestational hypertension
gestational proteinuria
gestational ring
gestational sac (GS)
gestational sac abnormality
gestational sac diameter
gestational size
gestational surrogacy
gestational surrogacy arrangements
gestational surrogate
gestational trophoblastic disease (GTD)
gestational trophoblastic neoplasia
  (GTN)
gestationis, herpes
gestator
gestodene low dose estrogen/progestin
  oral contraceptive
GFR (glomerular filtration rate)
GFS Mark II inflatable penile
  prosthesis
GH (growth hormone)
GI toxicity
giant anal wart
giant anorectal condyloma acuminatum
giant cell cirrhosis of the newborn
giant cell disease
giant cell formation
giant cell hepatitis
giant cell thyroiditis
giant chromosome
giant platelet syndrome, hereditary
giant tongue
Giemsa banding
Giemsa chromosome staining method
Giemsa stain
GIFT (gamete intrafallopian transfer)
GIFTT (gamete intrafallopian tube
  transfer)
gigantism
  acromegalic
  cerebral
  eunuchoid
  fetal
  hyperpituitary
  normal
  pituitary
  primordial
gigantomastia
GIH (growth hormone-inhibiting
  hormone)
Gilbert disease
Gilbert-Dreyfus syndrome
Gilford syndrome
Gilliam operation for retroversion of
  the uterus
Gilliam uterine suspension
GISH (genomic in situ hybridization)
Gittes repair for stress urinary incontinence
Gittes urethral suspension
gland (see also *glans*)
  adrenal
  anteprostatic
  areolar
  Bartholin
  body of mammary

gland *(cont.)*
  bulbourethral
  BUS (Bartholin, urethral, Skene)
  Cowper
  duct of bulbourethral
  endocervical
  endometrial
  excretory duct of seminal
  genital
  greater vestibular
  inflammation of vulvovaginal
  Littré
  mammary
  medial border of suprarenal
  medulla of suprarenal
  ovarian
  paraurethral
  periurethral
  pituitary
  prostate
  sebaceous
  Skene
  superior border of suprarenal
  suprarenal
  testes
  testicular
  thyroid
  urethral
  uterine
  vaginal
  venous circle of mammary
  vesical
  vulvovaginal
glands and stroma
glands of Littré
glandular endometritis
glandular hypospadias
glandular mastitis
glandular mucous membrane of cervix
glandularis cystitis
glandulopreputial lamella
glans (pl. glandes)
glans carcinoma
glans clitoridis
glans, corona of
glans of clitoris
glans penis
glans to cavernosum shunt
glans volume
glanular hypospadias
Glassman stone extractor
glaucoma, traumatic
Gleason score for carcinoma of prostate
Gleicher salpingography catheter
glimepiride
global sclerosis
globoid cell leukodystrophy
globular fundus
globulin
  ALG (antilymphocyte)
  antithymocyte
  gonadal steroid-binding
  sex hormone-binding globulin (SHBG)
  sex steroid-binding
  testosterone-estrogen-binding
  thyroxine-binding
globulinuria
GloFil-125 (sodium iothalamate I-125) renal function test
glomeriform arteriovenous anastomosis
glomeriform arteriovenular anastomosis
glomerular architecture
glomerular basement membrane (GBM)
glomerular capillary basement membrane (GCBM)
glomerular capillary endothelial cell
glomerular capillary permeability, altered
glomerular capillary wall of kidney
glomerular capsule
glomerular cyst
glomerular damage
glomerular derangement
glomerular disease

glomerular epithelial cells
glomerular fibrinoid necrosis
glomerular filtrate
glomerular filtration
glomerular filtration agent
glomerular filtration rate (GFR)
glomerular filtration surface
glomerular hypertrophy
glomerular mesangium
glomerular nephritis
glomerular obsolescence
glomerular permeability
glomerular syndromes
glomerular tip lesion
glomerular tuft
glomerule
glomerulitis
  chronic nephritis
  necrotizing
glomeruli (see *glomerulus*)
glomerulocapsular nephritis
glomeruloid formation
glomerulonephritic syndrome
glomerulonephritis (GN)
  acute
  acute crescentic
  acute hemorrhagic
  acute poststreptococcal (APSGN)
  acute proliferative
  ANCA-associated
  anti-basement membrane
  anti-GBM-antibody-mediated
  Berger focal
  chronic
  chronic hypocomplementemic
  crescentic
  de novo posttransplant
  diffuse
  diffuse proliferative
  endothelial
  exudative
  fibrillary
  focal

glomerulonephritis *(cont.)*
  focal embolic
  focal segmental (FSGN)
  hypocomplementemic
  hypocomplementemic persistent
  idiopathic
  idiopathic crescentic necrotizing
  IgA
  immune complex
  immune complex-mediated
  lobular
  lobulonodular
  local
  lupus
  malignant
  membranoproliferative (MPG, MPGN)
  membranous
  mesangial proliferative
  mesangiocapillary (MPGN)
  mesangioproliferative (MESGN)
  minimal change
  mixed membranous and proliferative
  necrotizing
  nodular
  nonstreptococcal acute
  pauci-immune
  pauci-immune crescentic
  pauci-immune rapidly progressive
  persistent
  PIGN (postinfectious)
  postinfectious (PIGN)
  postinfective
  poststreptococcal (PSGN)
  proliferative
  rapidly progressive (RPGN)
  renal limited
  renal limited ANCA-associated crescentic
  sclerosing membranous
  segmental
  segmental necrotizing
  subacute

glomerulonephritis with edema
glomerulopathy (pl. glomerulopathies)
  acute nephritic syndrome
  chronic nephritic/
  collapsing
  diabetic
  fibrillary
  focal sclerosing
  immunotactoid
  microtubular
  minimal change
  nephrotic syndrome
  postinfectious
  primary renal hematuric/proteinuric
    syndrome
  proteinuric syndrome
  renal ablation
glomerulopathy associated with
  bacterial endocarditis
glomerulopathy associated with infected
  prosthetic material
glomerulopathy associated with
  infectious hepatitis (HB_SAg-positive)
glomerulopathy associated with malaria
glomerulopathy associated with
  pneumonia
glomerulopathy associated with
  syphilis
glomerulopathy associated with
  varicella
glomerulopathy associated with
  visceral abscess
glomerulosclerosis
  collapsing
  diabetic (DGS)
  focal (FGS)
  focal segmental (FSGS)
  intercapillary
  nodular
  obliterative diabetic
  perihilar
glomerulus (pl. glomeruli)
  atrophic
  juxtamedullary

glomerulus *(cont.)*
  malpighian
  renal
  residual
  Ruysch
glomerulus of mesonephros
glossitis
glucagon
glucagon deficiency
glucagon injectable
glucagonoma
Glucochek Pocketlab II blood glucose
  system
glucocorticoids
Glucola
Glucometer DEX blood glucose
  monitor
Glucometer Elite R blood glucose
  monitor
Glucometer Elite R glucose monitor
Glucometer II blood glucose monitor
Glucophage (metformin)
GlucoProtein test
glucoronyl transferase deficiency
glucose administration, intravenous
glucose excursions, wide
glucose homeostasis
glucose in urine
glucose metabolism
glucose monitor (see *blood glucose
  monitor*)
glucose-galactose malabsorption
glucose-monitoring test strip, Excel GE
glucose-6-phosphate dehydrogenase
  (G6PD) deficiency
glucose tolerance test (GTT)
  one-hour
  impaired
glucosuria
glucosyl ceramide lysidosis
Glucovance (glyburide, metformin)
GlucoWatch blood glucose monitor
glutamic acid
glutaric aciduria I and II

glutaraldehyde cross-linked collagen
  injections
gluteal free flap
gluten-induced enteropathy
gluten intolerance
glutethimide
Glutose
glyburide
glycemic index
glycine
glycinuria, familial
glycogen disease of muscle
glycogenesis I-VIII
glycogen nephrosis
glycogen storage disease I-VIII (GSD)
glycoglycinuria
glycolic aciduria
glycolipid lipidosis
glycolylurea
glycolysis
glyconeogenesis
glycopenia
glycoprotein syndrome
glycosal diabetes test
glycosuria
  alimentary
  benign
  digestive
  nondiabetic
  nonhyperglycemic
  normoglycemic
  orthoglycemic
  pathologic
  phlorizin
  renal
glycosylated hemoglobin
glycuronuria
Glynase Pres Tab (glyburide)
Glyset (miglitol)
GM1 (gangliosidosis type 1)
GM2 (gangliosidosis type 2)
GN (glomerulonephritis)
gnathocephalus
GNG (generalized nephrographic)
  phase imaging
GnRH (gonadotropin-releasing
  hormone)
GnRH agonist
GnRH analog
GnRH and/or hCG stimulation tests
GnRH antagonist
goat's milk anemia
Goebel-Frangenheim-Stoeckel
  urethrovesical suspension
GOG (Gynecologic Oncology Group)
goiter
  aberrant
  adenomatous
  Basedow
  colloid
  congenital
  cystic
  diffuse
  diving
  endemic (colloid)
  euthyroid
  exophthalmic
  fibrous
  follicular
  iodide
  lingual
  lithiumogenic
  lymphadenoid
  multinodular
  multiple colloid adenomatous
  nodular
  nontoxic
  nontoxic diffuse
  nontoxic nodular
  parenchymous
  plunging
  simple
  substernal
  suffocative
  toxic
  toxic multinodular
  wandering

goitrogens
Golabi-Rosen syndrome
Goldberg-Maxwell syndrome
Goldblatt kidney
Goldenhar syndrome
gold-hole ureteral orifice
Goldman and Favre dystrophy
gold marker seeds
Goldstein Microspike approximator clamp
Goldstein sonohysterography catheter
Gomco circumcision clamp
gonad
  congenitally defective
  female
  indifferent
  male
  rudimentary
  streak
  streaked
  suspensory ligament of
gonadal agenesis
gonadal aplasia
gonadal cord
gonadal differentiation
gonadal dysgenesis (45,X)
gonadal hormones
gonadal mosaicism
gonadal mosaics
gonadal neoplasm
gonadal steroid-binding globulin
gonadal steroid production
gonadal steroids
gonadal streak
gonadectomy
gonadoblastoma
gonadopathy
gonadorelin
gonadotrope
gonadotroph
gonadotrophic cycle
gonadotropic
gonadotropin
  anterior pituitary
  chorionic (CG)
  human chorionic (hCG)
  human menopausal (hMG)
  pituitary
  placenta
gonadotropin concentration
gonadotropin-producing neoplasm
gonadotropin-releasing hormone (GnRH, GRH)
gonadotropin secretion
gonaduct
Gonal-F (follitropin alfa)
gonane
gonecyst
gonecystis
goniodysgenesis hypodontia
gonocide
Gono Kwik test
gonococcal arthritis
gonococcal cystitis
gonococcal infection
gonococcal orchitis
gonococcal perihepatitis
gonococcal prostatitis
gonococcal salpingitis
gonococcal stomatitis
gonococcal urethritis
gonococcal vulvar ulcer
gonococcus (pl. gonococci), chromosomally mediated resistant *Neisseria gonorrhoeae* (CMRNG)
gonorrhea (GC)
  endocervical
  rectal
  urethral
gonorrhea culture (GC)
gonorrheal arthritis
gonorrheal cervicitis
gonorrheal ophthalmia
gonorrheal rheumatism

gonorrheal salpingitis
gonorrheal urethritis
gonosome
gonotoxemia
gonotoxin
Goodell dilator
Goodell sign of early pregnancy
Goodell uterine dilator
Goodman syndrome
Goodpasture syndrome
good perinatal outcome
good vaginal support
good visualization
Gordon syndrome
Gore-Tex arteriovenous graft
Gore-Tex DualMesh Plus graft
Gore-Tex graft
Gore-Tex graft vein interposition
Gore-Tex MycroMesh Plus graft
Gorlin Chaudhry Moss syndrome
goserelin implant
Gottron syndrome
Gougerot-Carteaud syndrome
Goulian mammoplasty
gout, secondary
gouty nephropathy
gouty urine
GPA (gravida, para, abortus)
GPAL (gravida, para, abortions/ miscarriages, live births)
GPA terminology
GPMAL (gravida, para, multiple births, abortions/miscarriages, live births
graafian follicle
GraBag retrieval pouch
gracilis muscle transplant
grade, placental
gradient-limited renal tubular acidosis
gradient, concentration
graduated dilator
graft
    amnion
    aortorenal-saphenous vein bypass

graft *(cont.)*
    Bard Visilex mesh
    Composix mesh
    CryoVein SG vascular
    Diastat vascular access
    extended-survival
    FortaGen surgical mesh
    free fascial
    free nipple
    Gore-Tex
    Gore-Tex DualMesh Plus
    Gore-Tex MycroMesh Plus
    Graftpatch
    IMA (inferior mammary artery)
    Impragraft
    Impra Venaflo vascular
    Kugel Hernia Patch
    Marlex mesh
    Martius
    Perma-Seal dialysis access
    prosthetic woven Dacron
    PTFE
    Repliform tissue
    Sepramesh biosurgical composite
    seromuscular
    seromuscular intestinal patch
    Sperma-Tex preshaped mesh
    splenorenal arterial bypass
    Trelex mesh
    VacuLink vascular access
    vaginal wall
    vascular access (VAG)
    Vectra VAG (vascular access)
    Venaflo vascular
    Visilex mesh
graft necrosis
Graftpatch
graft rejection
graft slough
graft versus host disease (GVHD)
graft versus tumor activity
grain of sand
Gram stain from the cervix
gram-negative bacilli, coliform

gram-negative bacteria
gram-negative organism
gram-positive bacteria
gram-positive organism
Grams nylon nonabsorbable suture
Grams polypropylene nonabsorbable suture
Grams silk nonabsorbable suture
grand multipara (also "grand multip")
grand multiparity
grand multiparous patient
GraNee needle
Grantly Dick-Reed method
granular kidney
granular urethritis
granule
  juxtaglomerular
  seminal
granulin streak pattern
granuloma (pl. granulomas, granulomata)
  pulmonary necrotizing
  spermatocytic
  suture
  umbilical
  urethral
granuloma inguinale
granulomatosis, Wegener
granulomatous disease
granulomatous mastitis
granulomatous prostatitis
granulomatous thyroiditis
granulosa cells of ovary
granulosa-oocyte interaction
granulosa theca cell tumor
grapelike molar tissue
grasper
  Endo-Babcock
  Hasson
  MetraGrasp ligament
  100 series endoscopic
  Reddick-Saye suture
graph, Liley Rh sensitization
grasping forceps (see *forceps*)
grasping reflex
grasp reflex
gratification, sexual
Graves disease, congenital
Graves speculum
GRAVESPEC vaginal speculum
Graves vaginal speculum
Graves Wide View speculum
gravida (G) (number of pregnancies)
gravidae, hydrorrhea
gravidarum
  chorea
  hydrorrhea
  hyperemesis
  nausea
gravida, para, abortus (GPA)
gravidic
gravidism
graviditas
gravidity
gravid uterus
Gravindex
gravis
  icterus
  neonatal myasthenia
gravity drainage
gravity, specific
gray baby syndrome
gray exudate
Gray syndrome
greater vestibular gland
greatest length
great suprarenal vein
Grebe dysplasia
green discharge
Greene renal implant stent
Greene uterine curette
Greenfield umbrella/filter
Greenwald sound
Greig cephalopolysyndactyly syndrome (GCPS)
Greig polysyndactyly craniofacial dysmorphism syndrome
Grey Turner sign

gritty feel to uterine lining
groin dissection
groin mass
groin skin-flap technique
groove
  Blessig embryonic
  dental embryonic
  genital
  nasolacrimal embryonic
  pharyngeal embryonic
  primitive embryonic
  trigeminal embryonic
  urethral
Groshong catheter
gross blood on urination
gross edema
gross fetal anomaly
gross hematuria
gross reproduction
gross tumor involvement
group A beta-hemolytic streptococcal antigens
group B streptococcus (strep)
growing ovarian follicle
growing pains
growth
  excessive fetal
  poor fetal
  slow fetal
growth factor, vascular endothelial (VEGF)
growth hormone (GH)
growth hormone-inhibiting hormone (GIH)
growth hormone insensitivity syndrome (GHIS)
growth hormone-releasing hormone (GHRH, GH-RH)
growth retardation, intrauterine (IUGR)
growth retardation-Rieger anomaly
growth velocity
growth-retarded fetus
Gruber syndrome
grunting
grunting and retractions
GSI (genuine stress incontinence)
G6PD (glucose-6-phosphate dehydrogenase)
GTD (gestational trophoblastic disease)
GTG banding pattern
GTN (gestational trophoblastic neoplasia)
GTT (glucose tolerance test)
GU (genitourinary)
  GU infection
  GU system
  GU tract
guaiac-negative stool
guaiac-positive nipple discharge
guaiac-positive stool
guanethidine
guanine
guarding
  involuntary
  muscle
  voluntary
gubernaculum
gubernaculum testis
Guérin duct
Guérin-Stern syndrome
guidance
  sonographic
  ultrasound
guide
  Pilot suture
  trocar
guided needle biopsy
guidewire
  Amplatz Teflon-coated
  Conceptus Robust
  flexible-tip
  Teflon-coated
guidewire for needle localization
Guillain-Barre syndrome
guillotine blade
gumma, syphilitic
gummatous infiltration

gummatous lesion
gummatous necrosis
gummatous ulceration
Günter disease (also Guenter)
Gusberg hysterectomy clamp
gutters, pelvic
Guttmann retractor
Guttmann vaginal speculum
Guyon-Pean kidney clamp
Guyon sign
GVHD (graft versus host disease)
GVHD grading system
GYN, Gyn (gynecology)
gynandrism
gynandroblastoma
gynandromorphism
gynandromorphous
gynatresia
Gynazole-1 (butoconazole nitrate)
Gynecare GyneSys catheter system
Gynecare TVT tension-free support
Gynecare Verascope hysteroscope
gynecogenic
gynecoid distribution of body fat
gynecoid obesity
gynecoid pelvis
gynecologic examination
gynecologic neoplasm
gynecologic oncologist
gynecological
gynecologist
gynecology (GYN, Gyn)
gynecomania
gynecomastia
  male
  nutritional
  refeeding
gynecomasty
gynecoradiology
Gyne-Flo cannula, Leventhal
Gyne-Flo hysteroscopy irrigation system valve
GyneLase diode laser system
Gyne-Lite adjustable light
Gyne-Lotrimin 3 (clotrimazole)
Gyne-Moistrin vaginal lubricant
Gynepath biopsy needle
gynephilic sexual contact
gynephobia
Gyne-Pro hysteroscopic electrodes
Gyne-Rx vaginal cream
Gyne-Sulf vaginal cream
GyneSys cervical access catheter
GyneSys Dx diagnostic catheter system
GyneSys guidewire
GyneSys uterine cornual access catheter
GyneSys uterine ostial access catheter
Gyne-Tech B101-D colposcope
Gyne-Tech PPS
Gyne-T 200 IUD
Gyne-T 300 IUD
Gynex angle hook
Gynex Emmet tenaculum
Gynex endospeculum
Gynex extended-reach needle
Gynex iris hook
Gynogen L.A. 20
Gynogen L.A. 40
gynogenesis
Gynol II contraceptive cream
gynopathy
GynoSampler endometrial curette
Gyrus endourology system

H, h

Haas intrauterine insemination catheter
habenula, Haller
habenula urethralis
habitual aborter
habitual abortion
habitus
  body
  fetal
HAC (human artificial chromosome)
Haemonetics Cell Saver
Haemophilus ducreyi
Haemophilus influenza type B
Haemophilus vaginalis (see *Gardnerella vaginalis*)
Hageman factor deficiency
HAG3 (hydroxyacetyltriglycine)
Hailey-Hailey disease
hair growth, abnormal
haircut chancre
hairline, pubic
Hajdu-Cheney syndrome
Halban culdoplasty
Halcion (triazolam)
Hale obstetrical forceps
half-and-half nails
half-strength formula
Haller aberrant duct
Haller habenula
Hallerman-Streiff-Francois syndrome
Hallerman-Streiff syndrome
Hallervorden-Spatz disease
Hallgren syndrome
Hall-Pallister syndrome
hallux duplication, postaxial polydactyly, and absence of corpus callosum syndrome
halo of blanching
halo sign of hydrops
HALS (hand-assisted laparoscopic surgery)
Halsted radical mastectomy
hamartoma, renal
hamburger disease
hammock-type suspension
hamster free oocyte test
hamster zona-free ovum (HZFO) test
hand-assisted laparoscopic surgery (HALS)
hand-assisted laparoscopy (HAL)
handedness
hand exchange method for continuous ambulatory peritoneal dialysis
hand-heart syndrome
HandPort hand-assist device
handsewn anastomosis
Hanely-McDermitt pelvimeter

hanging panniculus
hanging stirrups
Hanhart syndrome
Hanks dilator
Hansel stain
Ha1A human monoclonal antibody
haploid
haploid number
haploinsufficiency
haplotype analysis
haploidentical
haplotype
happy puppet syndrome
hard calculi
harderoporphryrin
harderoporphyria
hard nodular urinary calculus
Hardy forceps
Hardy-Weinberg equilibrium
harelip
harlequin color change
harlequin fetus
harlequin ichthyosis
Harmonic scalpel
Hartley balloon catheter
Hartley breast implant
Hartnup disease
Hartnup syndrome
harvest
  organ
  total abdominal evisceration (TAE)
harvesting, fascia lata
Hashimoto struma
Hashimoto thyroiditis
Hasson blunt-end cannula
Hasson cannula
Hasson grasper
Hasson intrauterine cannula with inflatable balloon
Hasson laparoscopy cannula
Hasson SAC (stable-access cannula)
Hasson trocar
Hasson trocar and sleeve
hatching, assisted zonal (AZH)
Hawkins breast localization needle with FlexStrand cable
Hays-Wells syndrome
Hb (hemoglobin)
HB (hepatitis B)
HB_SAg (hepatitis B surface antigen)
HCA (hypothalamic chronic anovulation)
H-CAP (hexamethylmelamine, Cytoxan, Adriamycin, Platinol) chemotherapy protocol
hCFHrp (human complement factor H-related protein)
hCG (human chorionic gonadotropin)
  beta
  serum
HCO_3 (bicarbonate)
HCO_3 precursors
hCS, HCS (human chorionic somatomammotropin) hormone
Hct (hematocrit)
HCV (hepatitis C virus)
HD (hemodialysis)
HD (Huntington disease)
HDI 3000 ultrasound system
HDN (hemolytic disease of the newborn)
head
  aftercoming
  engaged
  fetal
  floating
  high
  molding of
  overriding
headache
  coital
  spinal
head birth
head circumference
head control, acquisition of
head kidney
head presentation
healed by primary intention

healed by secondary intention
healed per primam
healing by primary intention
healing by secondary intention
Healos synthetic bone-graft material
HealthCheck One-Step One Minute pregnancy test
Healthdyne apnea monitor
HealthShield wound drainage catheter
healthy appendix
Heaney-Ballentine hysterectomy forceps
Heaney clamp
Heaney forceps
Heaney hysterectomy forceps
Heaney hysterectomy retractor
Heaney-Mayo scissors
Heaney vaginal hysterectomy
hearing screen
heart-beating donor
heart block, congenital
heartburn during pregnancy
heart, fetal
heart-hand syndrome
heart murmur
heart rate, fetal (FHR)
heart-shaped uterus
heatstroke
heat-transmitting balloon catheter
heaviness of menstrual flow
heavy flow
heavy for dates infant
heavy leukorrhea
heavy menstrual flow
heavy particle radiation
heavy periods
heavy proteinuria
heavy uterine bleeding
heavy vaginal bleeding
Hecht syndrome
Hectorol (doxercalciferol; synthetic vitamin D prohormone)
Hedrocel bone substitute
heel stick hematocrit
heel-to-ear maneuver
Hegar dilator
Hegar sign
height, fundal
HeLa cells
helical suture
helicine artery of penis
helicine artery of uterus
heliX knot pusher
HELLP (hemolysis, elevated liver enzymes, and low platelet count) syndrome
helmet-molding therapy
helminthic disease
helper T cells
HEMA (hemophilia A)
Hemabate
hemagglutination inhibition/inhibiting (HI)
hemagglutination titers for MSA (microsomal antibodies)
hemangioma
hemangiomas-thrombocytopenia syndrome
hemangiomatosis chondrodystrophica
hemangiomatous branchial clefts-lip pseudocleft syndrome
hemangiopericytoma, renal
Hemasure r/LS red blood cell filtration system
hematocele, broad ligament
hematocolpos
hematocrit (Hct), heel stick
hematogenous dissemination of tumor
hematogenous dissemination of virus
hematogenous dissemination to distant organs
hematogenously disseminated candidiasis
hematogenous pyelitis
hematologic dyscrasia
  hemolytic-uremic syndrome
  Henoch-Schönlein purpura
  mixed IgG-IgM cryoglobinemia
  serum sickness

hematologic dyscrasia *(cont.)*
  thrombotic thrombocytopenic
    purpura
hematologic picture
hematoma
  broad ligament
  cord
  corpus cavernosum
  corpus luteum
  liver
  localized subdural
  penis
  perineal
  perinephric
  perirenal
  postoperative pelvic
  retromembranous
  scrotal
  subdural
  subepithelial
  subfascial
  testicular
  vaginal
  vulvar
hematometra
hematometrium
hematometrocolpos
hematomphalocele
hematopoietic stem cell
hematoporphyria, congenital
hematoporphyrin derivative (HPD)
hematosalpinx of ovary
hematospermia
hematuria
  asymptomatic
  benign familial
  benign recurrent
  endemic
  essential
  factitious
  false
  functional
  gross
  initial

hematuria *(cont.)*
  macroscopic
  microscopic
  nephrotic-range
  nonrenal
  painful
  persistent
  primary
  renal
  terminal
  total
  traumatic
  urethral
  vesical
HEMB (hemophilia B)
heme-negative stool
hemiacidrin
hemicardius
hemicervix
hemifacial atrophy
hemifacial microsomia
hemimegalencephaly
hemihypertrophy
hemimelia and scalp-skull defects
hemin
hemin and zinc mesoporphyrin
heminephrectomy
hemipelvis
hemisection of the spinal column
hemiscrotal incision
hemiscrotum
hemiuterus
hemivulvectomy, radical
hemizona assay test
hemizygous
Hemo-Cath catheter
Hemoccult II
hemochorial placenta
hemochromatosis, genetic
hemoconcentration
Hemocor HPH high-performance
  hemoconcentrator
hemodiafiltration, continuous venovenous

Hemo-Dial dialysate additives
hemodialysis (HD)
  LifeSite
  surgically implanted
  venovenous
hemodialysis access shunt
hemodialysis complication
hemodialysis-hemofiltration procedure
hemodialysis needle insertion, buttonhole puncture technique for
hemodialysis session
hemodialysis thrice weekly
hemodialyzer
  Altra Flux
  Altra Nova
  Altrex
  CAHP
  Centry system 3
  coil
  Fresenius
  Gambro
  Gambro Lundia Minor
  Gambro Polyflex
  hollow-fiber
  MCA
  parallel plate
  Primus
  PSN (polysynthane)
hemodynamic abnormality
hemodynamic and gas exchange improvement
hemodynamic stress
hemoendothelial placenta
hemofiltration
  continuous arteriovenous (CAVH)
  excess crystalloid removed by
  maintenance
hemofiltration circuit
hemofiltration connections
hemoglobin (Hb, Hgb)
  glycosylated
  postpartum
hemoglobin casts
hemoglobin C trait
hemoglobin electrophoresis
hemoglobinemia
  paroxysmal nocturnal
  puerperal
hemoglobinopathy
hemoglobinuria
  intermittent
  paroxysmal nocturnal
hemoglobinuric nephrosis
Hemolink blood substitute
hemolysis, intravascular
hemolytic anemia of newborn
hemolytic complications of pregnancy
hemolytic disease of newborn (HDN)
hemolytic-uremic syndrome (HUS)
hemopathy, maternal
hemoperfusion
hemoperfusion over charcoal (or resin)
hemophagocytic histiocytosis
hemophilia A (HEMA)
hemophilia B (HEMB)
Hemophilus ducreyi
hemorrhage
  accidental
  antepartum
  adrenal
  alveolar
  antepartum
  bladder wall
  cerebral
  concealed
  corpus luteum
  cutaneous
  dysfunctional uterine
  epicranial subaponeurotic
  external
  fetal-maternal
  fetomaternal
  functional uterine
  gastrointestinal
  intra-alveolar
  intracranial
  intraocular
  intrapartum

hemorrhage *(cont.)*
  intrarenal
  intratumoral
  intraventricular
  massive pulmonary
  neonatal intracranial
  peripartal vaginal
  perirenal
  postoperative
  postpartum
  profuse uterine
  prostatic
  renal
  renal artery
  retroperitoneal
  subarachnoid
  subdural
  third-stage
  umbilical
  uterine
hemorrhage from biopsy site
hemorrhage in ectopic pregnancy
hemorrhagic corpus luteum cyst
hemorrhagic cystitis
hemorrhagic disease of newborn
hemorrhagic dystrophic thrombocytopenia
hemorrhagic nephritis
hemorrhagic nodular purpura
hemorrhagic ovarian cyst
hemorrhagic pyelitis
hemorrhagic retinitis
hemorrhagic salpingitis
hemorrhagic telangiectasia, hereditary
hemorrhoid, hemorrhoids
  external
  internal
  mixed
  prolapsed
  strangulated
  thrombosed
hemosalpinx
hemosiderosis, pulmonary
hemospermia
hemospermia spuria
hemospermia vera
hemostasis
  complete
  ensure
  meticulous
hemostasis maintained with electrocautery
hemostasis obtained with electrocautery
Hemovac drain
Henle, loop of
Henoch-Schönlein nephritis
Henoch-Schönlein purpura
Henrotin weighted vaginal speculum
HEP (hematoerythropoietic porphyria)
heparin, beef lung
heparinize
heparinized solution
heparin lock (hep-lock)
heparin/protamine infusion
hepatic fibrosis
hepatic infantilism
hepatic insufficiency
hepatic vein thrombosis
hepatitis
  autoimmune
  cholestatic
  chronic active
  enterically transmitted non-A, non-B
  fetal
  giant cell
  infectious
  neonatal
  post-transfusion
  transfusion
  viral
hepatitis-associated antigen
hepatitis A virus
hepatitis B surface antigen (HB_SAg)
hepatitis B vaccine
hepatitis B virus (HBV)
hepatitis C virus (HCV)
hepatitis D virus
hepatitis E virus

hepatitis NANB (non-A, non-B) (now hepatitis C)
hepatolenticular degeneration
hepatophosphorylase deficient glycogenesis
hepatorenal glycogenesis
hepatorenal ligament
hepatorenal pouch
hepatorenal recess
hepatorenal syndrome (HRS)
hepatosplenic infestation
hep-lock (heparin lock)
herbal therapy
HercepTest
Herceptin (trastuzumab) anti-HER2 humanized monoclonal antibody
Hercules infant
Hercules Nd:YAG laser system
hereditary alkaptonuria
hereditary ataxia
hereditary benign tremor
hereditary breast cancer
hereditary cerebellar ataxia
hereditary chorea
hereditary disease
hereditary disorder
hereditary dystopic lipidosis
hereditary hemorrhagic telangiectasia
hereditary hyperuricemia
hereditary motor sensory neuropathy type 3
hereditary mutation
hereditary nephritis
hereditary nephropathy
hereditary nonpolyposis colon cancer
hereditary ovarian cancer
hereditary papillary renal cancer (HPRC)
hereditary prostate cancer
hereditary renal adysplasia
hereditary renal hypouricuria
hereditary sensory and autonomic neuropathy
hereditary sensory motor neuropathy
hereditary spastic paraplegia
hereditary syphilis
heredity
heredofamilial disease
heredofamilial nephrotic syndrome
heredopathia atactica polyneuritiformis
Herellea vaginicola
heritability
Heritage Panel genetic screening test for breast and ovarian cancer
herkogamy
Hermansky-Pudlak syndrome
hermaphrodite
hermaphroditism
- adrenal
- bilateral
- false
- female
- lateral
- male
- transverse
- true
- unilateral

hernia (pl. hernias, herniae)
- abdominal
- Barth
- Bochdalek
- cerebral
- congenital
- Cooper
- cul-de-sac
- diaphragmatic
- direct
- encysted
- epigastric
- external
- femoral
- gastroesophageal
- hiatal
- incarcerated
- incisional
- indirect
- inguinal
- inguinoscrotal

hernia *(cont.)*
  intersigmoid
  labial
  mesocolic
  Morgagni
  oblique
  omental
  ovarian
  pantaloon
  perineal
  pudendal
  scrotal
  sliding
  umbilical
  vesicle
hernia defect
hernial hydrocele
Herniamesh plug
hernia of bladder into vagina and introitus
hernia of broad ligament of the uterus
hernia of ovary
hernia repair
hernia sac
herniation
  bladder into vaginal canal
  bowel
  rectum into vagina
hernioplasty, LAP-TAPP (laparoscopic transabdominal preperitoneal)
herniorrhaphy
Herpasil
herpes
  genital
  labialis
  oral
herpes culture
herpes genitalis
herpes gestationis
herpes outbreak
herpes simplex
herpes simplex viral (HSV) infection
herpes simplex virus
  type 1 (HSV-1)
  type 2 (HSV-2)
herpesvirus
herpes zoster
herpetic infection of penis
Herrick kidney clamp
Hers disease
HER2/neu breast cancer gene marker
HER2/neu oncogene
HER2 protein receptor
Herxheimer reaction
hesitancy, urinary
HetaCool
heterochromatin
heterochromia of iris
heterochromosome
heteroduplex analysis
heteroduplex DNA
heteroduplexes
heterogeneity
heterogeneous deficiency of cosynthase oxidase activity
heterogenicity, genetic
heterograft arteriovenous (AV) fistula
heterokaryon
heterologous twins
heteroplasia, progressive osseous
heteroplastic
heterosexual precocity
heterosexual transmission of AIDS
heterosexuality
heterosome
heterostyly
heterotaxia
heterotopic pregnancies
heterotypical chromosome
heterozygosity
heterozygote
heterozygous deletion mutations
heterozygote
heterozygotic carrier
Hexalen (altretamine)
hexamethylmelamine
Hexastat (altretamine)
hexoprenaline sulfate
hexosaminidase A

Hextend blood plasma volume expander
Heyer-Schulte tissue expander
"H. flu" (slang for *Haemophilus influenzae*)
HFOV (high frequency oscillating ventilator)
HFV (high frequency ventilation)
HG-PIN (high grade prostatic intraepithelial neoplasia)
Hgb (hemoglobin)
H gene
HGSIL (high grade squamous intraepithelial lesion)
HHV-6 (human herpesvirus 6)
HHV-8 (human herpesvirus 8)
HI (hemagglutination inhibition/inhibiting) titer
Hib (*Haemophilus influenza* type B)
Hib vaccine
Hibbard technique
Hickman catheter
hidden penis
hidradenitis suppurativa
HIE (hyper IgE) syndrome
HIFU (high intensity focused ultrasound)
Higgins technique for ureterointestinal anastomosis
high biologic value protein content diet
high birth weight
high capacity bladder
high ceiling diuretic
high compliance bladder
high dose oral estrogen therapy
higher order pregnancy
high fluid requirements
high flux dialyzer
high forceps delivery
high frequency oscillating ventilator (HFOV)
high frequency ventilation (HFV)
high fundal insertion of IUD
high grade prostatic intraepithelial neoplasia (HG-PIN)
high grade squamous intraepithelial lesion (HSIL, HGSIL)
high head at term
high intensity focused ultrasound (HIFU)
high ligation of spermatic vein
high lithotripsy
highly conserved sequence
highly vascular vagina
high McCall vaginal vault suspension
high renal tolerance
high resolution chromosome studies
high resolution CT mammography
high resolution multicolor banding studies
high resolution multileaf collimator
high resolution ultrasonography
high resolution ultrasound
high-riding ballotable prostate
high-riding prostate
High Risk Hybrid Capture HPV test
high risk population
high risk pregnancy
high scapula
high vacuum extraction
high vaginal laceration
high vasal ligation
high viscosity fluid
high volume isovolemic hemofiltration
hila of kidney
Hildebrandt uterine hemostatic forceps
Hillis-Mueller maneuver
hilum of kidney
hilum (pl. hila), renal
hilus cells
hindbrain herniation
hindered transport
hip click
Hippuran I-123
hippuria
hippuric acid
Hirschsprung disease
hirsutism
histidase deficiency

histidinemia
histiocytosis
histone
histocompatibility
histocompatibility antigen, beta 2
  microglobulins
histocompatibility gene
histocompatibility leukocyte antigen
  (HLA)
histoincompatibility, maternal-fetal
histologic diagnosis
histologic involvement of axillary
  lymph nodes
histonuria
histopathologic injury
histopathology
history
  family
  menstrual
  past medical
  pregnancy
  prenatal
  sexual
  social
history and physical
hitchhiker gene
HIV (human immunodeficiency virus)
HIV-associated nephropathy
HIV etiology and pathogenesis
HIV-1E virus
HLA (histocompatibility leukocyte
  antigen) class I-II
HLA (human lymphocyte antigen)
HLA system
HLA-A
HLA-B
HLA-C
HLA-D
HLA-DR
HLA-G gene
HLP (hyperlipoproteinemia)
HMD (hyaline membrane disease)
HMG (human menopausal
  gonadotropins)
HM4 lithotriptor
HMFG1 (human milk fat globule 1)
HMG, hMG (human menopausal
  gonadotropin)
HMTV (human mammary tumor virus)
Hodge pessary
Hoehne sign of uterine rupture
Hofmeister biopsy curette
holandric gene
hollow fiber capillary dialyzer
hollow fiber dialyzer
hollow, muscular, retroperitoneal organ
hollow viscus
Holman aspiration needle
Holmes-Adie syndrome
holmium laser
holmium laser resection of the prostate
  (HoLRP)
holoprosencephaly
  alobar
  familial alobar
  semilobar
HoLRP (holmium laser resection of the
  prostate)
Holt-Oram syndrome
homaluria
Homans sign
Home Choice automated PD
  (peritoneal dialysis) system
HomeChoice Pro with PD Link home
  dialysis system
home delivery
home hemodialysis
home O_2
homeobox gene
homeostasis
  acid-base
  glucose
homeostatic balance of minerals
homeotic gene
home uterine activity monitor
home uterine monitoring
homocystinuria
homocarnosinosis

homocystinemia
homoduplex DNA
homoduplexes
homogeneous membrane
homogentisic aciduria
homokaryon
homolog (also homologue)
homologous chromosomes
homologous genes
homologous insemination
homologous recombination
homology
homophobia, internalized
homosexuality
  female
  latent
  male
  overt
  unconscious
homosexual rectal trauma
homosexual sex
homozygosity
homozygote
homozygous
honeymoon cystitis
hood
  dorsal
  persistent ventral
  ventral
hooded foreskin
hooded prepuce
hook
  Amniohook
  Emmet uterine tenaculum
  Gynex angle
  Gynex iris
  ramathibodi tubal
  Starion thermal cautery
hook-shaped ureter
Horizon nitinol temporary stent
horizontal incision
Horizon temporary urinary stent
hormonal adaptations
hormonal dilation during pregnancy
hormonal manipulation
hormonal substitution therapy
hormonal therapy
hormone
  adrenocorticotrophic
  antidiuretic
  Biotropin
  CGP (chorionic growth hormone-prolactin)
  chorionic gonadotropic
  counterregulatory
  ethinyl estradiol
  follicle-stimulating (FSH)
  follitropin alfa
  galactopoietic
  Genentech biosynthetic human growth
  gonadal
  gonadotropin-releasing (GnRH, GRH)
  goserelin
  growth (GH)
  growth hormone-inhibiting (GIH)
  growth hormone-releasing (GHRH, GH-RH)
  human chorionic somatomammotropic (HCS)
  human growth (hGH)
  human luteinizing
  Humatrope human growth
  hypothalamic luteinizing hormone-releasing
  inhibiting
  lactation
  lactogenic
  long-acting thyroid-stimulating (LATS)
  luteinizing
  luteinizing hormone-releasing (LH-RH, LHRH, LRH)
  mammotropic
  melanocyte-stimulating
  ovarian
  parathormone

hormone *(cont.)*
parathyroid (PTH)
placental growth (PGH)
pregnancy
progestational
ProLease encapsulated sustained-release growth
Protropin human growth
raging
releasing
reduced secretion of ovarian
sex
hormone production
hormone receptor site
hormone replacement therapy (HRT)
Alora (estradiol transdermal patch)
Cenestin (conjugated estrogen)
chlorotrianisene
Climara (estradiol)
CombiPatch (estradiol/norethindrone)
conjugated estrogens
Delestrogen (estradiol)
depGynogen (estradiol cypionate)
Depo-Estradiol Cypionate (estradiol)
DepoGen (estradiol)
Depo-Testadiol (estradiol)
Depotestogen (estradiol)
dienestrol (estrogen)
Duo-Cyp (estradiol)
Esclim (estradiol)
esterified estrogens
Estinyl (ethinyl estradiol)
Estrace (estradiol)
Estraderm (estradiol)
estradiol
estradiol cypionate
estradiol hemihydrate
Estradiol Transdermal System (estradiol)
estradiol valerate
Estra-L 40 (estradiol)
Estrasorb (estrogen)
Estratab (estrogen)

hormone replacement *(cont.)*
Estratest (estrogen; methyltestosterone))
Estratest H.S.
Estring
Estrogel (estrogen)
estrone
Estrone Aqueous (estrone)
estropipate
ethinyl estradiol
FemPatch (estradiol)
Gynogen L.A. 20 (estradiol)
Gynogen L.A. 40 (estradiol)
intravaginal ring (IVR)
Kestrone 5 (estradiol)
Menest (estrogen)
Menorest patch (estradiol)
mestranol
Oesclim patch (estradiol)
Ogen (estrone)
Ortho Dienestrol vaginal cream
Ortho-Est (estropipate)
Ortho-Prefest (17ß-estradiol/norgestimate)
PMS-Conjugated Estrogens
Premarin (estrogens)
Premarin with Methyltestosterone
Premphase (estrogen; methyltesterone)
Prempro (estrogen; medroxyprogesterone)
Prometrium (progesterone, micronized)
quinestrol
sodium estrone sulfate
TheraDerm-MTX (estradiol, testosterone)
TSH-01 transdermal tape with natural estrogen and 17-beta-estradiol
Vagifem vaginal tablets (estradiol)
Valergen 20 (estradiol)
Valergen 40 (estradiol)

hormone replacement *(cont.)*
  Valertest No. 1 (estradiol, testosterone)
  Vivelle (estradiol)
  Vivelle-Dot estradiol patch
hormone-refractory disease
hormone-refractory prostate cancer
hormone replacement therapy (HRT) patch
hormone-sensitive breast cancer
hormone-sensitive breast carcinoma
hormone-sensitive metastatic breast carcinoma
hormone-stimulated endometrial change
horn
  noncommunicating uterine
  rudimentary uterine
  uterine
horseshoe kidney
horseshoe placenta in twin pregnancies
HOS (hypo-osmotic swelling) test
Hospal Biospal dialyzer
host cell membrane
host constituent
host defense mechanisms
hostile mucus
host immune mechanisms
host immune responsiveness
host uterus
host uterus procedure
hot biopsy
hot flash (flashes)
hot flush (flushes)
hot sitz baths
hotspot mutation region
hourglass bladder
hourglass contraction of uterus
hourglass uterus
housekeeping gene
Houston muscle
HPA (hypothalamic-pituitary-adrenal) axis
HPD (hematoporphyrin derivative)
HPL (human placental lactogen)
HPRC (hereditary papillary renal cancer)
HPV (human papillomavirus)
HPV B19 (human parvovirus B19)
HRS (hepatorenal syndrome)
HRT (hormone replacement therapy) patch
H/S or HSG (hysterosalpingography) catheter
HSG (hysterosalpingogram)
HSIL, HGSIL (high grade squamous intraepithelial lesion)
HSSG (hysterosalpingosonography)
HSV (herpes simplex virus)
HSV-1 (herpes simplex virus, type 1)
HSV-2 (herpes simplex virus, type 2)
HTA (Hydro ThermAblator) system
H-TRON plus V100 insulin infusion pump
Hubner postcoital test
Hulka clip
Hulka clip applicator
Hulka ligating spring-loaded clip
Hulka uterine mobilizer
Hulka uterine tenaculum
Humalog insulin
Humalog Mix 50/50 insulin
Humalog Mix 75/25 insulin
Humalog Pen
human antimalignan antibody
human artificial chromosome (HAC)
human blastocyst implantation
human chorionic gonadotropin (hCG)
human chorionic somatomammotrophin (hCS, HCS) hormone
human complement factor H-related protein (hCFHrp)
human gene therapy
human genetics
human genome
Human Genome Initiative
Human Genome Project

human growth hormone
human homeobox gene
human herpesvirus 6 (HHV-6)
human herpesvirus 8 (HHV-8)
human homeobox gene
human immunodeficiency virus (HIV)
human islet allograft
human leukocyte antigen
human leukocyte group A (HLA)
human luteinizing hormone
human lymphocyte antigen (HLA)
human mammary tumor virus (HMTV)
human menopausal gonadotropin
 (HMG, hMG)
human papillomavirus (HPV),
 oncogenic
human parvovirus B19 (HPV B19)
human placental lactogen (HPL)
Human Surf
Humatro-Pen growth hormone delivery
 device
Humegon (menotropins for injection)
HUMI (Harris-Kronner Uterine
 Manipulator Injector)
HUMI cannula
HUMI inflatable uterine cannula
HUMI intrauterine cannula
HUMI uterine catheter
HUMI uterine manipulator
HUMI uterine manipulator/injector
humoral host defense mechanisms
humoral hypercalcemia of pregnancy
Humulin (human insulin)
Humulin R pen insulin delivery device
Humulin 70/30 pen insulin delivery
 device
hum, venous
hunger, air
Hunner (*not* Hunter) interstitial cystitis
Hunner (*not* Hunter) ulcer
Hunter syndrome
Huntington chorea
Huntington disease
Hurler-Scheie syndrome
Hurler syndrome
Hurwitz dialysis catheter
HUS (hemolytic-uremic syndrome)
Hutchinson-Gilford progeria syndrome
hutchinsonian molars
Hutchinson teeth
Hutterite syndrome, Bowen-Conradi-
 type
hyaline casts
hyaline membrane disease of newborn
hyalinization
hyalinosis, segmental
hyalinuria
hybrid
Hybrid Capture CMV DNA test
Hybrid Capture HPV DNA test
Hybrid Capture II test for human
 papillomavirus
hybridization, DNA
hybridizing
hybridoma
Hybritech free PSA test
Hybritech Tandem PSA ratio (free
 PSA/total PSA)
hydantoin syndrome
hydatid
 alveolar
 nonpedunculated
 sessile
 Virchow
hydatid cyst of Morgagni
hydatidiform mole
hydatid mole
hydatid of Morgagni
hydatid pregnancy
hydatid rash
hydramnion
hydramnios
 acute
 chronic
hydranencephaly
hydration
hydration and analgesia
hydraulic pressure gradient

hydraulic shock wave
hydraulic ultrafiltration
Hydrea (hydroxyurea)
hydrion paper
hydrion test
hydroanencephaly
HydroThermAblator (HTA) system
hydroa gestationis
hydroarthrosis
hydrocalycosis
hydrocarbon exposure
hydrocele
  chylous
  communicating
  congenital
  cord
  diffused
  Dupuytren
  encysted
  funicular
  hernial
  infected
  noncommunicating
  scrotal
  spermatic cord
  testicular
  tunica vaginalis
hydrocele colli
hydrocelectomy
hydrocele feminae
hydrocele renalis
hydrocephalic fetus
hydrocephalus
  acquired
  chronic
  communicating
  congenital
  obstructive
  posthemorrhagic
  primary
  tension
hydrocephalus ex vacuo
hydrocephaly
hydrochlorothiazide
hydrochromopertubation
hydrodissector, Trumpet Valve
HydroFlex HD (hysteroscopic
  distention) system
hydrogel coating
hydrogen bond
hydrogen ion concentration (pH)
hydrolyzed whey-based formula
hydrometrocolpos
hydronephrosis
  closed
  congenital
  mild
  moderate
  open
  primary
  proximal
  secondary
hydronephrosis due to ureteral
  obstruction
hydronephrotic kidney
hydroparasalpinx
hydrophilic-coated urologic stent
hydrophobic membranes of filters
hydropic nephrosis
hydropic villi
hydrops
  fetal
  idiopathic
  immune fetal
  nonimmune fetal
  nonimmunological fetal
hydrops amnii
hydrops fetalis
hydrops ovarii
hydrops tubae
hydrops tubae profluens
hydropyonephrosis
hydrorchis
hydrorrhea gravidae
hydrorrhea gravidarum
hydrosalpinx, intermittent
hydrostatic pressure
HydroSurg laparoscopic irrigator

HydroThermAblator system
hydrothionuria
hydrotubation
hydroureter, congenital
hydroureteronephrosis
hydrovarium
hydroxyacetyltriglycine (HAG3)
hydroxyprogesterone
hydroxystilbamidine
hydroxyurea
hygroma colli
hygroma, cystic
Hylagel Uro
Hylutin (hydroxyprogesterone)
hymen
  annular
  circular
  cribriform
  denticular
  falciform
  fenestrated
  imperforate
  intact
  lunar
  patent
  persistent
  rigid
  septate
hymen bifenestratus
hyman biforis
hymen subseptis
hymenal orifice patency
hymenal ring, tight
hymenal tear
hymenectomy
hymenitis
hymenoid
hymenorrhaphy
hymenotomy
hymen sculptetus
hyoscyamine sulfate
Hypaque contrast medium
Hypaque-Cysto contrast medium
Hypaque-M contrast medium
Hypaque Meglumine contrast medium
Hypaque Sodium contrast medium
hypazoturic nephropathy
hyperactivity of bladder
hyperacute rejection
hyperacute renal allograft rejection
hyperacute renal transplant rejection
hyperaldosteronism
hyperaldosteronism with hypokalemic alkalosis
hyperalimentation
hyperallantoinuria
hyperaminoaciduria
hyperammonemia
hyperandrogenic women with masculinization
hyperandrogenism
hyper-beta carnosinemia
hyperbilirulinemia
  hereditary
  neonatal
hyperbilirubinemia of prematurity
hypercalcemia
  familial hypocalciuric
  humoral (of pregnancy)
  idiopathic infantile
hypercalcemia-supravalvar aortic stenosis
hypercalcemic nephropathy
hypercalcinuria
hypercalciuria, idiopathic
hypercapnia
hypercatabolic patient
hypercatabolism
hypercellular glomeruli
hyperchloremia
hyperchloremic acidosis
hyperchloremic metabolic acidosis
hyperchloruria
hypercholesterolemia
  familial
  secondary
hyperchylomicronemia
hypercoagulable state

hypercorticoidism
hypercyesia
hypercyesis
hyperdense mass
hyperdiploid karyotype
hyperdynamic circulation of pregnancy
hyperdynamic precordium
hyperdynamic state
hyperechoic endometrium
hyperemesis
  persistent
  vicious
hyperemesis gravidarum
hyperemesis lactentium
hyperemia
  bladder
  pelvic
hyperesthesia of vulva
hyperexplexia
hyperfibrinolysis
hyperfunction, adrenal cortical
hypergalactosis
hypergenitalism
hyperglycemia
  diabetic
  symptomatic
hyperglycenemia and lactic acidemia, propionic-type
hyperglycinuria
hyperglycosuria
hypergonadism
hypergonadotropic amenorrhea
hypergonadotropic eunuchoidism
hypergonadotropic hypogonadism
hypergonadotropic pattern
hypergynecosmia
hyperhidrosis, primary
hyperimmunoglobulin E-recurrent infection syndrome
hyperimmunoglobulin E syndrome
hyperinsulinemia, fasting
hyper-IgE syndrome
hyper-IgM syndrome
hyperintense mass
hyperkalemia
hyperkalemic periodic paralysis (HYPOP)
hyperkaluresis
hyperkeratotic white patches of the vulvar epithelium
hyperketonuria
hyperlactation
hyperlipidemia
hyperlipoproteinemia (HLP), types 1-5
hyperlithuria
hyperlysinuria
hypermagnesemia
hypermastia
hypermenorrhea
hypermobile kidney
hypermobile urethra
hypermobility, urethral
hypernatremia
hypernephroid carcinoma
hypernephroma
hypersensitivity angiitis
hyperosmolality, fluid overload
hyperostosis corticalis
hyperovarianism
hyperoxaluria, primary
hyperparathryoidism
  primary
  secondary
  tertiary
hyperphosphatemia
hyperphosphaturia
hyperpituitary gigantism
hyperpituitarism
hyperplasia
  adenomatous
  adrenal cortical
  atypical
  atypical endometrial
  benign prostatic
  breast
  complex endometrial
  congenital adrenal
  congenital endometrial

hyperplasia *(cont.)*
- congenital renal
- cystic breast
- delayed virilized adrenal
- ductal
- endometrial
- endometrial cystic
- fetal congenital
- fibromuscular
- moderate ductal
- musculomucoid intimal
- polypoid lymphoid
- prostatic
- simple endometrial

hyperplasia of prostate
hyperplastic endometritis
hyperplastic prostate
hyperplastic vulvar dystrophy
hyperprolactinemia
hyperprolactinemic amenorrhea
hyperprolactinemic disorder
hyperprolinemia types 1-2
hyperreflexia
hyperreflexic bladder
hypersthenuria
hyperstimulation of ovaries
hypertelorism-hypospadias
hypertelorism, ocular
hypertension
- accelerated
- arterial
- benign essential
- chronic
- essential
- gestational
- left renal vein
- malignant
- maternal
- postpartum
- pregnancy-induced (PIH)
- pulmonary
- renal
- renal vascular (RVH)
- renovascular

hypertension *(cont.)*
- secondary
- transient

hypertension secondary to renal disease
hypertensive effects
hypertensive nephrosclerosis
hypertensive renal disease
hyperthecosis, stromal
hyperthermia in newborn
hyperthermia of anesthesia
hyperthyroidism
- apathetic
- Graves disease
- masked
- neonatal
- silent thyroiditis
- subacute thyroiditis
- thyrotoxicosis factitia
- toxic adenoma
- toxic diffuse
- toxic multinodular goiter
- transient

hyperthyroidism
hypertonic dysfunctional labor
hypertonic labor
hypertonic saline infusion
hypertonic state
hypertonic uterine contractions
hypertonic uterine dysfunction
hypertrichosis
hypertriglyceridemia, secondary
hypertrophic bladder
hypertrophic cardiomyopathy (HCM)
hypertrophic cervicitis
hypertrophic cervix
hypertrophic elongation of cervix
hypertrophic interstitial neuropathy
hypertrophic neuropathy of Refsum
hypertrophic obstructive cardiomyopathy
hypertrophied tissue
hypertrophy
- benign prostatic
- bilateral

hypertrophy *(cont.)*
- bladder
- breast
- clitoral
- compensatory renal
- corpus cavernosum
- glomerular
- labial
- massive pubertal
- penile
- physiologic
- renal
- trilobar
- unilateral
- vulvar

hyperuricemia
hyperuricemia-choreoathetosis-self-mutilation syndrome
hyperuricemia, hereditary
hyperuricemia-oligophrenia
hyperuricosuria
hyperuricuria
hypervalinemia
hypervascularity
hyperventilation syndrome
hyperviscosity
hypervolemia
hypoadrenalism
hypoalbuminemia
hypoaldosteronism
hypoaldosteronuria
hypoazoturia
hypobetalipoproteinemia
hypocalcemia
- cow's milk
- chronic
- phosphate-loading

hypocalcemia of newborn
hypocalcemic nephrosis
hypocalcemic tetany
hypocalciuria
hypochloremia
hypochloruria
hypochondrium
hypochondroplasia
hypocitricuria
hypocomplementemia
hypocomplementemic glomerulonephritis
hypocomplementemic persistent glomerulonephritis
hypocystotomy
hypodense mass
hypodontia
hypodynamic state
hypoechoic ultrasound
hypoestrogenemia
hypoestrogenic
hypoestrogenism, temporary
hypofibrinogenemia
hypofiltration
hypofunction, adrenal cortical
hypogalactia
hypogalactous
hypogammaglobulinemia
hypogastric artery
hypogastric artery ligation
hypogastric ganglion
hypogastric vessels
hypogenital dystrophy with diabetic tendencies
hypogenitalism
hypoglossal ganglion
hypoglycemia
- alcoholic
- alimentary
- autoimmune
- drug-induced
- fasting
- idiopathic
- ketotic
- leucine-induced
- neonatal
- postprandial
- reactive

hypoglycemic

hypogonadism
  familial hypogonadotropic
  hypergonadotropic
  hypogonadotropic
  hypothalamic
  male
  primary
  secondary
hypogonadism with anosmia
hypogonadotropic eunuchoidism
hypogonadotropic hypogonadism
hypokalemia
hypokalemic nephropathy
hypokalemic periodic paralysis (HYPP)
hypolactasia
hypoleydigism
hypomagnesemia of newborn
hypomagnesemic nephropathy
hypomastia
hypomelia-hypotrichosis-facial
  hemangioma syndrome
hypomenorrhea of hyperthyroidism
hypometabolism
hyponatremia
hypo-osmolar swelling test
hypo-osmotic swelling (HOS) test
hypo-ovarianism
hypoparathyroidism
  idiopathic
  neonatal
  pseudo-hypoparathyroidism
  transient
hypophosphatasia
hypophosphatemia
  acute severe
  chronic
hypophosphaturia
hypophysectomy
hypophysial amenorrhea
hypophysial infantilism
hypopituitarism and GH deficiency
hypoplasia
  breast
  cervical

hypoplasia *(cont.)*
  renal
  uterine
hypoplasia of the maxilla, primary
  familial
hypoplastic anemia
hypoplastic kidney
hypoplastic left heart syndrome
hypoproliferative anemia
hypoprothrombinemia
hyporeflexive bladder
hyporeninemic hypoaldosteronism
hypospadiac
hypospadias
  balanic
  coronal
  female
  glandular
  penile
  penoscrotal
  perineal
  pseudovaginal
  scrotal
  subcoronal
hypospadias-dysphagia syndrome
hypospadias repair
hypospermatogenesis
hypostasis
hypostatic
hyposthenuria
hypotelorism, ocular
hypotension, orthostatic
hypotension secondary to intravascular
  depletion
hypotensive (or hypertensive) effects
hypothalamic amenorrhea
hypothalamic chronic anovulation
    (HCA)
  exercise-associated
  malnutrition-associated
  mixed/unknown etiology
  psychogenic
hypothalamic dysfunction
hypothalamic hypogonadism

hypothalamic obesity with hypogonadism
hypothalamic or pituitary pathology
hypothalamic-pituitary-adrenal (HPA) axis
hypothalamic-pituitary unit
hypothalamic hamartoblastoma, hypopituitarism, imperforate anus, and postaxial polydactyly
hypothalamus, dysfunction of the
hypothermia of hypothyroidism
hypothermic perfusion
hypothermic storage
hypothyroid infantilism
hypothyroidism
  congenital
  fetal
  goitrous
  infantile
  pituitary
  post-therapeutic
  primary
  secondary
hypothyroid myopathy
hypotonia
  benign congenital
  detrusor
hypotonia-hypomentia-hypogonadism-obesity syndrome
hypotonic bladder
hypotonic infant
hypotonicity of bladder
hypotonic myometrium
hypotonic urine
hypotonic uterine dysfunction
hypotonic uterus
hypouricuria, hereditary renal
hypovarianism
hypovolemia
hypoxia
  intrapartum
  intrauterine
hypoxemia
hypoxemia and pulmonary hypertension
hypoxic nephrosis
Hyskon (dextran 70 in dextrose)
hysteralgia
hysteratresia
hysterectomy
  abdominal
  abdominovaginal
  Bell-Buettner
  Bonney abdominal
  CASH Semm
  cesarean
  classic abdominal Semm (CASH)
  complete
  conventional abdominal
  Döderlein (Doederlein) laparoscopic
  extrafascial total abdominal
  Freund total abdominal
  Heaney vaginal
  laparoscopic
  laparoscopically assisted vaginal (LAVH)
  Lash
  liposuction-assisted nerve-sparing radical (LANS-RH)
  modified radical
  paravaginal
  partial
  Porro
  primary vaginal
  radical
  Schauta radical vaginal
  Semm
  standard vaginal
  subtotal
  supracervical
  supravaginal
  TeLinde modified radical
  total abdominal (TAH)
  total abdominal with anterior vaginal colporrhaphy
  total abdominal with bilateral salpingo-oophorectomy (TAH/BSO)
  total vaginal (TVH)

hysterectomy *(cont.)*
- transabdominal
- transvaginal
- TVH (total vaginal)
- vaginal
- Wertheim radical

hysterectomy postpartum
hysterical pregnancy
Hysterocath
hysterocele
hysterocleisis
hysterocolposcope
hysterocystopexy
Hysteroducer
hysterodynia
hysterogram
hysterograph
hysterography
hysterolysis
hysterometer
hysteromyomectomy
hysteromyotomy
hystero-oophorectomy
hysteropathy
hysteropexy, abdominal
hysteroplasty
hysterorrhaphy
hysterorrhexis
hysterosalpingectomy
hysterosalpingogram
hysterosalpingography (H/S or HSG) catheter
hysterosalpingo-oophorectomy
hysterosalpingosonography (HSSG)
hysterosalpingostomy
hysteroscope (see also *endoscope*)
- ACMI
- Baggish
- Baggish contact panoramic
- Circon
- contact
- diagnostic
- flexible
- Galileo rigid

hysteroscope *(cont.)*
- Gynecare Verascope
- Hysteroser Contact
- Micro-H
- MicroSpan
- Olympus
- Olympus HYF-XP flexible
- OPERA STAR SL
- rigid
- rigid fiberoptic
- Storz
- USA series
- Valle

hysteroscopic catheter
hysteroscopic distention system, HydroFlex
hysteroscopic evaluation
hysteroscopic irrigation system
hysteroscopic lysis of adhesions
hysteroscopic myoma screw
hysteroscopic myomectomy
hysteroscopic polyp snares
hysteroscopic selective catheterization
hysteroscopic trocar
hysteroscopy
- media
- MicroSpan system

hysteroscopy electrodes, Gyne-Pro
hysteroscopy irrigation system
hysteroscopy sheath
Hysteroser contact hysteroscopy system
hysterosonogram
hysterosonography
hysterosonography catheter
hysterospasm
hysterothermometry
hysterotomy
- abdominal
- vaginal

hysterotrachelectomy
hysterotracheloplasty
hysterotrachelorrhaphy
hysterotrachelotomy
hysterotubogram

hysterotubography
Hy-Tape surgical tape
Hytrin (terazosin)
Hyzaar (losartan potassium)
HZA (hermizona) assay
HZFO (hamster zona-free ovum) test

I, i

I&D (incision and drainage)
I&O, I/O (intake and output)
iatrogenic fetal distress
iatrogenic ureteral injury
IBC (inflammatory breast cancer)
IBIDS (icthyosis, brittle hair, impaired intelligence, decreased fertility, and short stature) syndrome
IBM (inclusion body myositis)
IC (immune complex)
IC (interstitial cystitis)
I-Cath catheter
I cell disease
ICF (intracellular fluid)
ichthyosis fetalis
ichthyosis hystrix
ichthyosis linearis circumflexa
ichthyosis vulgaris
ICI (intracervical insemination)
IC reaction
ICSI (intracytoplasmic sperm injection)
icterohematuric
icterus gravis
icterus gravis neonatorum
icterus neonatorum
icterus, physiologic
ICU (intensive care unit)
IDDM (insulin-dependent diabetes mellitus)
ideal body weight
ideal separation factor
identical twins
identified, suture ligated, clamped, and cut
identity
idiopathic crescentic necrotizing glomerulonephritis
idiopathic edema
idiopathic fibrous retroperitonitis
idiopathic glomerular disease
idiopathic hydrops
idiopathic hypercalciuria
idiopathic hypoglycemia
idiopathic immune complex glomerulonephritis
idiopathic infantile hypercalcemia
idiopathic infantilism
idiopathic maternal thrombocytopenia
idiopathic membranous glomerular disease
idiopathic membranous nephropathy
idiopathic mesangioproliferative glomerulonephritis (MsPGN)
idiopathic neonatal hepatitis

idiopathic primary renal hematuric/
  proteinuric syndrome
idiopathic recurrent jaundice of
  pregnancy
idiopathic rapidly progressive
  glomerulonephritis
idiopathic respiratory distress syndrome
  (IRDS)
idiopathic retroperitoneal fibrosis
idiopathic RPGN
idiopathic tachypnea
IDM (infant of diabetic mother)
IFN-alpha 2 gene
IgA (immunoglobulin A)
  mesangial
  polymeric
IgA antigen complex
IgA glomerulonephritis
IgA nephropathy
IgE (immunoglobulin E)
IgE-mediated immune reaction type D
IgE-mediated injury
IGF-1 (insulin-like growth factor 1)
IgG (immunoglobulin G)
IgG 2A monoclonal antibody
Iglesias electrotome
Iglesias fiberoptic resectoscope
IgM (immunoglobulin M)
IgM nephropathy
IGR (intrauterine growth retardation)
ileal perforation
ILC (interstitial laser coagulation)
ileal conduit (*not* ileoconduit)
ileal loop urinary conduit diversion
ileal neobladder
ileal reservoir, inverted U-pouch ileal
  reservoir
ileal ureter
ileoanal pull-through
ileocecal area
ileocecal junction
ileocecocystoplasty
ileocolic arcade
ileocolic continent urinary diversion
ileocystoplasty
  Camey
  LeDuc-Camey
ileoproctostomy
ileostogram
ileostomy
  continent
  external ureteral
  Kock
  reservoir
  ureteral
ileus
  adynamic
  mechanical
  meconium
  paralytic
  transitory
ileus subparta
iliac nodes
iliac vein
iliococcygeus fascial attachment
ilioinguinal nerve
ill-defined mass
illegal abortion
illegally induced abortion
Illumina PROSeries laparoscopy system
illuminating catheter
IL-2 (interleukin-2, recombinant)
IMA (inferior mammary artery) graft
IMA (internal mammary artery)
  pedicle
IMAB (internal mammary artery
  bypass)
ImageChecker mammography
  detection system
ImageChecker M1000 computer aid
  device
imaging
  antegrade pyelography
  Aspen ultrasound system
  Aurora MR breast
  BAT (B-mode acquisition and
    targeting) system
  contrast epididymogram

imaging *(cont.)*
contrast vasogram
CRYOguide ultrasound system
cystourethroscopy
Delta 32 digital stereotactic system
Delta 32 TACT three-dimensional breast
DEXA scan
diuretic renal
EVII endoscopic video system
generalized nephrographic (GNG) phase
HDI 3000 ultrasound system
ImageChecker M1000 computer aid
LORAD full field digital mammography system
lymphoscintigraphy
magnetic resonance (MRI)
mammary ductogram
MammoReader system
Miraluma nuclear breast
nephrostogram
nephrotomography
Opdima digital mammography system
OptiVu HDVD (high definition video display) system
renal
renal circulation
retrograde cystography
retrograde ureteropyelography
scintirenography
Senographe 2000D digital mammography system
SenoScan mammography system
Sonablate 200 ultrasound system
SonoCT real-time compound imaging
Sonopsy 3-D ultrasound system
step-oblique mammography
Surgi-Vision prostate MRI microcoil
Synergy ultrasound system
T-Scan 2000 transpectral impedance scanner

imaging *(cont.)*
TDMS (Trex digital mammography system)
TechneScan MAG3 (^{99m}Tc mertiatide) renal diagnostic
Technos ultrasound system
terahertz waves
TransScan 2000 (TS2000)
Trex digital mammography system (TDMS)
TS2000 (TransScan 2000)
ureteral reflux
urethrocystography
urography
urologic
vaginogram
voiding cystourethrography
Xplorer 1000 digital x-ray

imaging agent
AngioMark
Combidex
Definity ultrasound
diatrizoate meglumine
gallium-67 citrate (^{67}GA)
Hippuran I-123
Hypaque
Hyskon
indigo carmine
iodamide meglumine
iodine-based
iopamidol
Iotrex
Levovist ultrasound
methylene blue
microbubble contrast
Miraluma (technetium Tc99m sestamibi kit)
NeoTect disease-specific
OncoScint OV103
osmolality of
osmolarity of
ProstaScint
radiolabeled peptide alpha-M2
RenoCal-76

imaging agent *(cont.)*
  Reno-Dip
  Renografin-60
  Reno-M-Dip (now Reno-Dip)
  Reno-M-30 (now Reno-30)
  Reno-M-60 (now Reno-60)
  Reno-30
  Reno-60
  Renovuc-Dip
  ReVele
  ^{99m}Tc-DMSA
  ^{99m}Tc-DTPA
  ^{99m}Tc-labeled HAG3
  ^{99m}Tc-labeled MAG3
  TechneScan DMSA
  TechneScan DTPA
  TechneScan MAG3
  technetium mercaptoacetyltriglycine
  technetium pentetic acid
  technetium pertechnetate
  Tru-Scint AD
  Urografin 290
  Visipaque (iodixanol)
  water soluble
  water soluble radiopaque
imaging artifact
imbalance
  electrolyte
  sex chromosome
imbricated
imbricating sutures
imbrication
Imferon
imipenem
imipramine
imiquimod cream
immaturity
  extreme
  pulmonary
immediate dialysis
immobilize, immobilization
immotile cilia syndrome
Immulite third-generation PSA assay
IMMULITE 2000 PSA test
immune complex (IC)
immune complex deposition
immune complex disease
immune complex glomerulonephritis
immune complex immune reaction, type 3
immune complex-mediated glomerulonephritis
immune complex nephritis
immune complex reaction
immune complex RPGN
immune derangement
  acquired
  congenital
immune fetal hydrops
immune inflammation
immune mechanisms, host
immune reactants
immune renal disease (IRD)
immune response
immune response gene
immune rubella titer
immune sera
immune system
immune thrombocytopenic purpura (ITP)
immune tubular interstitial disease
immunity
  antibody-mediated
  intrauterine
  maternal
  nonrubella
immunization
immunoassay
  Elecsys total PSA
  FastPack PSA
  urinalysis
immunobead antisperm antibody test
immunocompromised patient
ImmunoCyt bladder cancer test
immunodeficiency with ataxi telangiectasia
immunoelectrophoresis
immunofluorescence

immunofluorescence microscopy
immunofluorescence study
immunofluorescent microscopy
immunogenicity
immunoglobulin
immunoglobulin A (IgA)
immunoglobulin G (IgG)
immunoglobulin M
immunohistochemistry
immunoliposome
immunologically mediated disease
immunologic infertility
immunologic injury
immunologic insulin resistance
immunologic pregnancy test
Immuno 1 complex PSA (cPSA) test
immunoperoxidase study
immunosuppressant
immunosuppressant cocktail
immunosuppressant drugs
immunosuppression, intensified
immunosuppressive drugs
immunosuppressive therapy
immunotactoid glomerulopathy
immunotherapy
Immurait (IgG 2A monoclonal
  antibody)
Imodium, Imodium A-D (loperamide)
impacted fetus
impacted shoulders
impacted urethral stone
impaction
  fecal
  shoulder
  stone
impaired cellular defense mechanisms
impaired detrusor contraction
impaired embryonal development of
  immune system
impaired excretion
impaired fecundity
impaired glucose tolerance
impaired handling of autologous
  proteins
impaired humoral host defense
  mechanisms
impaired kidney function
impaired ovum pickup
impaired pressor response to
  angiotensin infusion
impaired renal excretion
impaired renal function
impaired route of excretion
impaired tubal transport mechanism
impaired voiding contraction
impairment
  acquired tubular
  congenital tubular
  functional tubular
  renal function
impairment in renal concentrating
  capacity
impairment of neuromuscular
  transmission
imperfecta, osteogenesis
imperfect fungus
imperforate anus
imperforate anus with urinary bladder
  opening into anus
imperforate aperture
imperforate hymen
impetigo, bullous
impetigo neonatorum
Implanon contraceptive implant
implant (see also *device; prosthesis*)
  adjustable saline breast
  Alpha 1 penile
  anatomically shaped silicone breast
  BEBIG iodine-125 seed
  Becker breast
  Biocell RTV saline-filled breast
  BioDimensional breast
  bladder neck support
  breast
  complex intracavitary radium
  Contigen
  Contour Profile silicone breast
  double-lumen breast

implant *(cont.)*
endometrial
fetal tissue
goserelin
Greene renal
Implanon contraceptive
Introl bladder neck support
islet cell
leuprolide
mammary
NovaGold
NovaSaline inflatable saline breast
NovaSaline pre-filled breast
palladium (^{103}Pd) prostate
penile (also see *penile implant*)
prostate
radioactive seed
radium needle
removal of intact mammary
Restore orthobiologic soft-tissue
retropectoral mammary
silicone
single-lumen breast
single-lumen silicone breast
testicular
Trilucent breast
ureteral reimplantation
Zoladex (goserelin)
implantable urinary prosthesis
implantable vascular valve system
implantation
endometrial
human blastocyst
ovarian tissue
percutaneous transperineal seed
implantation of inflatable cylinders
implantation theory of endometriosis
impotence
erectile
female
organic
psychological
impotence of organic origin
impotency
impotent
Impra graft
Impra Venaflo vascular graft
impregnate
impregnated ovum in cervical canal
impregnated vaginal packing
impregnation
Impress Softpatch foam pad
Impress Softpatch urinary incontinence device
imprinting
improved hemodynamics
IMRT (intensity-modulated radiotherapy treatment)
Imuran (azathioprine)
inability to get an erection
inability to maintain an erection
inability to sustain an erection
inactivated polio vaccine (IPV)
inadequate circulating blood volume
inadequate luteal phase
inadequate neovaginal size
inadequate ovarian function
inadequate renal perfusion
inadequate visualization
inadvertent dissection of ureter
inadvertent perforation of vessels
inadvertent subdural tap
inappropriate gonadotropin secretion
inappropriate increase in LH:FSH ratio
inappropriate steroid feedback
inappropriate uterine bleeding
inborn errors of metabolism
inborn errors of urea synthesis
inbreeding
inbreeding coefficient
inbreeding depression
INCA (infant nasal cannulae assembly)
incapacitating pain
incarcerated gravid uterus
incarcerated hernia
incarcerated placenta
incarceration of inguinal hernia
Incert implantable sponge

incest
incest barrier
In Charge diabetes control system
incidental appendectomy
incipient acute renal failure
incision
  chevron
  circumareolar
  circumferential
  circumlinear
  classic longitudinal uterine
  classic uterine
  colpotomy
  cruciate
  curvilinear
  Duhrssen
  elliptical
  flank
  horizontal
  infraclavicular
  inframammary
  infraumbilical
  infraumbilical skin
  inguinal
  intraperitoneal
  Kerr low transverse
  keyhole
  Krohnig low vertical midline
  lazy S
  longitudinal
  longitudinal lower segment uterine
  low segment
  low vertical
  Maylard
  McBurney
  midline
  minilaparotomy
  muscle-splitting
  oblique
  paramedian
  paraumbilical
  Penduloff
  penoscrotal
incision *(cont.)*
  periareolar
  periumbilical
  Pfannenstiel
  puncture
  right flank
  Rockey-Davis
  saber cut
  semilunar
  skin crease
  smile
  stab
  subcostal
  subumbilical
  suprapubic
  supraumbilical
  thoracoabdominal
  through-and-through
  transverse
  transverse abdominal
  transverse lower segment uterine
  transverse Pfannenstiel
  U-shaped
  uterine
  vertical
  vertical fundal
  vertical midline Pfannenstiel
incisional biopsy
incisional hernia
incision and drainage (I&D)
incision and drainage of abscess
incision biopsy
incision extended laterally
incision extended superiorly and inferiorly
incision made from xiphoid to umbilicus
incision site
inclusion
  fetal
  tubal reticular
inclusion body myositis
inclusion cell disease

incompatibility
  ABO
  fetal-maternal
  maternal and fetal blood group
  maternal-fetal
  maternal-fetal histoincompatibility
  renal
  Rh
incompetence
  cervical
  pelvic fundus
  urinary sphincter
incompetent cervical os
incompetent cervix
incomplete AB (abortion)
incomplete bladder emptying
incomplete conjoined twins
incomplete dominance
incomplete emptying of bladder
incomplete filling
incomplete foot presentation
incomplete knee presentation
incomplete penetrance
incomplete placenta previa
incomplete spermatogenic arrest
incomplete spontaneous abortion
incomplete testicular feminization
incomplete voiding
incompletus, coitus
incontinence (see also *incontinence devices; urinary incontinence devices; urinary incontinence treatment*)
  active
  bladder
  bowel
  chronic
  detrusor-sphincter incoordination with urinary
  dribbling
  drip
  electrode
  environmental
  fecal

incontinence *(cont.)*
  genuine stress (GSI)
  indurative nephritis
  intermittent
  mild urge
  mixed-type
  overflow
  paradoxical
  paralytic
  passive
  postprostatectomy
  psychogenic
  short-term
  stool
  stress
  stress urinary (SUI)
  total
  urge
  urgency
  urge urinary
  urinary
  urinary exertional
  urinary stress
incontinence device (see also *urinary incontinence device*)
  Autocath 100 bladder-control
  Avina female urethral plug
  barrier
  BioSling urethral sling
  CapSure continence shield
  Carlesta skin treatment for urinary incontinence
  Cunningham clamp for male urinary incontinence
  Depend pads for incontinence
  Dumontpallier pessary
  Duth pessary
  Emmet-Gelhorn pessary
  fat injection
  FemSoft insert urinary
  Findley folding pessary
  Gariel pessary
  Gelhorn pessary
  Guhrung pessary

incontinence device *(cont.)*
  Gynecare TVT tension-free
  Hodge pessary
  Impress Softpatch urinary
  InnoSense urinary
  InterStim implantable continence-control therapy
  Introl bladder neck support prosthesis
  Macroplastique implantable
  Mayer pessary
  Medworks urinary
  Menge pessary
  Miniguard
  NeoControl
  On-Command catheter for
  Pelvic Flex
  PerQ SANS urge
  Persist system
  pessary
  Prentif pessary
  Prochownik pessary
  Reliance Urinary Control Insert
  ring pessary
  SANS (Stoller afferent nerve stimulation)
  stiff ring
  Stoller afferent nerve stimulation (SANS)
  Suspend sling
  TriAngle sling
  UroMed incontinence patch
  woven sling
  Zwanck pessary
  Z-stitch bladder neck stabilization
incontinence monitoring, anal EMG
  PerryMeter sensor
incontinence of urine
incontinence procedure (see also *operation; sling; urethral sling*)
  anterior colporrhaphy
  anterior plication
  Benderev bone fixation for stress urinary incontinence (SUI)
incontinence procedure *(cont.)*
  biofeedback for incontinence
  Burch colposuspension for stress incontinence
  Burch iliopectineal ligament urethrovesical suspension
  Burch retropubic urethropexy
  collagen injection
  electrical stimulation
  fat injection
  Kelly
  Kelly-Kennedy urethral
  Kelly-Stoeckel urethral plication
  Marshall-Marchetti-Krantz
  needle urethropexy
  Oxford
  periurethral collagen injection
  promontofixation
  pubovaginal repair
  pubovaginal sling
  sling
  urethral sling
incontinence ring (see *urinary incontinence device*)
incontinence training
incontinence treatment (see *incontinence device; incontinence procedure; urinary incontinence treatment)*
incontinent external stoma
incontinentia pigmenti (IP)
incontinent ileal conduit
incontinent of stool
incontinent of urine
incoordinate uterine contractions
increased androgen secretion
increased erythropoietin activity
increased libido
increased maternal age
increased peritoneal macrophage activity
increased peritoneal prostaglandin production
increased protein catabolism

increased red cell mass
increased renin secretion
increased testicular pressure
increased venous capacitance
 in pregnancy
increase in urine volume
increase of filtered proteins
increase in the serum creatinine level
increasing pulmonary infiltrates
incrusted cystitis
incubation, urine
incubator
 double-walled
 Forma in vitro
 Forma water-jacketed
 single-walled
incudiform uterus
indentation of fundus of uterus
index (pl. indices)
 AFI (amniotic fluid)
 amniotic fluid (AFI)
 apoptotic
 American Urological Association
 (AUA) Symptom
 body mass (BMI)
 Doppler Perfusion
 fetal-pelvic
 free/total PSA (prostate-specific
 antigen)
 glycemic
 Gravindex
 mean amniotic fluid
 Mengert pelvimetry
 Pearl
 penile brachial pressure (PBPI)
 prostate-specific antigen (PSA)
 free/total index
 renal failure
 renal resistive
 umbilical coiling
 vaginal maturation
index case
Indiana urinary pouch procedure
indicanuria syndrome
indications for prenatal diagnosis
indicator, prognostic
indifferent genitalia
indifferent gonad
indigo carmine dye
Indigo LaserOptic treatment system
indirect Coombs test
indirect diuretic
indirect IBT (immunobead test)
indirect maternal death
indoluria
indomethacin
induced abortion
induced labor
induced termination of pregnancy
induction
 medical
 menstrual cycle
 postdate
induction and delivery
induction of anesthesia
induction of labor
indurated prostate
induration
 breast
 parametrial
 prostate
 skin
 urethral
induratio penis plastica
indwelling catheter in bladder
indwelling Foley catheter
indwelling ureteral stent
indwelling urinary bladder catheter
inertia
 primary uterine
 secondary uterine
 true uterine
 uterine
inevitable abortion
Infalyte
infant (see also *baby; newborn*)
 appropriate for gestational age
 (AGA)

infant *(cont.)*
- extremely low birth weight (ELBW)
- heavy for dates
- Hercules
- high birth weight
- jittery
- large for dates
- LBW (low birth weight)
- liveborn
- living
- low birth weight (LBW)
- micropreemie
- nonviable
- postmature
- post-term
- premature
- preemie
- preterm
- small for gestational age (SGA)
- stillborn
- stimulation of
- term
- very low birth weight (VLBW)
- viable

infant cystoscope

infant death

infant formula
- Alimentum
- Alsoy
- amino acid based
- Carnation Follow-Up Formula
- Carnation Good Start
- casein hydrolysate
- cow's milk-based
- Elecare
- Enfamil
- Enfamil Human Milk Fortifier
- Enfamil Premature Formula
- Enfamil Premature Formula with Iron
- Enfamil 22
- Enfamil with Iron
- Gerber Baby Formula with Iron
- Gerber Soy Formula

infant formula *(cont.)*
- hydrolyzed whey-based
- Isomil
- Isomil DF
- Isomil SF
- Lactofree
- LBW
- L-Emental
- Lofenalac
- Neocate
- Neosure
- Nursoy
- Nutramigen
- PM 60/40
- Portagen
- Preemie SMA 20
- Preemie SMA 24
- Pregestimil
- preterm
- ProSobee
- RCF
- SCF 24
- Similac Improved
- Similac Lactose Free
- Similac Natural Care Human Milk Fortifier
- Similac PM 60/40
- Similac Special Care 20
- Similac Special Care 24
- Similac Special Care with Iron 24
- Similac 13
- Similac 20
- Similac 24
- Similac 27
- Similac with Iron 20
- Similac with Iron 24
- SMA 13
- SMA 20
- SMA 24
- SMA 27
- SMA Lo-Iron 13
- SMA Lo-Iron 20
- SMA Lo-Iron 24
- soy

infant formula *(cont.)*
  Soyalac
  Vivonex
infanticide
infantile acute hemorrhagic edema of skin
infantile autism
infantile beriberi
infantile celiac disease
infantile cerebral palsy
infantile hypercalcemia syndrome, idiopathic
infantile hypothyroidism
infantile myofibromatosis
infantile nephrotic syndrome
infantile neuronal degeneration
infantile phytanic acid storage disease
infantile progressive spinal muscular atrophy
infantile purulent conjunctivitis
infantile Refsum disease
infantile spasms
infantile subacute necrotizing encephalopathy of Leigh disease
infantile uterus
infantilism
  Brissaud
  dysthyroidal
  hepatic
  hypophysial
  hypothyroid
  idiopathic
  Lorain-Lévi
  myxedematous
  pancreatic
  pituitary
  proportionate
  renal
  sexual
  static
  tubal
  universal
infant mortality
infant mortality rate
infant nasal cannulae assembly (INCA)
infant of diabetic mother (IDM)
infant respiratory distress syndrome (IRDS)
Infant Star ventilator
infant was suctioned on the perineum
infarcted appendix epididymidis
infarcted testis
infarction
  cerebral
  fallopian tube
  maternal floor
  ovarian
  placental
  prostatic
  renal
  testicular
  therapeutic
infarct, placental
In-Fast bone screw for urinary sling procedure
In-Fast bone screw system used in cystourethropexy
Infasurf (calfactant) intratracheal suspension
infected abortion
infected decidua
infected hydrocele
infected megaureter
infected placental fragments
infection
  amniotic sac
  anaerobic
  asymptomatic urinary tract
  bacterial
  bladder
  chlamydial
  clostridial
  congenital cytomegalovirus
  Escherichia coli (E. coli)
  falciparum
  fungal
  genital tract
  gonococcal

infection *(cont.)*
- herpes simplex viral
- intra-amniotic
- Listeria
- navel cord
- neonatal Candida
- neonatal urinary tract
- nipple
- occult urinary tract
- opportunistic
- parasitic
- placental
- puerperal
- relapsing
- relapsing-remitting
- rickettsial
- secondary
- sexually transmitted
- systemic
- umbilical stump
- ureaplasmal
- urinary tract (UTI)
- vaginal
- vaginal yeast
- viral
- yeast

infection calculus
infection secondary to instrumentation
infectious avian nephrosis
infectious disease
infectious hepatitis
infective mastitis
infective pneumonia
infecundity
INFeD (iron dextran injection)
inferior central pedicle reduction augmentation mammoplasty
inferior collecting system
inferior epigastric vessels
inferior mammary artery (IMA) graft
inferior margin of vesical neck
inferior mesenteric artery
inferior pedicle of breast
inferior pedicle technique reduction mammoplasty
inferior pole of kidney
inferior rectal vascular system
inferior vena cava
inferior venacavography
inferior vesical artery
inferolateral surface of prostate
infertile male syndrome
infertility
- abnormal tubal function
- absolute
- drug therapy
- ovulatory dysfunction
- primary
- radiation
- secondary
- unexplained
- unidentified

infestation, parasitic
infibulation ("pharaonic circumcision")
infiltrate, mononuclear interstitial
infiltrating ductal carcinoma of breast
infiltration
- gummatous
- interstitial
- lymphomatous

infiltrative dermopathy
infiltrative ophthalmopathy
inflammation
- adnexa uteri
- Bartholin gland
- bladder
- cell-mediated immune
- chronic
- immune
- perivesical
- tubulointerstitial
- urinary tract
- vulvovaginal

inflammatory breast cancer (IBC)
inflammatory breast carcinoma
inflammatory carcinoma of breast

inflammatory cytokines
inflammatory fibroid polyp
inflammatory response to sperm
  leakage
inflatable penile prosthesis (IPP)
inflation pistol
inflow
influenza A vaccine
Inform HER2/neu gene-based test for
  recurrent breast cancer
infraclavicular incision
infraclavicular lymph nodes
inframamillary
inframammary approach in
  augmentation mammoplasty
inframammary crease
inframammary incision
inframammary scar
inframammary sulcus
infrarenal stenosis
infraumbilical incision
infraumbilical skin incision
infraumbilical trocar
infrequent ovulation
infiltrate, recovery of
inflatable silicon vaginal stent
In-Flow intraurethral valved catheter
informatics
informed consent
in-frame mutation/deletion
infundibulo-ovarian ligament
infundibulopelvic ligament
infundibulum (pl. infundibula)
infundibulum of kidney
infundibulum of uterine tube
infusion
  hypertonic saline
  isotonic
infusion of balanced electrolyte
  solution
inguinal canal
inguinal exploration
inguinal hernia
inguinal hernia repair
inguinal herniorrhaphy
inguinal incision
inguinal lymphadenectomy
inguinal nodes
inguinal orchiectomy
inguinal ring
  external
  internal
inguinolabial
inguinoscrotal hernia
inheritance
  alternative
  codominant
  complemental
  cytoplasmic
  dominant
  extrachromosomal
  holandric
  homochronous
  homotropic
  intermediate
  mandelian
  maternal
  mitochondrial
  monofactorial
  multifactorial
  polygenic
  quantitative
  quasidominant
  recessive
  sex-influenced
  sex-limited
  sex-linked
  X-linked
  Y-linked
inherited
inherited breast and ovarian cancer
inherited dominant gene mutation
inhibiting hormone
inhibition of prostaglandin synthesis
inhibition, labor
inhibitor
  angiotensin-converting enzyme
    (ACEI)

inhibitor *(cont.)*
  cartilage-derived (CDI)
  CDI (cartilage-derived)
  MAO
  prostaglandin synthetase
  uterine
iniencephaly
initial apnea
initial genital reconstruction
initial hematuria
initial morning urine
initiation of labor
injected fertility drugs
injection
  Bard flexible endoscopic
  botulinum-A toxin
  collagen (for incontinence)
  fetal umbilical vein
  glutaraldehyde cross-linked collagen
  intra-amniotic
  intramuscular fetal
  intraperitoneal fetal
  intravenous fetal
  periurethral collagen
injection of prostaglandin into amniotic sac
injection procedure for mammary ductogram or galactogram
injection therapy with intralesional steroids
injection tube (see *catheter*)
injector
InjecTx customized cystoscope
injured kidney
injured tubular epithelium
injury (pl. injuries)
  bilateral incomplete ureteral
  bladder
  cold
  direct endothelial cell
  iatrogenic ureteral
  IgE-mediated
  immunologic
  maternal

injury *(cont.)*
  obstetrical
  perinatal
  renal
  urethral
injury during parturition
inlet contraction of pelvis
inlet, pelvic
inlet shoulder dystocia
inner symphyseal cartilage
innervation, extracorporeal magnetic (ExMI)
innocent murmur
Innofem (estradiol)
InnoSense urinary incontinence device
Innova home therapy system for urinary incontinence
Innovo insulin delivery device
inoculum, marrow
INOmax (nitric oxide) inhalation for newborns
InPath cervical cancer screening test
INR (International Normalized Ratio)
Insemini-Cath catheter
insemination
  artificial
  donor
  homologous
  intrauterine
  Makler
  therapeutic
insemination catheter (see *catheter*)
insemination cup
insert
  FemSoft Insert
  Reliance Urinary Control Insert
insertion
  penile prosthesis
  ureteral
insertion sequence (IS) element
in silico
insipidus
  diabetes
  nephrogenic diabetes

in situ
in situ breast cancer
in situ, carcinoma
in situ culture
in situ hybridization
in situ urethral sling
in situ vaginal wall sling for stress urinary incontinence
in situ vascular reconstructive techniques
inspissated bile syndrome
inspissated milk
instability, detrusor
instill
instillation
  amniotic
  antibiotic solution
  medication
instillation therapy
instilled
instrumentation, urethral
instrument holder, Bookler swivel-ball
instruments were removed under direct vision
insufficiency
  acquired renal
  placental
  renal
  uterine
  uteroplacental
insufflate
insufflation
  blind needle
  gas
  tubal
  uterotubal
insufflator
  automatic
  Karl Storz N_2O Endoflator
  laparoscopic
Insuflon indwelling device for delivering insulin
insulin
  AC137 analog
  exogenous
  Humalog
  Humalog Mix50/50
  Humalog Mix75/25
  Humulin
  insulin glargine
  intermediate-acting
  Lente
  long-acting
  neutral protamine Hagedorn (NPH)
  NPH (neutral protamine Hagedorn)
  Oralgen oral aerosol
  protamine zinc (PZI)
  rapid-acting
  regular
  Semilente
  short-acting
  Ultralente
  Velosulin BR
  Velosulin BR human buffered regular
insulin allergy
insulinase manufactured by placenta
insulin clearance
insulin deficient
insulin delivery device
insulin-dependent diabetes mellitus (IDDM)
insulin glargine
insulin-like growth factor 1 (IGF-1)
insulinopathy
insulinotardic
insulinotropin
insulin preparation
insulin pump
  Felig
  H-TRON plus V100 infusion
insulin reaction
insulin resistance, immunologic
insulin resistance in gestational diabetes

insulin resistance syndrome
insulin resistant
insulin-resistant diabetes mellitus associated with acanthosis nigricans
insulin-secreting cells
insulin tolerance test
insulin treatment
Insul-Sheath
inSync miniform menstrual device
In-Tac bone anchor for urinary sling procedure
intact amniotic sac
intact hymen
intact membranes
intact placenta
intake and output (I&O, I/O)
intellectual property rights
intended parents
intensified immunosuppression
intensive care nursery
intensive care unit (ICU)
intensivist
interaction, granulosa-oocyte
intercapillary glomerulosclerosis
Interceed absorbable adhesion barrier
Interceed TC7
Intercept prostate microcoil
Intercept urethra microcoil
intercostal nerve
intercostal nerve block
intercostal retractions
intercostal vessels
intercourse
  anal
  pain during
  sexual
  vaginal
intercurrent illness
interfamilial variability
interference
interferon alfa-n3
interkinesis
interleukin-1
interleukin-1b
interleukin-2, recombinant (IL-2)
interleukin-3, recombinant, human (IL-3)
interleukin 4 (IL-4)
interleukin-6 (IL-6)
interleukin-10 (IL-10)
interleukin-11 (IL-11)
interlobar veins of kidney
interlobular artery
interlobular artery of kidney
interlobular veins of kidney
intermediate allele
intermediate fetal death
intermediate part of male urethra
intermediate spinal muscular atrophy
intermenstrual bleeding
intermenstrual interval
intermenstrual pain
intermenstrual spotting
intermittency of urination
intermittent androgen withdrawal
intermittent ataxia with pyruvate dehydrogenase deficiency
intermittent drainage
intermittent excess of fluid weight gain
intermittent hemodialysis
intermittent hemodialysis filters
intermittent hemoglobinuria
intermittent hydrosalpinx
intermittent peritoneal dialysis (IPD)
intermittent proteinuria
intermittent self-catheterization
intermittent urinary frequency
intermittent urinary stream
internal calcification of kidney
internal cephalic version
internal female genital organs
internal fetal monitor
internal hemorrhoid
internal iliac artery
internal iliac node
internalized homophobia
internal jugular vein
internal male genital organs

internal mammary artery bypass (IMAB)
internal mammary lymph node
internal monitoring
internal oblique muscle
internal os
internal os sphincter
internal podalic version
internal pudendal artery
internal pudendal vein
internal ring
internal spermatic artery
internal spermatic fascia
internal spermatic vein
internal sphincter
internal urethral meatotomy
internal urethral orifice
internal urethral sphincter
internal urethrotomy
internal urinary diversion
International Federation of Gynecology and Obstetrics (FIGO)
International Prostate Symptom Score (IPSS)
International Register of Lithium Babies
International Society for the Study of Vulvar Disease (ISSVD)
International System of Units (SI)
interphase
interposition, Gore-Tex graft vein
interrenal stenosis
interrupted coitus
intersex abnormality
intersex anomaly
intersex children
intersex disorder
Intersex Society of North America
intersexual
intersexuality
intersigmoid hernia
inter-simple sequence repeat (ISSR)
InterStim implantable continence-control therapy
InterStim urinary neurostimulation device
interstitial cell
interstitial cystitis (IC)
interstitial deletion
interstitial disease
interstitial edema
interstitial emphysema
interstitial fibroid
interstitial implants
interstitial infiltration
interstitial laser coagulation (ILC)
interstitial mastitis
interstitial nephritis
interstitial pregnancy
interstitial pulmonary fibrosis of prematurity
interstitial salpingitis
interstitial X chromosome deletion
interstitium
  cortical
  medullary
  renal
intertriginous folds
intertrigo
intertuberous diameter
interureteral
interureteric crest
interureteric fold
interureteric ridge
interval between periods
interval, intermenstrual
interval sterilization
intervening myometrium
intervillous space
intestinal atresia
intestinal endometriosis
intestinal glucose transport
intestinal perforation
intestinal pouch
intestinal pseudo-obstructions
intestinal reconfiguration, Yang-Monti concept of
intestinal stenosis

intestinal ureter, construction of
intestinal urinary conduit
intestine, endometriosis of
intestinoureteral fistula
intestinouterine fistula
intestinovaginal fistula
intestinovesical fistula
in toto
intra-abdominal adhesion
intra-abdominal bleeding
intra-abdominal endoscopic procedure
intra-abdominal irritation
intra-abdominal IUD
intra-abdominal ligation
intra-abdominally
intra-abdominal pressure
intra-abdominal reservoir
intra-abdominal vascular prosthesis
intra-access blood flow
intra-alveolar hemorrhage
intra-amniotic infection in fetus
intra-amniotic injection
intra-anal wart
intracavernous injection for erectile dysfunction
intracavernous injection test
intracavitary irradiation
intracavitary prostate ultrasonography
intracavitary prostate ultrasound
intracellular anion
intracellular buffer system
intracellular diplococci
intracellular enzymes
intracellular fluid (ICF)
intracellular PO_4 depletion
intracervical insemination (ICI)
intracervical tent
intracorporal (also intracorporeal)
intracorporeal injections for impotence
intracorporeal lithotripter
intracranial calcification
intracranial hemorrhage
intracranial venous sinus thrombosis
intractable metabolic acidosis
intractable pain
intracytoplasmic bacilli
intracytoplasmic sperm injection (ICSI) fertilization
IntraDose gel (purified bovine collagen, cisplatin, and epinephrine)
intraductal carcinoma of breast
intraductal papilloma
intraepithelial carcinoma of cervix
intraepithelial cervical dysplasia
intraepithelial endometrial cancer
intrafallopian transfer, gamete
intrafallopian transfer zygote
intrafamilial variability
intragenic marker
intrafimbrial bridging
intrahepatic cholestasis of pregnancy
intraligamentary pregnancy
intraligamentous pregnancy
intraluminal adhesions
intraluminal foreign body
intraluminal pressure gradient
intramammary lymph nodes
intramammary node
intramammary sulcus
intramembranous dense deposit disease
intramural fibroid
intramural portion of distal ureter
intramural pregnancy
intramuscular fetal injection
intramuscular narcotics
Intran disposable intrauterine pressure measurement catheter
intranuclear inclusion
intraoperative bladder drainage
intraoperative high dose rate (IOHDR) brachytherapy
intraoperative lymphatic mapping
intrapartal care
intrapartum anoxia
intrapartum complication
intrapartum events
intrapartum fetal bradycardia
intrapartum hemorrhage

intrapartum hypoxia
intraperitoneal bleeding
intraperitoneal fetal injection
intraperitoneal incision
intraperitoneal IUD
intraperitoneal palpation
intraperitoneal pregnancy
intraperitoneal transplantation of ureters
intrarenal artery
intrarenal coagulation
intrarenal hemorrhage
intrarenal hyperdense mass
intrarenal hypodense mass
intrarenal precipitation
intrarenal reflux
intrarenal tubular blockade
intrarenal tubular blockade with urates
intrascrotal temperature
IntraStent DoubleStrut renal artery stent
IntraStent DoubleStrut XS renal artery stent
intratesticular mass
intrathecal
intratrigonal ridge
intratubal
intratumoral hemorrhage
intraurethral coil
intraurethral coils and springs
intraurethral spring
intrauterine insemination (IUI)
intrauterine short stature
intrauterine adhesions
intrauterine cardiac failure
intrauterine catheter (see *catheter*)
intrauterine cavity
intrauterine coil
intrauterine contraceptive device
intrauterine cytomegalic inclusion disease
intrauterine death
intrauterine demise
intrauterine device (see also *IUD*)
  bow "T"
  coil
intrauterine device *(cont.)*
  Copper 7
  Cu-Safe 300
  Dalkon Shield
  Lippes loop
  loop
  lost
  TCu380A
intrauterine fetal death
intrauterine fetal demise
intrauterine fetal surgery
intrauterine fetal transfusion, ultrasonic guidance for
intrauterine fetus
intrauterine fossa
intrauterine fracture of fetus
intrauterine gestation
intrauterine growth retardation (IGR, IUGR)
intrauterine heart failure
intrauterine hypoxia
intrauterine immunity
intrauterine injection catheter (see *catheter*)
intrauterine insemination
intrauterine insemination catheter (see *catheter*)
intrauterine life
intrauterine passage of meconium
intrauterine pregnancy (IUP)
intrauterine pressure catheter (IUPC)
intrauterine pressure determination procedure
intrauterine probe
intrauterine protuberance
intrauterine resuscitation
intrauterine sac
intrauterine sepsis of fetus
intrauterine synechiae
intrauterine thermal balloon ablation
intrauterine thrombocytopenia
intrauterine transfusion
intravaginal radium treatment
intravaginal ring (IVR) hormone replacement therapy

intravaginal torsion
intravascular blood transfusions
intravascular dehydration
intravascular depletion
intravascular fetal transfusion
intravascular hemolysis
intravenous (I.V., IV)
intravenous fetal injection
intravenous fluids
intravenous hydration
intravenous pyelogram or pyelography (IVP)
  antegrade
  retrograde
intravenous sedation
intravenous urogram or urography (IVU) (see also *intravenous pyelogram* or *pyelography*)
intravenous urography (IVU)
intraventricular hemorrhage (IVH)
intravesical bacillus
intravesical crushing of bladder calculi
intravesical irrigation
intravesical lesion
intravesical obstruction
intravesical pathology
intravesical pressure
intravesical stone
intravesical ureter
intravesicular pressure
intrinsic genitourinary disease
intrinsic mass
intrinsic rejection factor
intrinsic renal cause of acute renal failure
intrinsic renal concentration defect
intrinsic renal disease
intrinsic renal failure
intrinsic sphincter deficiency (ISD)
intrinsic urinary system disease
introducer
  Foley catheter
  laparoscopic
  LapSac
introducer *(cont.)*
  needle
  P.D. Access peel-away needle
  suprapubic
  transcervical
  Vascu-Sheath
introducer/extractor
introital dyspareunia
introital stenosis
introitus
  marital
  parous
  tight
  vaginal
  virginal
Introl bladder neck support prosthesis
intromission
intromittent organ
Intron A (interferon alfa-2b, recombinant)
intronic mutation
intubate
intubation, endotracheal
intussuscepted appendiceal mucosa
in utero
in utero fetal structural abnormality
in utero fetal surgery
in utero repair of neural tube defect
in utero surgery
invaginata
invaginate
invagination
InVance male sling procedure
invasion
  bladder wall
  metastatic
  stromal
invasive adenocarcinoma
invasive bladder cancer
invasive breast cancer
invasive breast carcinoma
invasive carcinoma
invasive lesion
invasive malignancy

invasive mole
invasive neoplasm
invasive procedure
invasive squamous cell carcinoma
invasive vulvar carcinoma
inverse polymerase chain reaction (IPCR)
inversion
  nipple
  paracentric
  pericentric
inverted duplicated marker
inverted nipples
inverted repeat
inverted sutures
inverted U-pouch ileal reservoir
inverted uterus
Investa suture
investigation, urologic
Invicorp (phentolamine mesylate)
in vitro
in vitro fertilization (IVF)
in vitro fertilization of human embryos
in vitro sensitivity assay
in vivo
in vivo fertilization by artificial insemination
in vivo urethral sling
involuntary contraction of detrusor muscle
involuntary discharge of urine during sleep
involuntary loss of urine during intercourse
involuntary muscle of corpus of uterus
involuntary urination
involuted uterus
involution, senile
INVOS 2100 test for breast cancer
Ioban drape
Ioban Vi-Drape
iodamide meglumine imaging agent
iodide goiter
iodides
  organic
  protein
iodinated contrast dye
iodinated contrast medium
iodine
iodine-based contrast media
iodine-125 brachytherapy
Iodoflex dressing
Iodoform gauze dressing
Iodoform gauze pack
Iodosorb dressing
IoGold radioactive seeds
IOHDR (intraoperative high dose rate) brachytherapy
ion bombardment
ionic concentration of interstitial fluid
ion-selective membrane
iopamidol
iopamidol injection
Iotec flexible cannula
Iotec trocar
iothalamate clearance
Iotrex radiation liquid
Iotrex radioisotope
Iowa membrane forceps
Iowa trumpet
Iowa trumpet needle guide
I-OXY (intravesical oxybutynin)
IPCR (inverse polymerase chain reaction)
IPD (intermittent peritoneal dialysis)
I-Plant brachytherapy seeds
I-Plant iodine-125 seeds
I-Plant radioactive iodine-125 seeds
IPP (inflatable penile prosthesis)
iproplatin
ipsilateral arm
ipsilateral breast
ipsilateral iliac fossa
ipsilateral internal mammary lymph node
ipsilateral pneumoscrotum

ipsilateral vascular access
IPSS (International Prostate Symptom Score)
IPV (inactivated polio vaccine)
IRD (immune renal disease)
IRDS (idiopathic respiratory distress syndrome)
IRDS (infant respiratory distress syndrome)
irideremia
iridogoniodysgenesis with somatic anomalies
irritable bowel in children
irritable bowel syndrome (IBS)
IRIS (Intensified Radiographic Imaging System)
iron-deficiency anemia
iron dextran
iron overload
iron overload syndrome
iron-resistant microcytic anemia
iron, serum
iron storage disease
iron sucrose
irradiation
  bladder
  breast
  gonad
  intracavitary
  prostate
  vaginal cone
  whole pelvis
irradiation cystitis
irregularity of uterus
irregular kidney
irregular labor
irregular menstrual cycles
irregular periods
irregular uterine bleeding
irregular uterine contractions
irreparable obstructive azoospermia
irreversible anuria
irreversible chronic graft rejection
irreversible renal disease
irrigant, Renacidin
irrigating syringe, Toomey
irrigation
  bladder
  copious
  tissue
  urinary tract
irrigator
  End-Flo laparoscopic
  Hi-Flo irrigator/aspirator
  HydroSurge laparoscopic
  hysteroscopic
  Lap Vacu-Irrigator
  Pathfinder urologic
  StrykeFlow suction
  suction
irritability, cerebral
irritable bowel in children
irritable bowel syndrome
irritable breast
irritant, bladder
irritation, peritoneal
Irving tubal ligation
ischemia
  kidney
  penile
  renal
  vasospastic
ischemic necrosis
ischemic penile gangrene
ischial spine
ischiocavernous muscles
ischiospongiosus muscle of penis
ischiovaginal
ISD (intrinsic sphincter deficiency)
IS (insertion sequence) element
island tensor fasciae latae flap
islet cell antibodies
islet cell autoantibody
islet cell allografting
islet cell implant
islet cryopreservation
Isletest and Isletest-ICA kits for detection of islet cell autoantibodies

isochromosome
isodense
isodensity
isoechoic
isoelectric focusing
isoelectric point
isoenzyme
isoforms
isograft
isoimmune neutropenia
isoimmunization
  ABO
  Rhesus
Isojima antisperm antibody test
isolated adrenocorticotropic hormone deficiency
isolated birth defect
isolated chordee
isolated clustered calcifications of breast
isolated gonadotropin hormone deficiency
isolated lissencephaly
isolated pituitary hormone deficiency
isolated prolactin deficiency
isolated proteinuria
isolated tetrasomy
isolated thyroid stimulating hormone deficiency
Isolette infant warmer
Isomil DF infant formula
Isomil SF infant formula
isosexual virilization
isosthenuria
isotonic replacement fluid
isotonic saline
isotonic solution
isotope
isotretinoin
isovaleric acidemia CoA dehydrogenase deficiency
isovaleryl-CoA carboxylase deficiency
isozyme
ISSR (inter-simple sequence repeat)
ISSVD (International Society for the Study of Vulvar Disease)
isthmica nodosa, salpingitis
isthmus
  cervical
  kidney
  renal
  tube
  uterine
itching
  penile
  perineal
  vaginal
  vulvar
IUD (see *intrauterine device*)
IUD embedded in uterus
IUD extractor
IUD string
IUGR (intrauterine growth retardation)
IUI (intrauterine insemination)
IUP (intrauterine pregnancy)
IUPC (intrauterine pressure catheter)
I.V., IV (intravenous)
I.V. administration of fluids
I.V. administration of medications
Ivemark syndrome
IVF (in vitro fertilization) egg donor
IVF-ET (in vitro fertilization-embryo transfer)
I.V. fluids
I.V. glucose administration
IVH (intraventricular hemorrhage)
I.V. hydration
I.V. hyperalimentation
I.V. KVO (keep vein open)
ivory bones
I.V. piggyback
I.V. push
IVP (intravenous pyelogram)
IVP (intravenous pyelography)
IVR (intravaginal ring)
IVU (intravenous urogram)
IVU (intravenous urography)

J, j

Jackson-Pratt drain
Jackson retractor
Jacobs cannula
Jacobson hemostatic forceps
Jacquemier sign of pregnancy
Jadassohn-Lewandowsky syndrome
Jakob-Creutzfeldt disease
Jameson scissors
janiceps
Janosik embryo
Jansen-Anderson intrauterine catheter
Jansen forceps
Jarcho-Levin syndrome
Jarcho uterine cannula
Jarish-Herxheimer reaction
Jarit cystoscope
jaundice
  breast milk
  neonatal
  perinatal
  physiologic
jaundice of newborn
jaw length, forceps
JDM (juvenile diabetes mellitus) (now type 1)
jejunal atresia
Jeliffe formula/equation
Jello sign
jelly
  K-Y
  Wharton
  Xylocaine
Jenest-28 oral contraceptive
Jeune syndrome
Jeune thoracic dystrophy
jeweler forceps
Jewett bladder carcinoma classification
J-hook deformity of distal ureter
jittery baby
jittery infant
Jobst breast support dressing
Job syndrome
Jod-Basedow phenomenon
JODM (juvenile onset diabetes mellitus) (now type 1)
jogger's amenorrhea
Johnson stone basket
Jonas Graves vaginal speculum
Jonas penile prosthesis
Jorgenson scissors
Joseph disease
Joubert syndrome
journal
  bladder
  urination
JT1001 prostate cancer vaccine

Juberg-Marsidi syndrome
jumping gene
jumping Frenchmen of Maine
jumping translocation
junction
- cervicovaginal
- corticomedullary
- ileocecal
- pelviureteral
- pelviureteric
- penoscrotal
- squamocolumnar
- ureteropelvic (UPJ)
- ureterovesical (UVJ)
- urethrovesical
- uterotubal
- UV (ureterovesical)
- UVJ (ureterovesical)

juvenile arthritis
juvenile diabetes mellitus (JDM) (now type 1)
juvenile gout-choreoathetosis-mental retardation syndrome
juvenile nephronophthisis
juvenile onset diabetes mellitus (JODM) (now type 1)
juvenile spinal muscular atrophy
juxta-articular adiposis dolorosa
juxtaglomerular apparatus of kidneys
juxtaglomerular body
juxtaglomerular complex
juxtaglomerular granule
juxtamedullary glomerulus
juxtapositioned
juxtavesical
J-wire

K, k

K (potassium)
Kabuki makeup syndrome
kallikrein excretion
Kallmann syndrome
kaluresis
kangaroo care
Kanner syndrome
Kaposi sarcoma
  penile
  penoscrotal
  testicular
Kapp-Beck serrations
Karl Storz Calcutript
Karl Storz flexible ureteropyeloscope
Karl Storz N_2O Endoflator
Karnofsky rating scale
Karsch-Neugelbauer syndrome
Kartagener syndrome
karyotype (see also *syndrome*)
  fetal
  45,XO
  46,XX
  46,XY
  47,XXY
  47,XY
  47,XYY
  48,XXXX
  48,XXXY
karyotype *(cont.)*
  48,XXYY
  49,XXXYY
  hyperdiploid
  spectral (SKY)
karyotype determination
karyotyping
Kasabach-Merritt syndrome
Kast syndrome
Katamaya hysteroscopic catheter
Kato-Asch coaxial needle
Kaye Lap-Wand
Kaye tamponade nephrostomy balloon
Kayexalate (sodium polystyrene
  sulfonate)
kb (kilobase)
KDF-2.3 intrauterine catheter
K-Dur (potassium chloride)
Kearns-Sayre syndrome (KSS)
Kegel exercises
Kelly anterior colporrhaphy
Kelly clamp
Kelly correction of retroverted uterus
Kelly correction of urinary stress
  incontinence
Kelly-Kennedy urethral operation
Kelly placenta forceps
Kelly plication of urethra

Kelly-Stoeckel urethral plication procedure
Kelly sutures
Kelly tissue forceps
Kelly vulsellum forceps
keloid formation
keloid scar
keloid tissue
keratinization
keratitis-ichthyosis-deafness (KID syndrome)
keratoconus
keratolysis neonatorum
keratosis follicularis
keratosis follicularis spinulosa decalvans
kernicterus, fetal
Kerr low transverse incision
Kestrone 5
ketoacidosis
- alcoholic
- benign dietary
- diabetic

ketoaciduria
ketoconazole
ketones in urine
ketonuria
ketorolac tromethamine
ketosis
ketosis-prone diabetes mellitus
ketosis-resistant diabetes mellitus
KetoSite test for status of ketoacidosis
ketotic hypoglycemia
ketotic hyperglycinemia
Kevorkian-Younge curette
keyhole incision
keyhole limpet hemocyanin
keyhole mastopexy
key-in-lock rotation of fetal head
Key-Med dilator
keystone mastopexy
Kibrick antisperm antibody test
kick counts
kidney
- abdominal
- absence of

kidney *(cont.)*
- abscess
- afferent vessels of
- amyloid
- arcuate artery of
- Armanni-Ebstein
- arteriolosclerotic
- arteriosclerotic
- artificial
- Ask-Upmark
- atrophic
- autotransplantation of
- bilateral small
- biopsy of
- blunt trauma to
- cadaveric
- cake
- carbuncle of
- cicatricial
- clear cell of
- congenital absence of
- congested
- contracted
- contralateral
- cortical scarring of
- cow
- crossed ectopic
- crush
- cyanotic
- cystic
- decapsulation of
- decortication of
- dialysis
- disk
- displacement of
- distended
- donor
- double
- doughnut
- dromedary
- duplex
- duplication of left
- duplication of right
- dysfunctional
- ectopic

kidney *(cont.)*
edematous
enlarged
fatty
fibrotic
fibrous capsule of
flea-bitten
floating
Formad
fracture of
fused
Gambro Lundia Minor artificial
Goldblatt
granular
head
hila of
hilum of
horseshoe
hydronephrotic
hypermobile
hypoplastic
infundibulum of
injured
interlobar veins of
interlobular artery of
interlobular veins of
irregular
ischemic
lacking
large red
lateral border of
lobe of
lobulated
long axis of
lower pole of
lumbar
malacoplakia of
medial border of
medulla of
medullary cystic
medullary sponge
middle
mobile
mortar

kidney *(cont.)*
movable
multicystic dysplastic
mural
myelin
myeloma
native
nonfunctioning
pancake
pelvic
pelvis of
pole of
polycystic
porous
ptotic
putty
pyelonephritic
Rose-Bradford
sacciform
scarred
sclerotic
shriveled
sigmoid
small
small atrophic
solitary
solitary functioning
sponge
stab wound to
straight veins of
supernumerary
suspension of
tenderness over
thoracic
transplanted
tuberculosis of
unilateral small
venous segments of
wandering
water-bottle
waxy
wedge resection of
kidney adhesions
kidney and ureter tenderness

kidney arteriovenous fistula
kidney atrophy
kidney bar
kidney biopsy
kidney calculus
kidney carbuncle
kidney carcinoma
kidney donor
kidney failure, chronic
kidney function study
kidney function test
kidney hypertrophy
kidney imaging agent (see *imaging agent*)
kidney internal splint/stent (KISS) catheter
kidney laceration
kidney lobe
kidney machine
kidney medulla
kidney pain
kidney-pancreas transplant
kidney parenchma
kidney pinked up immediately
kidney pole
kidney rest
kidney scan
KidneyScreen At Home test
kidney shadow
kidney-shaped placenta
kidney stone
kidney stone forceps
kidney stone, passing of
kidney tenderness
kidney tomography
kidney transplant
kidney transplantation
kidney transport anomaly
kidney tubule
kidney tumor
kidneys, ureters, and bladder (KUB)
KID (keratitis-ichthyosis-deafness) syndrome
Kielland forceps
Kielland obstetrical forceps
Kielland rotation of fetal head
Killian syndrome
kilobase (kb)
kilogram
kilovolt (kV)
Kimmelstiel-Wilson disease
kindred
kinetic modeling
kinetochore
kinked ureter
kinking
kinking at ureteropelvic junction
kinking of graft
kinking of ureter
kinky hair disease
Kiricuta breast reconstruction
Kisbourne syndrome
Kish urethral illuminating catheter
KISS (kidney internal splint/stent) catheter
kit
- athVysion HER-2 DNA probe kit
- BabyStart ovulation prediction
- B-D Basal Thermometry
- CLA
- Cycle Check ovulation prediction
- Euro-Collins multiorgan perfusion
- Fortel ovulation prediction
- Lady-Q saliva ovulation prediction
- Matritech NMP22 test
- Metra PS procedure
- Ovuplan ovulation prediction
- OvuQuick ovulation prediction
- OvuSign midstream ovulation prediction
- Preven emergency contraceptive
- Vesica sling

Kitano knot
Kitner clamp (also Kittner)
Kitner dissector (also Kittner)
Kitner retractor (also Kittner)
Kitner tip wand (also Kittner)
Kjelland (see *Kielland*)

Klebsiella oxytoca
Klebsiella pneumoniae
Kleeblattschadel deformity
Kleenspec disposable vaginal speculum
Kleihauer test of fetal-maternal hemoglobin
Kleihauer-Betke stain
Kleihauer-Betke test
Klein-Waardenburg syndrome
Kleppinger bipolar forceps
KLH-ImmuneActivator
Klinefelter syndrome
Klintmalm clamp
Kliovance oral contraceptive
Klipper-Feil syndrome
Klipper-Trenaunay syndrome
Klipper-Trenaunay-Weber syndrome
Klumpke palsy
Klumpke paralysis
knee-chest position
knee presentation
knife
  Cobalt Knife
  fistula
  Foerster capsulotomy
  Lorenz PC/TC scissors ultrasharp
  Selikowitz endoscopic
knitted fabric
knockout
knot
  Aberdeen
  convertible slip
  Kitano
  Roeder loop
  Topel
knot in cord
knotless suture anchor
knot pusher
  Clarke-Reich
  heliX
  MetraTie
  Tuason endoscopic
knot-pushing notch
knot tied with throws
knuckle of fallopian tube
Koala intrauterine pressure catheter
Kocher bladder spatula
Kocher clamp
Koch-Mason dressing
Kock ("coke")
Kock continent ileostomy pouch
Kock ileostomy
Kock modified pouch procedure
Kock nipple valve
Kock U-shaped urinary pouch
Kogan endocervical speculum
Kogan endospeculum
KOH (potassium hydroxide)
KOH colpotomizer system
KOH prep
KOH stain
KOH test
koilocytosis
Kollmann urethral dilator
Kontrast U radiopaque medium
Kopans breast lesion localization needle
Kormex II contraceptive cream
Krabbe disease
K-ras gene
kraurosis of penis
kraurosis of vulva
kraurosis vulvae
Kreiselman infant warmer
Kristeller maneuver for fundal pressure
Krivitski method
Krohnig low vertical midline incision
Kroner tubal ligation
Kronner Manipujector uterine manipulator
Kropp bladder neck reconstruction
Krukenberg tumor of ovary or breast
KryMed FO-101 colposcope
KTP laser
KTP/532 laser system
Kt/V or KT/V ratio
KUB (kidneys, ureters, bladder) x-ray
Kugelberg-Welander disease
Kugel hernia patch

Kun colocolponeopoiesis
Kun colocolpopoiesis
Kurzrok postcoital fertility test
Kussmaul-Landry paralysis
Kussmaul respiration
kV (kilovolt)
KVO (keep vein open)-type I.V.
Kwart AQ Retro-Inject stent
Kwart Retro-Inject stent
kwashiorkor
K-Y jelly
kyphotic pelvis
K-Y Silk-E vaginal moisturizer
K-Y vaginal lubricant

L, l

Laband syndrome
Labcath catheter
labetalol
Labhart-Willi syndrome
labia
  caruncle of
  hypertrophy of
labial (adj.)
labial agglutination
labial folds
labial hernia
labialis herpes
labial lips
labial swelling
labial tear
labia majora
labia majus pudendi
labia minora
labia minus pudendi
labia plexus (pl. labiae plexae)
labia uteri
labiocervical
labiocrural folds
labioscrotal folds
labium (pl. labia)
labium majorus
labium minorus
labium urethrae

labor
  active
  active phase of
  arrest of
  artificial
  atonic
  augmentation of
  complicated
  delayed
  desultory
  dry
  dyscoordinate
  dysfunctional
  early
  failed trial of
  false
  first stage
  habitual
  hard
  hypertonic
  induced
  instrumental
  irregular
  latent phase of
  mechanical induction of
  mimetic
  missed
  multiple

labor *(cont.)*
  obstructed
  Pitocin induction of
  placental stage
  postmature
  postponed
  precipitate
  precipitous
  premature
  preterm
  primary dysfunctional
  prodromal
  prolonged
  protracted
  rapid second stage of
  second stage
  slow slope active phase of
  spontaneous
  stages of
  third stage
  threatened
  threatened premature
  trial of (after cesarean section)
labor and delivery (L&D)
labor and delivery room
labor and delivery suite
labor augmentation
labor curves
labor inhibition
labor initiation
labor pains
labyrinthine placenta
labyrinthine syndrome
labyrinth, renal
lacerated perineum
laceration
  anal sphincter
  bladder
  bowel
  broad ligament
  central
  cervical
  first degree
  first degree perineal

laceration *(cont.)*
  fourth degree
  fourth degree perineal
  high vaginal
  kidney
  pelvic floor
  perineal
  perineal muscle
  periurethral
  second degree perineal
  third degree perineal
  uterine
  vaginal
lacking kidneys
lack of adequate water intake
lacrimal duct, congenital obstruction of
lacrimoauriculodentodigital (LADD) syndrome
Lact-Aid STARTrainer Nursing System
lactate
lactate dehydrogenase (LDHA) deficiency
lactating adenoma
lactating breast
lactation
  abnormal
  failure of
  suppressed
lactational mastitis
lactation amenorrhea
lactation consultant
lactation hormone
lactation letdown response
lactation specialists
lactation suppression
lacteal fistula
lactentium, hyperemesis
lactescent sera
lactic acidosis
lactic and pyruvate acidemia with carbohydrate sensitivity
lactic and pyruvate acidemia with episodic ataxia and weakness
lactic dehydrogenase (LDH)

lactiferous duct
lactifuge
lactigenous
lactobacillus (pl. lactobacilli)
lactocele
Lactofree infant formula
lactogenesis
lactogen, human placental (HPL)
lactogenic hormone
lactometer
lactorrhea
lactoscope
lactose intolerance
lactosuria
lactotropin
lacuna (pl. lacunae)
  blood
  intervillous
  penis
  trophoblastic
  urethral
lacunae urethrales
lacuna of Morgagni
lacus (pl. lacus)
lacus seminalis
LADD (lacrimoauriculodentodigital)
  syndrome
Lady-Q saliva ovulation prediction kit
Lahey clamp
Lahey forceps
Lahey tenaculum
lake, seminal (lacus seminalis)
La Leche League
LAL (*Limulus amoebocyte* lysate) test
LAM (lymphangioleiomyomatosis)
Lamaze method
Lambda (lanthanum carbonate)
Lambert-Eaton myasthenic syndrome
Lambert-Eaton syndrome (LES)
lamella (pl. lamellae)
lamella, glandulopreputial
lamellar body number density
lamellar ichthyosis
  autosomal dominant
  recessive
lamina (pl. laminae)
lamina densa
  multilamination of
  spikes of
laminaria
laminaria cervical dilator
Laminaria digitata
laminaria sulfate
laminaria tent
lamina, basal
lampbrush chromosome
LANCET needle
Landau-Kleffner syndrome
L&D (labor and delivery)
Landing ascending paralysis
landmarks, bony
Landouzy-Dejerine atrophy
Landouzy-Dejerine dystrophy
Langer-Giedion syndrome
Langmuir-Blodgett (LB) membrane
LANS-RH (liposuction-assisted nerve-
  sparing radical hysterectomy)
lanthanum carbonate
Lantus (insulin glargine)
lanugo
laparoamnioscopy
Laparofan
laparohysterectomy
laparohysteropexy
laparohysterotomy
Laparolift gasless laparoscopy system
laparomyomectomy
Laparosac obturator and cannula
laparosalpingectomy
laparosalpingo-oophorectomy
laparoscope (see also *endoscope*)
  ACMI rigid
  Adler Eagle Vision
  Adler P.L.U.S.
  Arthrotek rigid
  Bryan rigid
  Cabot rigid
  Circon rigid
  Comeg rigid
  Concept rigid

laparoscope *(cont.)*
- CorTek semirigid microlaparoscope
- Cuda
- Demir rigid
- diagnostic
- Dyonics
- Eder
- Effner
- Endolap rigid
- Endolase rigid
- flexible video
- Foroblique optic
- Henke-Sass rigid
- Henke-Sass Wolf
- Illumina PROSeries
- Inspex rigid
- InstrumentMakar
- Jacobs-Palmer
- Jarit
- Karl Storz rigid
- laser
- Linvatec
- Marlow rigid
- Marlow video
- Medilas
- micro
- MicroLap Gold microlaparoscope
- MiniSite
- Olympus
- operating
- operative
- Optik rigid
- Pilling rigid
- REI rigid
- Schoelly
- Semm rigid
- Solos rigid
- Storz
- Storz Hopkins
- Stryker
- Surgitech
- Surgiview
- 3Dscope

laparoscope *(cont.)*
- Transvaginal Hydro (THL)
- VerreScope microlaparoscope
- VideoHydro
- V. Mueller rigid
- Weck-Baggish rigid
- Wisap
- Wolf Lumina
- Wolf rigid
- Wolf operative
- Zimmer rigid

laparoscope camera
laparoscopic access sheath
laparoscopically assisted vaginal hysterectomy (LAVH)
laparoscopic-assisted vaginal hysterectomy (LAVH)
laparoscopic basket
laparoscopic bilateral tubal coagulation
laparoscopic biopsy device
laparoscopic bladder neck suture suspension
laparoscopic bladder suspension
laparoscopic fenestration
laparoscopic fulguration of pelvic endometriosis
laparoscopic hysterectomy (LAVH)
laparoscopic instrument pouch
laparoscopic insufflator
laparoscopic intracorporeal ultrasound (LICU)
laparoscopic introducer
laparoscopic knot pusher
laparoscopic laser ablation of endometriosis
laparoscopic laser-assisted auto-augmentation
laparoscopic lysis of adhesions
laparoscopic mini-retractor
laparoscopic myoma screw
laparoscopic nephrectomy
laparoscopic nephropexy
laparoscopic pelvic lymph node dissection

laparoscopic pelvic lymph node dissection and extraperitoneal pelvioscopy
laparoscopic pneumodissection
laparoscopic port closure needle
laparoscopic pyeloplasty
laparoscopic radical prostatectomy
laparoscopic resection of uterosacral ligaments
laparoscopic sleeve
laparoscopic transcystic duct exploration
laparoscopic transcystic lithotripsy (LTCL)
laparoscopic transcystic papillotomy
laparoscopic trocar
laparoscopic trocar and trocar sleeve
laparoscopic tubal ligation
laparoscopic ultrasound (LUS)
laparoscopic urethral sling
laparoscopic urinary diversion
laparoscopic uterine nerve ablation (LUNA)
laparoscopic uterosacral nerve ablation
laparoscopy
  diagnostic
  double-puncture
  gasless
  hand-assisted (HAL)
  laser
  LULA (laparoscopy under local anesthesia)
  needle
  second-look
  single-port
  single-port, double-puncture
  single-puncture
  video
laparoscopy under local anesthesia (LULA)
LaparoSonic coagulating shears for autograft harvesting
laparotomy
  abdominal
  exploratory
  exploratory pelvic
laparotomy *(cont.)*
  mini-
  open
  pelvic
  second-look
laparotomy pad, sponge, and needle count
laparotomy pad, Weck
Lapontre syndrome
lap pad (laparotomy pad)
Lapro-Clip ligating clip system
LapSac introducer
lap, sponge, and needle count
lap tape (pad or sponge)
LAP-TAPP (laparoscopic transabdominal preperitoneal) hernioplasty
LapTie endoscopic knot-tying instrument
Lap Vacu-Irrigator
Lapwall laparotomy sponge and wound protector
large bladder capacity
large bladder rupture
large-capacity bladder
large cell carcinoma
large clots
large for dates
large for date fetus
large for dates infant
large for dates uterus
large for gestational age (LGA)
large loop excision of transformation zone (LLETZ) of cervix
large postvoid residual
large red kidney
large residual urine
large sharp curet
large single copy
large-surface dialyzer
Laron dwarfism
Laroyenne operation for pelvic suppuration
Larsen syndrome

laser
- argon
- ClearView CO_2
- CO_2
- Cooper
- coumarin pulsed-dye
- erbium:YAG
- ErCr:YAG
- flash lamp-pulsed dye
- flashlamp-pulsed Nd:YAG
- GyneLase diode
- He-Ne
- Hercules Nd:YAG
- holmium
- Indigo LaserOptic system
- KPT
- KTP/532
- Lightstic 180 fiberoptic
- Lightstic 360 fiberoptic
- Medilas-H holmium
- Medilas-H pulsed holmium:YAG
- MultiPulse
- neodymium:yttrium-aluminum-garnet (Nd:YAG)
- OmniPulse-MAX holmium
- Opmilas 144 Plus Nd:YAG
- Prostalase
- Pulsolith
- UltraStat 10
- Urolase
- Urolase fiber
- VersaPulse Select holmium
- Xanar 20 Ambulase CO_2 laser

laser ablation of endometriosis
laser ablation of prostate
laser Adson forceps
laser Allis forceps
laser arm drape
laser-assisted tissue welding technique for bladder augmentation
laser Auvard weighted speculum
laser Backhaus towel clamp
laser Bozeman forceps
laser bra procedure
laser Campion forceps
laser Clemetson forceps
laser cone biopsy
laser conization
laser depth ruler
laser fulguration of bladder tumor
laser Graves speculum
laser Jackson retractor
laser Kogan endospeculum
laser laparoscopy
laser lithotripsy
laser mammography system
laser plume
laser Potts-Smith forceps
laser reduction mammoplasty
laser resection of prostate
laser Rochester-Pean forceps
laser scalpel and quartz rod
LaserSonics EndoBlade
LaserSonics Nd:YAG LaserBlade scalpel
LaserSonics SurgiBlade
laser therapy
Laserthermia
LaserTripter MDL 3000
laser uterosacral nerve ablation (LUNA)
laser vaporization of endometrial implants
laser wand
laser wand clamp
laser welding
Lasette finger stick device
Lash hysterectomy
Lash internal cervical os repair
Lasix (furosemide)
last menstrual period (LMP)
last normal menstrual period (LNMP)
latching on
latch on
late anemia
late benign syphilis
late decelerations
late fetal death

late first pregnancy
late latent syphilis
late luteal phase dysphoria
late luteal phase dysphoric disorder (LLPDD)
late menarche
late menopause
late metabolic acidosis of newborn
late neonatal death
latent homosexuality
latent phase of labor
latent syphilis
late onset disorders
late onset Tay-Sachs
lateral angle of uterus
lateral border of kidney
lateral circumflex femoral artery
lateral decubitus position
lateral extension of laceration
lateral films
lateral fornix
lateral hermaphroditism
lateral lithotripsy
lateral lobe hyperplasia
lateral lobe hypertrophy
lateral lobe of prostate
lateral mammary branch
lateral part of vaginal fornix
lateral pelvic wall
lateral placenta previa
lateral recumbent obstetric position
lateral recumbent position
lateral slit of prepuce
lateral transverse thigh flap
lateral vaginal fornices
lateral vaginal retractor
lateral vaginal wall smear
lateral wall of urinary bladder
late replicating chromosome
late-replicating X-chromosome
lateroversion
late syphilis
late vomiting of pregnancy
latex balloon probe
latex condom
latex sensibility
latissimus dorsi flap
latissimus dorsi flap procedure
latissimus dorsi island flap
latissimus dorsi muscle
latissimus dorsi myocutaneous flap
LATS (long-acting thyroid-stimulating) hormone
Latzko cesarean section
Latzko vesicovaginal fistula repair
Laufe divergent obstetrical forceps
Laufe-Piper obstetrical forceps
Laufe uterine polyp forceps
Laurence-Moon-Bardet-Biedl syndrome
Laurence-Moon-Biedl syndrome
Laurence-Moon syndrome
lavage
  bladder
  pelvic
  peritoneal
  uterine
LAVH (laparoscopic-assisted vaginal hysterectomy)
LAVH (laparoscopically assisted vaginal hysterectomy)
Lawrence Add-A-Cath trocar
Lawrence SupraFoley catheter
laxative
  bulk
  osmotic
layer
  subcutaneous
  subcuticular
lay midwife
lazy S incision
LBW (low birth weight)
LBW (limb-body wall) complex
LBW 24 infant formula
LCAD (long chain acyl-CoA-dehydrogenase deficiency)
LCIS (lobular carcinoma in situ)
LCMV (lymphocytic choriomeningitis virus)

LCx probe system
LDH (lactic dehydrogenase)
LDHA (lactate dehydrogenase) deficiency
LDR (labor, delivery, and recovery) room
LE (lupus erythematosus)
Leadbetter-Politano submucosal tunnel
Leadbetter-Politano ureteral advancement
Leadbetter-Politano ureteroneocystotomy
leading bar
Leading Lady breast implant
Leading Lady breast prosthesis
lead wires
League, La Leche
leakage from endometrioma
leakage into peritoneal cavity
leakage of dialysate
leakage of urine
leak, dialysate
leaking water
leak point pressure in bladder
leapfrog position
LeBag ileocolic urinary reservoir
Leber congenital amaurosis
Leber optic atrophy
lecithin/sphingomyelin (LS) ratio
Leder stain
LeDuc anastomosis for ureteral reimplantation
LeDuc-Camey ileocystoplasty
Lee ganglion
LEEP (loop electrosurgical excision procedure)
Lee-Ray aspiration biopsy needle
leflunomide
LeFort colpocleisis
LeFort urethral sound
LeFort uterine prolapse repair
left CVA (costovertebral angle) tenderness
left frontoanterior (LFA) position
left frontoposterior (LFP) position
left frontotransverse (LFT) position
left internal mammary artery (LIMA)
left lower quadrant (LLQ)
left lower quadrant tenderness
left mentoanterior (LMA) position
left mentotransverse (LMT) position
left occipitoposterior (LOP) position
left ovarian vein
left renal vein hypertension
left sacroposterior (LSP) position
left-sided bladder diverticulum
left-sided ureteral colic
left testicular vein
left umbilical vein
left upper quadrant (LUQ)
left ureter
left ureterolithiasis
leg abduction and support
legal abortion
legal father
legally induced abortion
legal mother
legal parents
leg cramps
Legg-Calve-Perthes
Legionella bozemanae
Legionella dumoffii
Legionella feeleii
Legionella gormanii
Legionella jordanis
Legionella longbeachae (serogroups 1 and 2)
Legionella micdadei
Legionella pneumophila
legionellosis
legionnaires disease
Leica colposcope
Leigh disease
Leigh necrotizing encephalopathy
leiomyofibroma
leiomyoma (pl. leiomyomata)
  parasitic uterine
  uterine

leiomyoma uteri
leiomyomata uteri
leiomyomatosis
leiomyomectomy
leiomyosarcoma
leishmaniasis
LeJeune syndrome
Lejour-type breast reduction, modified
Lembert suture
L-Emental infant formula
lemon sign
length
  crown-heel (CH, CHL)
  crown-rump (CR, CRL)
  greatest
Lennox-Gastaut syndrome
lens
  foroblique
  right-angle
Lente insulin
lenticular degeneration, progressive
Lenz micro-ophthalmia syndrome
Leonard Arm
Leopold maneuver
LEOPARD (multiple lentigines, electrocardiographic conduction abnormalities, ocular hypertelorism, pulmonic stenosis, abnormal genitalia, retardation of growth, and sensorineural defects) syndrome
leprechaunism
leptomeningeal angiomatosis
leptotene
Leriche syndrome
Leri pleonosteosis
Leri-Weill syndrome
Leroy disease
LES (Lambert-Eaton syndrome)
lesbian
Lesch-Nyhan disease
lesion
  ablation
  aneurysmal
  Antopol-Goldman

lesion *(cont.)*
  areolar
  cystic renal
  extracapillary
  fluctuant
  fungating
  genital
  glomerular tip
  gummatous
  high grade squamous intraepithelial (HGSIL)
  intravesical
  invasive
  LGSIL (low grade squamous intraepithelial)
  Lohlein-Baehr
  low grade squamous intraepithelial (LGSIL)
  malignant
  mass
  metaphyseal
  mucocutaneous
  neoplastic
  neurologic bladder
  neuropathic GU tract
  nipple
  preinvasive
  premalignant
  renal mass
  resectable
  SIL (squamous intraepithelial)
  solid renal
  sonolucent cystic
  squamous intraepithelial (SIL)
  stellate
  stenotic
  treated premalignant
  tubulointerstitial
  ulcerative
  vascular
lesion of rapidly progressive glomerulonephritis
lesion with poorly defined margins
letdown reflex

lethal gene
lethal neoplasm
lethargy
letrozole
leucine-induced neonatal hypoglycemia
leucinuria
leukemia, myelomonocytic
Leukeran (chlorambucil)
leukocyte
leukocyte esterase determination
leukocyte esterase dipstick test
leukocyte hexosaminiside assay
leukocytes, radionuclide-labeled
leukocytosis of the newborn
leukocyturia
leukodystrophy
leukokraurosis
leukoplakia
  cervical
  penile
  vulvar
leukoplakia vulvae
leukoplasia of vulva
leukorrhagia
leukorrhea
  heavy
  menstrual
  purulent-appearing
  yellow
Leung coaxial catheter
Leuprogel (leuprolide)
leuprolide acetate for depot suspension
leuprolide acetate implant
Leuvectin
Levant stone basket
levator ani muscle
levator muscle
levator muscle sling
LeVeen shunt
level
  air-fluid
  basal prolactin
  circulating androgen
  peak and trough

level *(cont.)*
  prolactin
  uric acid
level of ischial spines
level of nipple
Leventhal Gyne-Flo cannula
Levlen oral contraceptive
Levlite (levonorgestrel/ethinyl estradiol) oral contraceptive
levobupivacaine
levonorgestrel
levonorgestrel/ethinyl estradiol oral contraceptive pill
Levora (levonorgestrel/ethinyl estradiol)
levothyroxine sodium
Levovist ultrasound contrast agent
Levoxyl (levothyroxine sodium)
Levret forceps
Levulan (5-aminolevulinic acid)
Levulan photodynamic therapy (PDT)
Levy-Hollister syndrome
Leydig cells
Leydig duct
LFA (left frontoanterior) position
LFP (left frontoposterior) position
LFS (Li-Fraumeni syndrome)
LFT (left frontotransverse) position
LFT (liver function tests)
LGA (large for gestational age)
LGSIL, LSIL (low grade squamous intraepithelial lesion)
LGV (lymphogranuloma venereum)
LH-RH (luteinizing hormone-releasing hormone)
LH-RH agonist
  goserelin
  leuprolide
LH-RH receptors
LH (luteinizing hormone) surge
liarozole fumarate
Liazal (liarozole fumarate)
libido
  decreased
  diminished
  increased

libido hormones
library
licensure
Lich-Gregoire repair in kidney transplant surgery
Lich technique in neobladder construction
Lich ureteral implantation in transplantation surgery
lichen planus
lichen sclerosus et atrophicus
lichen simplex chronicus
LICU (laparoscopic intracorporeal ultrasound)
Liddle syndrome
lidocaine
lie (also see *position*)
  fetal
  longitudinal
  oblique
  posterior
  transverse
  unstable
lienorenal ligament
life
  postnatal
  prenatal
life events
LifeSign1 midstream pregnancy test
LifeSite Dialysis Access System
LifeSite hemodialysis access system
life-span development
life span, fertilizable
lifestyle
life-threatening hyperkalemia
Li-Fraumeni cancer syndrome
Li-Fraumeni syndrome (LFS)
L.I.F.T. (laser-assisted internal fabrication) of breast
Ligaclip
ligament
  abscess of broad
  broad
  cardinal

ligament *(cont.)*
  colosplenic
  Cooper
  epididymal
  falciform
  fallopian
  genital
  genitoinguinal
  hepatorenal
  infundibulo-ovarian
  infundibulopelvic
  lienorenal
  median umbilical
  ovarian
  polyp of broad
  Poupart
  pubocervical
  puboprostatic
  pubovesical
  round
  sacrospinous
  sacrouterine
  splenorenal
  superior epididymal
  suspensory breast
  Treitz
  umbilical
  uterine
  utero-ovarian
  uterosacral
  uterovesical
  vesicoumbilical
  vesicouterine
ligaments were clamped, cut, and suture ligated
LigaSure vessel sealing system
ligated
  doubly
  staple-
ligation
  intra-abdominal
  Kroner tubal
  penile vein
  Pomeroy tubal
  tubal

ligation and division of fallopian tubes
ligator, Suture Lok vessel
ligature (see also *suture*)
  Endoloop
  slipped umbilical
  suture
ligature carrier
  Rereyra-Raz
  Raz double-prong
light for dates
light microscope
light microscopy
LightSheer SC diode laser hair removal system
Lightstic 180 fiberoptic laser
Lightstic 360 fiberoptic laser
lightening
Lignac-Fanconi syndrome
Liley graphs for Rh sensitization
Lilly Pen for insulin
LIMA (left internal mammary artery)
limb-body wall (LBW) complex
limb-girdle muscular dystrophy
limb malformations-dentodigital syndrome
limit dextrinosis
limited, supervised, judicially-guided surrogacy
limiting current density
limbus fossae ovalis
limited renal diluting capacity
Limitrol-DM (*Trigonella foenum-graecum* [fenugreek])
Limulus amoebocyte lysate (LAL) assay
Lindau disease
Linder-Golomb SP introducer sound
line
  anterior axillary
  blood outflow
  Brödel white
  dentate
  embryonic
  Farre white
  mammary
line *(cont.)*
  mammary milk
  mammillary
  neonatal
  nipple
  Poupart
  pubic hair
  relaxed skin tension
  Rolando
  simian
  subcostal
  suture
  Sydney
  Toldt
  Toldt white
linea alba
linea nigra
linear calcification
linear deposition of IgG
linear epidermal nevus
linear salpingostomy
linear skull fracture
linear sperm velocity
line infection
line of demarcation
line of Toldt, white
lingual goiter
linguine sign in breast
linkage
linkage analysis
linkage disequilibrium
linkage equilibrium
linkage group
linkage map
lip
  cervical
  cleft
lipemia
lipid-associated sialic acid in plasma (LASA-P) test
lipid granulomatosis
lipid histiocytosis
lipid-laden macrophages

lipid-laden modified tubular epithelial cells
lipid nephrosis
lipid storage disease
lipiduria
lipoatrophic diabetes
lipodystrophy
lip of cervix
lipogranulomatosis
lipoid nephrosis
lipoma of cord
lipoprotein-lipase deficiency
liposomal anthracyclines
liposomal daunorubicin
liposomal doxorubicin
liposome encapsulated doxorubicin citrate complex
liposuction-assisted nerve-sparing radical hysterectomy (LANS-RH)
Lippes loop intrauterine device
lip pseudocleft-hemangiomatous branchial cyst syndrome
liquefied argon gas
liquid, Iotrex radiation
liquid membrane
liquid phase
liquor, meconium in
LIS1 (lissencephaly 1) gene
lissencephaly 1 gene (LIS1)
lissencephaly syndrome
Listeria infection
Listeria monocytogenes
listeriosis, congenital
lithiasis
  bladder
  renal
  ureteral
lithium
lithiumogenic goiter
lithoclast, Swiss
lithogenicity of bile
litholapaxy
lithonephritis
lithopedian
Lithospec intracorporeal lithotripter
Lithostar lithotriptor
Lithostar multiline lithotripter
lithotome
lithotomist
lithotomy
  bilateral
  high
  median
  mediolateral
  perineal
  prerectal
  rectal
  rectovesical
  renal
  suprapubic
  transurethral ureteroscopic
  uric acid
  urinary
  vaginal
  vesical
  vesicovaginal
lithotomy position
lithotresis
lithotripsy
  electrohydraulic (EHL)
  electrohydraulic shock wave (ESWL)
  extracorporeal shock wave (ESWL)
  high
  laparoscopic transcystic (LTCL)
  laser
  lateral
  Medstone STS-T transportable
  shock wave (SWL)
  suprapubic
  transurethral ureteroscopic
  tubeless
  ultrasonic
  ureteral stone
  waterbath
lithotripsy bath
lithotripter (see *lithotriptor*)
lithotriptic

lithotriptor (also *lithotripter*)
  Calcutript
  DoLi S extracorporeal shock wave
  Dornier
  Dornier HM3
  Econolith
  electrohydraulic
  EMS Swiss lithoclast intra-
    corporcal
  EPL (extracorporeal piezoelectric)
  Genestone 190
  HM4
  intracorporeal
  Lithospec intracorporeal
  Lithostar multiline
  LithoTron
  LT.01
  LT.02 piezoelectric
  Medstone STS shock wave generator
  Medstone STS-T transportable
  Modulith SL 20
  Piezolith-EPL (extracorporeal piezo-
    electric lithotriptor)
  Pulsalith
  Pulsolith laser
  Sonolith Praktis portable
  Sonolith 3000
  Sonolith 4000
  Sonolith 4000+
  Swiss lithoclast
lithotriptor gantry system
lithotriptoscopy
lithotrite
lithotrity (pl. lithotrities)
LithoTron lithotripsy machine
lithuresis
lithuria
Littles disease
Littré gland abscess
Littré, glands of
live birth
liveborn child
liveborn infant
livedo reticularis
liver
  renal impression on
  rupture of
liver and spleen were congested
liver disorders
liver function tests (LFT)
liver phosphorylase deficiency
liver edge
liver hematoma
liver, spleen, and kidneys (LKS)
living donor, unilateral
living infant
living-related donor (LRD)
living-related donor transplant
living-related transplant (LRT)
living will
LKS (liver, kidneys, and spleen)
LLETZ (large loop excision of transformation zone)
Llorente dissecting forceps
Lloyd-Davis stirrups
LLPDD (late luteal phase dysphoric
  disorder)
LLQ (left lower quadrant)
LMA (left mentoanterior) position
LMP (last menstrual period)
LMT (left mentotransverse) position
LNCap
LNMP (last normal menstrual period)
LOA (left occipitoanterior)
loading dose
lobar atrophy
lobar holoprosencephaly
lobe
  fetal
  kidney
  mammary gland
  placental
  prostatic
  renal
  succenturiate
Lobstein disease type 1
lobster-claw deformity
lobular carcinoma

lobular carcinoma in situ (LCIS)
lobular carcinoma of breast
lobular glomerulonephritis
lobular neoplasia
lobulated kidney
lobulated mass
lobulation, fetal
lobule of mammary gland
lobule of testis
lobulonodular glomerulonephritis
local anesthesia
local edema
local glomerulonephritis
localization
localization of infection
localization studies
localization, placental
localize
localized prostate cancer
localized subdural hematoma
localizer, breast
location, ureter
lochia
lochia alba
lochia cruenta
lochia purulenta
lochia rubra
lochia sanguinolenta
lochia serosa
lochial
lochiometra
lochiometritis
lochiorrhagia
lochiorrhea
loci (plural of locus)
lock
  English
  Luer
  sliding
locked twins
locomotor ataxia
Loc-Sure single-pass catheter
locus heterogeneity
locus of HLA (A, B, C, D, or DR)
locus of HLA (human leukocyte antigen)
locus of HLA (written HLA-C8, HLA-DR2, etc.)
locus of infection
locus (pl. loci)
  sex-linked
  X-linked
  Y-linked
LOD score (logarithmic odds ratio "log of the odds")
Loeb deciduoma
Loestrin oral contraceptive
Lofenalac infant formula
LOH (loss of heterozygocity) analysis of prostate tumors
Lohlein-Baehr lesion
loin pain hematuria syndrome (LPHS)
Loken-Senior syndrome
lollipop mastopexy
Lomac stone basket
lomefloxacin
Lone Star retractor
long-acting thyroid-stimulating (LATS) hormone
long axis of kidney
long cervix
long chain acyl-CoA-dehydrogenase deficiency (LCAD)
Long hysterectomy forceps
longitudinal incision
longitudinal lie
longitudinal studies
long tensor fasciae latae
long tensor fasciae latae neurovascular island flap
long-term access for hemodialysis
long-term access to circulation
long-term catheter drainage
long-term hemodialysis
long-term prophylaxis
long-term radiation effects
long-term side effects of chemotherapy
long-term vascular access

long thoracic nerve
loop
  bipolar cutting
  bipolar urological
  Cordonnier ureteroileal
  Henle
  lyodura
  PEARL (physiologic endometrial ablation/resection)
  vessel
loop colostomy
loop cutaneous ureterostomy
loop diuretic
looped ureter
loop electrosurgical excision procedure (LEEP)
loop excision for removing dysplastic cells
loop IUD (intrauterine device)
loop of Henle
loopogram
loop resection
Lo/Ovral oral contraceptive
LOP (left occipitoposterior) position
Lorabid (loracarbef)
loracarbef
LORAD full field digital mammography system
LORAD StereoGuide stereotactic breast biopsy system
Lorain-Lévi infantilism
Lorenz PC/TC scissors ultrasharp knife
losartan potassium
loss
  bladder elasticity
  estrogen
  fetal blood
  urine
loss of heterozygocity (LOH) analysis of prostate tumors
loss of normal posterior urethrovesical angle
loss of pars
loss of performance of a membrane
loss of semen phobia
loss of urine with changing position
loss of urine with coughing
loss of urine with sneezing
loss of urine with straining
LOT (left occipitotransverse) position
Lou Gehrig disease
Louis-Bar syndrome
Louis mastopexy
lover
low birth weight (LBW) infant
low bladder compliance
low capacity bladder
low current electrocautery
low cervical cesarean section
low density beta lipoprotein deficiency
low dose film mammographic technique
low dose mammogram
low dose mammography using Egan technique
Lowe-Bickel syndrome
lower genital tract
lower inner quadrant of breast
lower lateral quadrant of breast
lower medial quadrant of breast
lower nephron nephrosis
lower outer quadrant of breast
lower pole calix (calyx)
lower pole collecting system
lower pole heminephrectomy
lower pole of kidney
lower pole of renal pelvis
lower pole of testis
lower pole ureter
lower segment cesarean section
lower tract localization culture
lower tract obstruction
lower tracts
lower ureteral stone
lower urinary tract infection
lower urinary tract symptoms (LUTS)
lower uterine segment
lower uterine segment cesarean section

lower uterine segment transverse cesarean section
Lowe syndrome
Lowe-Terrey-MacLachlan syndrome
low fat diet
low flap vertical cesarean section
low forceps
low forceps delivery
low grade fever
low grade neoplasm
low grade squamous intraepithelial lesion (LSIL, LGSIL)
low implantation of placenta
low-lying placenta
Low-Ogestrel (norgestrel/ethinyl estradiol) oral contraceptive
low pressure, adequate capacity bladder
low pressure urinary bladder
low profile catheter retention system
low segment incision
low-set ears
Lowsley prostatic tractor
low sodium diet
low sperm count
low transverse cesarean section
low urethral pressure (LUP)
low vertical cesarean section
low vertical incision
LPD (luteal phase deficiency)
L-phenylalanine mustard
LPHS (loin pain hematuria syndrome)
LRD (living-related donor)
LRT (living-related transplant)
LSe Kwart Retro-Inject stent
LSIL (low grade squamous epithelial lesion)
LSP (left sacroposterior) position
L/S (lecithin/sphingomyelin) ratio
LT.01 lithotripter
LT.02 piezoelectric lithotripter
LTCL (laparoscopic transcystic lithotripsy)
lubricant
  K-Y Silk-E vaginal moisturizer
  K-Y vaginal
  Lubrin vaginal
  Silken Secret vaginal moisturizer
lubricating jelly
lubrication, vaginal
Lubri-Flex urologic stent
Lubrin vaginal lubricant
Lubs syndrome
Lucey-Driscoll syndrome
Luer locks
Luer-Lok syringe
Luer slip syringe
lues
Lugol solution (iodine; potassium iodide)
Luikart obstetrical forceps
Luikart-Simpson forceps
Lukens PGA synthetic absorbable suture
LULA (laparoscopy under local anesthesia)
LuMax cystometry system
lumbar epidural anesthesia
lumbar kidney
lumbar nephrectomy
lumbar vein
lumbo-ovarian
lumen (pl. lumina)
lumen of tube
lumpectomy mastectomy
lumpectomy of breast
lumpiness in breast
"lumpy-bumpy" microscopic appearance of glomerulus
"lumpy-bumpy" pattern
LUNA (laparoscopic uterine nerve ablation)
LUNA (laser uterosacral nerve ablation)
lunar hymen

Lunelle (formerly Cyclofem and Cyclo-Provera) injectable contraceptive
lung endometriosis
lung maturity profile
LUP (low urethral pressure)
Lupron, Lupron Depot (leuprolide)
Lupron Depot-4 Month (leuprolide acetate for depot suspension)
lupus anticoagulant
lupus erythematosus (LE)
  cutaneous
  discoid (DLE)
  neonatal
  systemic
lupus glomerulonephritis
lupus-like syndrome
lupus nephritis
  diffuse membranous
  focal mesangial
lupus obstetric syndrome
LUQ (left upper quadrant)
LUS (laparoscopic ultrasound)
Luschka, foramen of
Lustra (hydroquinone)
luteal phase
luteal phase deficiency (LPD)
luteal phase lysis of adhesions
luteal phase of menstrual cycle
lutein cyst
luteinization
luteinized unruptured follicle
luteinized unruptured ovarian follicle syndrome
luteinizing hormone (LH)
luteinizing hormone-releasing hormone (LH-RH, LRH)
luteohormone
luteolysin
luteolysis
luteolytic
luteoma
luteoma pregnancy
luteotropic
Lutrepulse (gonadorelin)
Lutrin (lutetium texaphryin)
LUTS (lower urinary tract symptoms)
LUTS (lower urinary tract syndrome)
lymphadenectomy
  bilateral inguinofemoral
  pelvic
lymphadenoid goiter
lymphadenopathy
  axillary
  infraclavicular
  inguinal
  supraclavicular
  pedal
lymphangioleiomyomatosis (LAM)
lymphangioma cavernous
lymphangiosarcoma
lymphangitis of breast
lymphapheresis
lymphatic channel
lymphatic compression
lymphatic cyst
lymphatic drainage
lymphatic flow
lymphatic mapping, intraoperative
lymphatics
  abdominal
  inguinal
  mediastinal
  pelvic
  perineural
  perirectal
Lymphazurin dye
Lymphedema Alert Bracelet
lymphedema, hereditary
lymph in urine
lymph node
  axillary
  femoral
  fixed axillary
  infraclavicular
  inguinal
  matted axillary
  para-aortic

lymph node *(cont.)*
paramammary
parauterine
paravaginal
paravesical
pelvic
superficial inguinal
supraclavicular
retroperitoneal
lymph node dissection
lymph node metastasis
lymph node positive
lymph node survey
lymphocele
lymphocyte
lymphocyte immune globulin, antithymocyte
lymphocytic choriomeningitis
lymphocytic choriomeningitis virus (LCMV)
lymphocyturia
lymphogranuloma inguinale
lymphogranuloma venereum (LGV)
lymphogranuloma, venereal
lymphoid follicle
lymphokines
lymphoma
lymphomatous infiltration
lymphopathia venereum
lymphoproliferative disorder
lymphoscintigraphy
lymph vessels of prostate
Lynch syndrome
lyodura loop
lyonization
lyophilized collagenase
lypressin (lysine-8-vasopressin)
Lyrelle patch
lysate
lyse
lysed
lysis of adhesions
lysis of intraluminal adhesions
lysis of pelvic and abdominal adhesions
lysis of perirenal adhesions
lysis of perivesical adhesions
lysis, transurethral
lysomal alpha-D mannosidase deficiency
lysomal alpha-glucosidase deficiency
lysozymes
lysozymuria

M, m

MAAP (multiple arbitrary amplicon profiling)
MAb monoclonal antibody
MAb-170 monoclonal antibody
macerated fetus
Machado-Joseph disease
machinery murmur in patent ductus arteriosus
Maciol laparoscopic suture needle set
macrencephaly
macrocephaly
macroscopic hematuria
Macritonin (calcitonin)
macroamylasemia
Macrobid (nitrofurantoin)
macrocyclic lactone
macrocytic anemia of pregnancy
Macrodantin (nitrofurantoin)
macroevolution
macroglossia
macrogyria
macroorchidism
macrophages
  lipid-laden
  stimulated
Macroplastique implantable urinary continence device
macrorestriction map
macroscopic hematuria
macrostomia ablepheron syndrome
macrostomia, fetal
macula (pl. maculae)
macula gonorrhoica
macular degeneration, polymorphic
maculopapular rash
MAD (myoadenylate deaminase deficiency)
Madayag biopsy needle
Madelung deformity
Madigan prostatectomy
Madlener tubal sterilization
Maestro fluid-management system
Maffucci syndrome
Magendie, foramen of
magnesium (Mg)
magnesium loading dose
magnesium sulfate infusion
magnesium sulfate ($MgSO_4$)
magnetic resonance imaging (MRI)
magnetic resonance mammography (MRM)
magnetic resonance urography (MRU)
magnetic retriever
magnification mammography
magnification, power (measured in loupes)

magnifying loupe
MAGPI (meatal advancement, glanuloplasty, penoscrotal junction meatotomy) operation
MAGPI hypospadias repair
Magrina-Bookwalter vaginal retractor
MAG3 (mercaptoacetyltriglycine)
Maher elevator
maieusiophobia
main d'accoucheur ("obstetrician's hand")
Mainstay urologic soft tissue anchor
maintain urinary continence
maintenance dialysis
maintenance hemofiltration
Mainz pouch urinary reservoir
Mainz urinary pouch
Majoli uterine manipulator/injector
major calices
major causes of genetic disorders
majora, labia
making water
Makler insemination device
malabsorption, glucose-galactose
malacoplakia of kidney
maladaptive coping behavior in dialysis patients
malaise and fever
malaria
  congenital
  falciparum
  quartan
Malassezia furfur pustulosis of newborn
male
  genetic human
  XX
  XXY
  XYY
male body habitus
male breast
male breast cancer
male choriocarcinoma
Malecot catheter
Malecot wings
male escutcheon
male external genitalia
male factor infertility
male genital tissue
male germ cell
male, gestating
male gonad
male gynecomastia
male hermaphroditism
male homosexuality
male hypogonadism
male infertility
male internal genitalia
male libido
male menopause
male pattern alopecia
male pseudohemaphrodite
male pseudohemaphroditism
male reproductive cell
male reproductive system
male sterility
male to female sex reassignment surgery
male to female transsexual
male Undies
male urethra
male urethra stricture
malformation
  Arnold-Chiari
  arteriovenous of uterus
  cystic adenomatoid
  Dandy-Walker
  fetal
malformation syndrome
malfunctioning urinary bladder
malignancy
  bladder
  cervical
  endometrial
  invasive
  kidney
  metastatic
  penile
  prostatic

malignancy *(cont.)*
  renal
  uterine
  vulvar
malignancy-associated nephropathy
malignant breast mass
malignant fever
malignant glomerulonephritis
malignant hyperphenylalaninemia
malignant hyperpyrexia
malignant hyperthermia (MH)
malignant hydatidiform mole
malignant hypertension
malignant lesion
malignant melanoma
malignant nephroangiosclerosis
malignant nephrosclerosis
malignant ovarian teratoma
malignant renal neoplasm
malignant teratoma
malignant transformation
malignant-type calcification
Malis forceps
malleable mass
malleable obturator
malleable retractor
Mallory-Weiss syndrome
Malmstrom cup
Malmstrom vacuum extraction
malnutrition, fetal
malodorous
malpighian corpuscles
malpighian glomerulus
malpighian stigmas
malpositioned fetus
malposition of fetus
malposition of uterus
malpresentation of fetus
malrotation of the intestine
Maltese crosses
Mamex DC mammography
mamillary (see *mammillary*)
mamma (pl. mammae)
mamma erratica
mammalation
mammalgia
mamma masculina
mammaplasty (see *mammoplasty*)
mammary abscess
mammary aspiration specimen (MAS)
  cytology test
mammary aspiration specimen cytology
  test (MASCT)
mammary atrophy
mammary calculus
mammary cyst
mammary duct
mammary duct ectasia
mammary duct obstruction
mammary ductal ectasia
mammary ductogram
mammary ductogram imaging
mammary dysplasia
mammary ectasia
mammary fistula
mammary galactogram
mammary gland
  lobes of
  lobule of
mammary implant
mammary line
mammary milk line
mammary neuralgia
mammary ptosis
mammary ridge
mammary souffle
mammastatin protein
mamma virilis
mammectomy
Mammex TR computer-aided
  mammography diagnosis system
mammiform
mammilla (pl. mammillae)
mammillaplasty
mammillary (also mamillary)
mammillary body
mammillary fistula
mammillary line

mammillate
mammillation
mammilliform
mammillitis
mammilopeduncular tract
mammilotegmental tract
mammilothalamic tract
mammogram, mammography
  annual
  baseline
  bilateral
  computed tomographic
  computed tomography laser (CTLM)
  contoured tilting compression
  CT laser (CTLM)
    digital
  ductographic
  Dynamic Optical Breast Imaging System (DOBI)
  Egan
  full-field digital
  GE Senographe 20001 digital
  high resolution CT
  laser
  LORAD full field digital
  low dose
  magnetic resonance (MRM)
  magnification
  Mamex DC
  Mammex TR computer-aided
  Mammomat B
  Mammo QC
  MammoReader system
  microfocal spot
  nonpalpable mass on
  Opdima digital
  Palpagraph
  prebiopsy
  radionuclide
  repeat
  retromammary space view in
  scintimammography
  screen-film

mammogram *(cont.)*
  screening
  Senographe 2000D digital
  SenoScan
  SoftScan laser
  step-oblique
  tag of Spence
  tail of breast in
  Trex digital mammography system (TDMS)
  ultra-high magnification (UHMM)
  ultrasound augmented
  xeromammogram
  XMG (x-ray mammogram)
  x-ray (XMG)
mammogram-guided core biopsy
mammographer
mammographically guided needle localization
mammographic features
mammographic findings
mammographic-histopathologic correlation
mammographic measurement
mammographic parenchymal patterns, Wolfe
mammographic system, Lorad M-II D
mammographic technique, low dose film
mammographic view, retromammary space view
mammography (see *mammogram*)
Mammography Quality Standards Act (MQSA)
Mammomat B mammography
mammoplasty (also mammaplasty)
  augmentation
  axillary approach in augmentation
  axillary endoscopic reduction
  BAMBI (breast augmentation mammoplasty by injection)
  "belly button" augmentation
  breast augmentation mammoplasty by injection (BAMBI)

mammoplasty *(cont.)*
- central cone technique reduction
- "cleavoplasty" augmentation
- "cross-the-heart" augmentation
- en bloc augmentation
- endoscopic-assisted transumbilical
- endoscopic transaxillary augmentation
- free nipple transposition technique reduction
- Goulian
- inferior central pedicle reduction
- inferior pedicle technique reduction
- inframammary approach in augmentation
- laser reduction
- LeJour technique of reduction
- "mega-pocket" augmentation
- nonrigid technique reduction
- owl incision technique reduction
- pedicle technique reduction
- periareolar augmentation
- reconstructive
- reduction
- short-scar tumescent reduction
- subglandular augmentation
- transaxillary subpectoral
- vertical bipedicle flap technique reduction
- vertical reduction
- videoendoscopic augmentation
- wet-technique reduction
- Wise areola mastopexy breast augmentation (WAMBA)

Mammo QC mammography
MammoReader system
MammoSite RTS (radiation therapy system) catheter
mammosomatotroph cell adenoma
Mammotest breast biopsy system
Mammotest Plus breast biopsy system
Mammotome handheld breast biopsy device
Mammotome probe
Mammotome ultrasound system
mammotomy
mammotropic factor
mammotropic hormone
management, expectant
Manchester colpoperineorrhaphy
Manchester vaginal operation for prolapse of the uterus
Mandrin catheter guide
maneuver (also see *operation; technique*)
- all-fours
- Barlow
- Baudelocque
- bimanual
- Bracht
- Brandt-Andrews
- Braxton Hicks
- Bruhat
- cephalic
- corkscrew
- Credé
- Cushieri two-hand
- DeLee
- ECV (external cephalic version)
- extreme lithotomy
- Gastaldo
- Gaskin shoulder dystocia
- heel-to-ear
- Hibbard
- Hicks
- Hillis-Mueller
- Kristeller
- Leopold
- Mariceau
- Mattox
- Mauriceau-Smellie-Veit
- McDonald
- McRoberts
- modified Prague
- Mueller-Hillis
- Ortolani hip
- Pajot
- Pinard

maneuver *(cont.)*
  Potter
  Prague
  Prentice
  Ritgen
  Rubin
  Saxtorph
  Saxtorph-Pajot
  Scanzoni
  Schatz
  Sellick
  Smellie-Veit
  Valsalva
  Veit
  Westbury
  Wigand
  Woods corkscrew
  Woods screw
  Zavanelli
mandibulofacial dysostosis
mandibulofacial dysostosis with epibulbar dermoids
mandibulo-oculofacial dyscephaly
mandibulo-oculofacial dystrophy
manifold assembly
manipulate
manipulation
  fetal
  stone
manipulation of hypothalamic-pituitary-testicular axis
manipulator/injector
  HUMI (Harris-Kronner uterine manipulator injector)
  Kronner Manipujector
  RUMI uterine
  suprapubic
  uterine
  ZUMI (Zinnanti uterine manipulator injector)
mannosidosis
mannitol
mannitol solution
Mannuti sampling needle
manual assisted delivery
manual CPD
manual exploration
manual intermittent peritoneal dialysis (IPD)
manual pelvimetry
manual removal of retained placenta
manual rotation of fetal head
manual urinalysis
manual vacuum device
MAO (monoamine oxidase) inhibitor
maple leaf flap
maple syrup odor of urine
maple syrup urine
maple syrup urine disease (MSUD)
MA (mentoanterior) position
mapped gene/phenotype
mapping
  chromosome
  functional anatomic
mapping device, Palpagraph breast
marble bones
Marcaine (bupivacaine)
Marcus Gunn phenomena
Marden-Walker syndrome
Marfan syndrome
Margolin HSG (hysterosalpingogram) catheter
Marie-Sainton disease
Marinesco-Sjögren-Gorland syndrome
Marinesco-Sjögren syndrome
marginal necrosis of flap
marginal placenta
marginal placenta previa
marginal sinus
marimastat
marital counseling
marital introitus
marked fetal bradycardia
marker (see also *genetic marker; tumor marker*)
  AFP (alpha-fetoprotein)
  CEA (carcinoembryonic antigen)
  Freeman cookie cutter areola

marker *(cont.)*
  genetic
  nicked-free beta subunit of hCG
  nipple
  oncofetal
  PLAP serum
  polymorphic genetic
  PSA (prostate-specific antigen)
  tumor
marker chromosome
marker X syndrome
Markov simulation model
Marlex mesh
Marlex mesh graft
Marlex PerFix plug
marmorata, cutis
Marogen (epoetin beta)
Maroteaux-Lamy syndrome
marrow inoculum
marrow purging ex vivo pretransplant
Marrs intrauterine catheter
Marrs laparoscopic catheter
Marshall and Tanner pubertal staging
Marshall-Marchetti-Krantz (MMK) modified procedure
Marshall-Marchetti-Krantz operation for urinary stress incontinence
Marshall-Marchetti procedure for bladder repair
Marshall-Marchetti test
Marshall-Smith syndrome
Marshall syndrome
Marshall test
Marsupial adjustable belt with attachable pouch
marsupial drain pouch
marsupialization of Bartholin cyst
marsupialization of cyst
marsupialization of kidney lesion
marsupialization of ovarian cyst
Marsupial pouch drainage system
marsupium
Martin-Bell syndrome
Martin cutting needle
Martin pelvimeter
Martius flap and fascial sling
Martius graft
Martius labial fat pad flap
Maryland dissector
MAS (mammary aspiration specimen) cytology test
MAS (meconium aspiration syndrome)
MASA syndrome
MASCT (mammary aspiration specimen cytology test)
masculine secondary sex characteristics
masculine uterus
masculinity-femininity scale
masculinization
masculinization of external genitalia
masculinum, ovarium
mask of pregnancy
mass (pl. masses)
  adnexal
  bilateral adnexal
  calcified
  calcified bladder
  cavitary
  conical
  cordlike
  cystic
  discrete
  dominant
  elongated
  encapsulated
  enhancing
  expansile
  extraovarian
  fecal
  firm
  fixed
  fleecy
  fluctuant
  fluid
  fluid-filled
  focal
  freely movable
  friable

mass *(cont.)*
- fungating
- groin
- hyperdense
- hyperintense
- hypodense
- ill-defined
- intrarenal hyperdense
- intrarenal hypodense
- intratesticular
- intrinsic
- lobulated
- malignant
- malleable
- nodular
- ovarian
- palpable
- pelvic
- perirenal
- polypoid calcified irregular
- renal
- retroareolar
- saccular
- scrotal
- sex chromatin
- soft tissue
- solid
- solitary
- sonolucent cystic
- space-occupying
- spherical
- stonelike
- stony
- suspicious
- testicular
- tissue

massage
- prostatic
- uterine

mass effect
Massengill vaginal douche
mass in uterus, fluid-filled
massive edema
massive effusion
massive embolism
massive enlargement of ovaries
massive genital prolapse
massive hemorrhage from renal artery and veins
massive pubertal hypertrophy of breast
massive pulmonary hemorrhage
massive vaginal eversion
mass lesion
mass-like configuration
mastadenitis
mastadenoma
mastalgia
mast cells
mastectomy (pl. mastectomies)
- Auchincloss modified radical
- axillary node dissection
- bilateral
- breast-sparing
- complete
- extended radical
- Halsted radical
- lumpectomy
- McWhirter simple
- modified radical
- partial
- Patey modified radical
- preventive
- prophylactic
- quadrantectomy
- radical
- "scarless"
- segmental
- simple
- skin-sparing
- subcutaneous
- total
- two-stage technique of
- Urban extended radical
- Willy Meyer incision for

mastectomy for gynecomastia
Masters-Allen syndrome

Masterson endometrial sampling device
mastitis
  chronic cystic
  cystic
  gargantuan
  glandular
  granulomatous
  infective
  interstitial
  lactational
  neonatal infective
  noninfective
  noninfective neonatal
  nonpurulent
  parenchymatous
  periductal
  plasma cell
  puerperal
  purulent
  retromammary
  stagnation
  submammary
  suppurative
mastitis neonatorum
mastocytosis
mastodynia
mastoid
mastoid fontanelle
mastoiditis
mastopathia chronica cystica
mastopathy
  cystic
  diffuse cystic
mastopexy
  anchor
  areolar
  augmentation
  Benelli
  Benelli lollipop
  Benelli pursestring
  Benelli round block
  Biesenberger technique of
  breast-lift
  central technique of

mastopexy *(cont.)*
  circumareolar
  concentric
  crescent
  donut
  double skin
  endoscopic-assisted
  full
  keyhole
  keystone
  LeJour
  lollipop
  Louis
  modified
  modified Benelli round block
  periareolar
  pursestring
  reduction
  Regnault type B
  round block technique of
  short-scar technique of
  simple
  vertical
  Wise
mastoplasia
mastoplasty
mastoptosis
mastorrhagia
mastosyrinx
mastotomy
mastotomy with abscess drainage
masturbate
masturbation
material
  atheromatous
  cheesy
  genetic
  mucoid
  preservation of solid
  scant mucoid
maternal abdominal pressure
maternal and fetal blood group
  incompatibility
maternal antibodies

maternal aunt/uncle
maternal bleeding diathesis
maternal blood clot patch therapy
maternal bradycardia
maternal cell contamination
maternal contamination in chorionic villi sampling
maternal cotyledon
maternal death
  direct
  indirect
maternal death rate
maternal decidua
maternal determination
maternal diabetes
maternal distress
maternal dystocia
maternal-fetal histoincompatibility
maternal-fetal incompatibility
maternal-fetal medicine
maternal-fetal transfusion
maternal floor infarction
maternal grandmother/grandfather
maternal health
maternal health problems
maternal hemopathy
maternal hydrops fetalis
maternal hypertension
maternal hypotension
maternal hypotension syndrome
maternal hypovolemia
maternal immunity
maternal inheritance
maternal injury
maternal insulin-like growth factor-1
maternal morbidity
maternal mortality
maternal mortality rate
maternal obesity syndrome
maternal parvovirus fetalis
maternal pelvis
maternal placenta
maternal pyrexia
maternal rights and responsibilities
maternal rubella
maternal screening
maternal sequelae, serious
maternal serum alpha-fetoprotein (MSAP, MSAFP)
maternal systemic circulation
maternal tachycardia
maternity pad
maternity testing
maternal thyroid dysfunction, postpartum
maternal transfer neutropenia
mathematical genetics
mating
mating frequency
mating system
mating type
matricide
matrilineal
Matritech NMP22 test kit for bladder cancer
matrix metalloprotease (metalloproteinase) enzyme
matrix metalloprotease (metalloproteinase) inhibitor (MMPI)
matrix (pl. matrices)
  mesangial
  protein
matroclinous inheritance
Matsner median episiotomy and repair
matted lymph nodes
Mattox maneuver
mattress sutures
maturation arrest at spermatid state
maturation of germ cells
maturation, premature accelerated lung (PALM)
mature fistula
mature messenger RNA
mature male germ cell
mature ovarian follicle
mature ovum
maturing ova

maturity
 fetal lung
 pulmonary
 sexual
maturity of fetus
maturity onset diabetes mellitus (MODM)
maturity onset diabetes of the young (MODY)
Mauriceau method of delivery
Mauriceau-Smellie-Veit maneuver
Maxaquin (lomefloxacin)
maxillofacial dysostosis
maxillonasal dysplasia, Binder type
maximum urethral closure pressure (MUCP)
Maxipime (cefepime)
Mayer pessary
Mayer-Rokitansky-Küster-Hauser syndrome
Mayer-Rokitansky syndrome
May-Hegglin anomaly
Maylard incision
Mayo culdoplasty
Mayo-Guyon kidney pedicle clamp
Mayo needle
Mayo noncutting needle
Mayo-Russian tissue forceps
Mayo scissors
mazoplasia
Mb (megabase)
MCA hemodialyzer
MCA (multiple congenital anomaly) syndrome
MCAD (medium chain acyl-CoA dehydrogenase deficiency)
MCAG (multiple colloid adenomatous goiter)
McArdle disease
MCAS (modular clip application system)
MCB (multicolor banding) studies
McBurney incision
McCall culdoplasty
McCall modified posterior culdoplasty
McCall posterior culdoplasty
McCall vaginal vault suspension, high
McCarthy panendoscope
McCraw gracilis myocutaneous flap for vaginal reconstruction
McCune-Albright syndrome
MCD (minimal change disease)
McDonald cervical cerclage procedure
McDonald maneuver
McDonald measurement
McDougal prostatectomy clamp
M cell genesis
McGhan breast implant
MCGN (minimal change glomerulonephritis)
McGraw gracilis myocutaneous flap vaginal reconstruction
MCH (mean corpuscular hemoglobin)
MCHC (mean corpuscular hemoglobin concentration)
McIndoe development of neovagina
McIndoe vaginal construction
McKusick-type metaphyseal chondrodysplasia
McLane-Tucker-Kielland obstetrical forceps
McLane-Tucker-Luikart obstetrical forceps
McLane-Tucker obstetrical forceps
McPherson forceps
McRoberts maneuver
MCTD (mixed connective tissue disease)
MCV (mean corpuscular volume)
MCV (methotrexate, cisplatin, vinblastine) chemotherapy protocol
McWhirter simple mastectomy
MD (muscular dystrophy)
MD (myotonic dystrophy)
M.D. Anderson clamp
MEA (microwave endometrial ablation)
MEA (multiple endocrine adenomatosis)

mean amniotic fluid index
mean birth weight
mean corpuscular hemoglobin (MCH)
mean corpuscular hemoglobin concentration (MCHC)
mean corpuscular volume (MCV)
mean length of gestation
measles-mumps-rubella (MMR) vaccine
measurement
 access flow
 bone density
 bone mass
 McDonald
meatal advancement, glanuloplasty, penoscrotal junction meatotomy (MAGPI) operation
meatal-based skin flap
meatal stenosis
 acquired
 congenital
meatal stricture
meatoplasty, urethral
meatotomy
 internal urethral
 ureteral
 urethral
meatus
 pinhole
 urethral
MEB (muscle-eye-brain disorders)
mechanical dysmenorrhea
mechanical ileus
mechanical induction of labor
mechanical ultrafiltration
mechanism
 counterregulatory
 immune
 transcription control
Meckel diverticulum
Meckel-Gruber syndrome
Meckel syndrome
meclizine
meconiorrhea
meconium
 delayed passage of
 intrauterine passage of
 thick
meconium aspiration
meconium aspiration below vocal cords
meconium aspiration syndrome
meconium below the cords
meconium blockage syndrome
meconium ileus
meconium in liquor
meconium obstruction
meconium peritonitis
meconium plug
meconium plug syndrome
meconium pneumonitis
meconium stain
meconium staining
meconium staining of amniotic fluid
meconium-stained amniotic fluid
Mectra Tissue Sample Retainer
Medela breast pump
media hysteroscopy
medial border of kidney
medial border of suprarenal gland
medial umbilical fold
median bar of prostate
median furrow of prostate
median length of survival
median lobe of prostate
median raphe of scrotum
median ridge of prostate
median umbilical ligament
mediastinal lymphatics
medical castration
medical genetics
medical induction of labor
medical induction of uterine contractions
medicated urethral system for erection (MUSE) urethral suppository

medications (including pharmaceuticals, natural substances, imaging agents, and prescription and over-the-counter drugs)
abarelix-depot M
abetimus sodium
acarbose
AccuSite injectable gel
Accutane (isotretinoin)
acetaminophen
acetaminophen-codeine combination
Acticoat burn dressing
Action-II (pimagedine)
Activella (estradiol/norethindrone
Actonel
Actos (pioglitazone)
acyclovir
Adcon-L gel
Adipex-P
Adriamycin
Advil
AGT (aminoglutethimide)
AIDSvax
Alasulf (sulfanilamide and aminacrine)
albumin, human sonicated
Albunex (albumin, human sonicated)
Aldara Cream 5%
Aldara (imiquimod) cream
aldesleukin
Aldurazyme (iduronidase)
alendronate
Alesse (levonorgestrel/ethinyl estradiol) oral contraceptive
alfacalcidol
Alferon LDO (interferon alfa-n3)
Alferon N Gel (interferon alfa-n3)
alfuzosin
Alibra (alprostadil/prazosin)
Alista (alprostadil)
Alkeran (melphalan)
allopurinol

medications *(cont.)*
Aloe Vesta perineal foam
Alora (estradiol) transdermal patch
alpha$_1$-adrenergic blockers
alpha blockers
alpha-calcidiol
alprostadil for injection
alprostadil/prazosin
Alprox-TD (alprostadil)
Alredase (tolrestat)
altretamine
aluminum carbonate gel
aluminum hydroxide
aluminum hydroxide gel
Amaryl (glimepiride)
Amen (medroxyprogesterone)
Amerge (naratriptan)
amikacin
amiloride
aminacrine
aminobenzoate potassium
aminobiphosphonates
Amino-Cerv pH 5.5 cervical cream
aminoglutethimide
Amoxil (amoxicillin)
amoxicillin
Amphojel (aluminum hydroxide)
ampicillin
ampicillin and gentamicin ("amp and gent")
anagestone
Anandron (nilutamide)
anastrozole
Ancef
Andractim (dihydrotestosterone gel)
Androderm testosterone transdermal patch
Androsorb
AngioMark MRI contrast medium
annamycin
Anovlar oral contraceptive
Anovulatorio oral contraceptive
Antagon (ganirelix)
antestrogen drug

medications *(cont.)*
- anti-human thymocyte immuno-immunoglobulin, rabbit
- antispasmodic
- antithymocyte globulin, rabbit
- Antivert
- Antizol (fomepizole)
- Aphrodyne (yohimbine)
- A.P.L. (chorionic gonadotropin)
- apomorphine
- Apra (CT-2584 mesylate)
- Apri (desogestrel and ethinyl estradiol) tablets
- aqueous procaine penicillin G
- aqueous vasopressin
- Aranesp (darbepoetin alfa)
- Arimidex (anastrozole)
- Aromasin (exemestane)
- aromatase inhibitors
- Aroplatin
- arzoxifene
- Astroglide personal lubricant
- Atgam (antithymocyte globulin)
- atrasentan
- Atrosept (methenamine)
- AuraTek FDP (fibrin/fibrinogen degradation products)
- Avandia (rosiglitazone)
- AVC vaginal cream
- Aviane-28 (levonorgestrel and ethinyl estradiol)
- Avicidin
- Avicine
- Aygestin (norethindrone)
- azathioprine
- azidothymidine (AZT)
- azithromycin
- azodicarbonamide
- Azo-Gantrisin
- Azo-Sulfisoxazole (sulfisoxazole)
- azothioprine sodium
- bacitracin ointment
- Bactrim
- Bactrim DS

medications *(cont.)*
- Bactroban (mupirocin)
- basiliximab
- BCI-Immune Activator
- BEBIG iodine-125 seed implant
- beclomethasone
- Belzer solution
- Benadryl
- benzathine penicillin G
- Betadine
- Betadine gel
- betaine anhydrous
- betamethasone suspension
- betamethasone sodium phosphate
- bethanechol chloride
- bicalutamide
- Bicarbolyte
- Bicitra
- BioHy
- biopirimine
- botulinum-A toxin
- BrachySeed
- Brevicon oral contraceptive
- Brevinor 21 or 28 oral contraceptive
- Bricanyl (terbutaline)
- bromocriptine mesylate
- Brethine (terbutaline)
- Broxidine (broxuridine)
- broxuridine
- bryostatin
- bumetanide
- Bumex (bumetanide)
- busulfan
- butoconazole nitrate
- cabergoline
- CAF (cyclophosphamide, Adriamycin, fluorouracil)
- Cafcit (caffeine citrate) oral solution
- CAFTH (cyclophosphamide, Adriamycin, fluorouracil, tamoxifen, Halotestin)
- Calcijex (calcitriol)
- calcitonin
- calcitriol

medications *(cont.)*
calcium
calcium gluconate
calusterone
Camptosar (irinotecan)
Canasa (mesalamine)
Candistroy
Candistat-G
capecitabine
Capoten (captopril)
captopril
carbimazole
Carlesta skin treatment
CarraVex injectable
Casodex (bicalutamide)
Cataflam (diclofenac)
Caverject (prostaglandin E1, PGE1, alprostadil)
CEB (carboplatin, etoposide, bleomycin)
CEF (cyclophosphamide, epirubicin, fluorouracil)
cefadroxil
cefazolin
cefepime
Cefobid
cefotaxime
cefpodoxime proxetil
ceftazidime
ceftriaxone
CellCept (mycophenolate mofetil)
Celsior organ preservation solution
Cenestin (conjugated estrogen)
Cenogen-OB prenatal formula
Centara (priliximab)
cephalosporin
Certican (everolimus)
Cervidil (dinoprostone) vaginal insert
cetrorelix
Cetrotide (cetrorelix)
Chemet (succimer)
Chirocaine (levobupivacaine)

medications *(cont.)*
chlorambucil
chlorotrianisene
chlorpropamide
cholestyramine
Chondrogel tissue augmentation material
Chorex 10 (chorionic gonadotropin)
Chorex-5 (chorionic gonadotropin)
Choron-10 (chorionic gonadotropin)
choriogonadotropin
Chromagen OB prenatal vitamins
Cialis
Ciclovulan oral contraceptive
cidofovir gel
cimetidine
Cinobac (cinoxacin)
cinoxacin
Cipro
ciprofloxacin
cis-platinum (now cisplatin)
cisplatin
Claforan
clarithromycin
clavulanate
Cleocin (clindamycin phosphate) vaginal cream
Cleocin vaginal ovules
Climara (estradiol transdermal system) patch
Climara Pro estrogen replacement patch
clinidamycin
clodronate
clofibrate
Clomid (clomiphene)
clomiphene citrate
clonidine
clotrimazole vaginal cream
CMFP (cyclophosphamide, methotrexate, fluorouracil, prednisone)
CMFPT (cyclophosphamide, methotrexate, fluorouracil, prednisone, tamoxifen)

medications *(cont.)*
CMFVP (cyclophosphamide, methotrexate, fluorouracil, vincristine, and prednisone)
Coagulin-B
codeine
Colace
colchicine
CombiPatch (estradiol/norethindrone) transdermal
Compliance Pak
Comprecin (enoxacin)
Condylox (podofilox) gel
conjugated estrogens
ConXn (recombinant human relaxin)
corticosteroids
co-trimoxazole
Coumadin
Crinone bioadhesive progesterone gel
cryoprecipitate
CT-2584 mesylate
Curosurf (poractant alfa)
Curretab (medroxyprogesterone)
Cyclessa (desogestrel/ethinyl estradiol)
Cyclofem (now Lunelle) injectable contraceptive
cyclophosphamide
cyclosporine
Cycrin (medroxyprogesterone)
CyPat
cyproterone
Cystadane (betaine anhydrous)
Cystagon (cysteamine bitartrate)
cysteamine bitartrate
Cystex (methenamine)
Cystistat (sterile sodium hyaluronate solution)
Cytadren (aminoglutethimide)
CytoGam (cytomegalovirus immune globulin)
Cytolex (pexiganan)
cytomegalovirus immune globulin

medications *(cont.)*
CytoTAb
Cytovene (oral ganciclovir)
Cytovene-IV (ganciclovir sodium for injection)
Cytoxan
dacliximab (also daclizumab)
daclizumab (also dacliximab)
dactinomycin
Dalgan (dezocine)
danazol
darbepoetin alfa
darifenacin
Darvocet
Darvocet-N 100
DaunoXome (liposomal daunorubicin)
Dayto Himbine
D-chiro-inositol
DDAVP (desmopressin)
Decadron (dexamethasone)
Deflux
Delaprem (hexoprenaline sulfate)
Delestrogen (estradiol)
Delfen foam
Demadex (torsemide)
Demerol
Demulen
depGynogen (estradiol cypionate)
Depo-Estradiol Cypionate (estradiol)
DepoGen (estradiol)
Depo-Provera (medroxyprogesterone)
Depo-Testadiol (estradiol)
Depotestogen (estradiol)
DES (diethylstilbestrol)
desferoxamine mesylate
deslorelin
desmopressin
Desogen (ethinyl estradiol, desogestrel)
desogestrel
desogestrel/ethinyl estradiol
Detrol, Detrol LA (tolterodine)

medications *(cont.)*
dexamethasone
dextran 10
dextran 70
dezocine
DHE (dihematoporphyrin ether)
DHPG (dihydroxypropoxymethyl-guanine)
DiaBeta (glyburide)
Dialose Plus
dialysate
Dibenzyline
diclofenac
Didronel (etidronate)
dienestrol (estrogen)
diethylstilbestrol
diethylstilbestrol diphosphate
Diflucan (fluconazole)
digoxin
dihematoporphyrin ether (DHE)
dihydrotestosterone gel
dihydroxypropoxymethylguanine (DHPG)
Dilantin
Dilapan
dinoprostone cervical gel
Diovan HCT (valsartan and hydrochlorothiazide)
dipyridamole
Ditropan
Ditropan XL (oxybutynin chloride)
docetaxel
Dolsed (methenamine)
dopamine
dospirenone/ethinyl estradiol oral contraceptive
Dostinex (cabergoline)
doxazosin mesylate
doxercalciferol
Doxil (doxorubicin)
doxorubicin
doxycycline
droloxifene

medications *(cont.)*
DRYalysate
Dulcolax suppositories
Dulcolax tablets
Duo-Cyp (estradiol)
Durasphere
Duricef
Duvoid (bethanechol)
Dynepro (gene-activated erythropoietin)
EchoSeed (iodine-125) brachytherapy seed
Edex (alprostadil)
eflornithine
Eligard (leuprolide acetate)
Elipten (aminoglutethimide)
Ellence (epirubicin)
Elmiron (pentosan polysulfate sodium)
Emcyt (estramustine phosphate sodium)
Emko foam
Empirynol Plus contraceptive gel
enalapril
Enfamil Natalins Rx prenatal vitamins
enisoprost
enoxacin
Enpresse (levonorgestrel/ethinyl estradiol tablets)
ERxinol tablets
epirubicin
epoetin alfa
Epogen (epoetin alfa)
Eprex (recombinant human erythropoietin)
Ergoset (bromocriptine mesylate)
ERxin
erythromycin
erythropoietin, recombinant human
Esclim (estradiol transdermal system)
Estinyl (ethinyl estradiol)

medications *(cont.)*
- Estraderm (estradiol)
- estradiol
- estradiol cypionate and medroxy-progesterone
- estradiol hemihydrate
- estradiol/norethindrome patch
- estradiol/norgestimate
- Estradiol Transdermal System patch
- estradiol valerate
- Estra-L 40 (estradiol)
- Estratab
- Estratest
- Estratest H.S.
- estramustine
- estramustine phosphate sodium
- Estrasorb (17-beta-estradiol) cream
- Estrasorb transdermal patch
- Estratab tablets
- Estrinor oral contraceptive
- Estrogel
- estrogen
- estrone
- Estrone Aqueous
- Estrophasic
- estropipate
- Estrostep
- ethacrynic acid
- ethinyl estradiol
- ethinyl estradiol/levonorgestrel
- Ethmozine (moricizine)
- ethoglucid
- ethynodiol diacetate/ethinyl estradiol oral contraceptive
- Ethyol (amifostine)
- etidronate
- etoglucid
- etoposide
- etretinate
- Eulexin (flutamide)
- Eulexin plus LHRH-A
- Evacet (doxorubicin [liposomal])
- everolimus
- Evista (raloxifene)

medications *(cont.)*
- exemestane
- Exosurf Neonatal (colfosceril palmitate)
- Extraneal (7.5% icodextrin) peritoneal dialysis solution
- Factive (gemifloxacin)
- Factrel (gonadorelin)
- famciclovir
- Famvir (famciclovir)
- Fareston
- Faslodex (ZD 9238)
- Fasturtec (rasburicase)
- FCAP (fluorouracil, cyclophos-phamide, Adriamycin, Platinol)
- FEC (fluorouracil, epirubicin, cyclophosphamide)
- Femara (letrozole) tablets
- femhrt or FemHRT (norethindrone and ethinyl estradiol)
- FemPatch (transdermal estrogen replacement)
- Femprox (alprostadil)
- Femstat 3 (butoconazole nitrate 2%) vaginal cream
- Femstat One (butoconazole nitrate)
- fenretinide
- fentanyl
- Ferrimin 150
- Ferrlecit (sodium ferric gluconate complex)
- ferrous sulfate
- Fertinex (urofollitropin)
- finasteride
- 5-alpha-reductase inhibitors
- 5-aminolevulinic acid
- 5′-DFUR
- 5-fluorouracil (5-FU)
- Flagyl
- Flagyl ER (metronidazole)
- Flexeril
- Flomax (tamsulosin)
- Floxin (ofloxacin)
- fluasterone

medications *(cont.)*
fluconazole
flucytosine
fluoexitine
fluorine-18-deoxyglucose (FDG)
fluorouracil cream
fluoxetine
flutamide
Folex PFS
Follistim (follitropin beta)
follitropin alfa
follitropin beta
fomepizole
Forvade (cidofovir gel)
Fosamax (alendronate)
foscarnet
fosfomycin tromethamine
furosemide
ganciclovir sodium injection
ganciclovir triphosphate
ganirelix
Gantrisin
Garamycin
gatifloxacin
gemcitabine
gemfibrozil
gemifloxacin
Gencept oral contraceptive
Gengraf (cyclosporine)
Genora oral contraceptive
gentamicin
Geocillin
Geref (sermorelin)
gestodene low dose estrogen/progestin
glimepiride
glomerular filtration agent
glucagon injectable (rDNA origin)
Glucophage (metformin hydrochloride)
Glucovance (glyburide, metformin)
Glutose
glyburide
glycine

medications *(cont.)*
Glynase Pres Tab (glyburide)
Glyset (miglitol)
gonadotropin, chorionic human recombinant
Gonal-F (follitropin alfa)
goserelin implant
Gynazole-1 (butoconazole nitrate)
Gyne-Lotrimin 3 (clotrimazole)
Gyne-Moistrin vaginal lubricant
Gyne-Pro vaginal cream
Gyne-Sulf vaginal cream
Gynogen L.A. 20
Gynogen L.A. 40
HAG3 (hydroxyacetyltriglycine)
Halcion
Hectorol (doxercalciferol; synthetic vitamin D prohormone)
Hemabate
hemiacidrin
hemi and zinc mesoporphyrin
hemin
heparin
Herceptin (trastuzumab)
Herpasil
Hexalen (altretamine)
hexamethylmelamine
Hexastat
hexoprenaline sulfate
HMFG1 (human milk fat globule 1)
HMG (human menopausal gonadotropin)
Humalog Mix 50/50 insulin
Humalog Mix 75/25 insulin
Humegon (menotropin)
Hydrea (hydroxyurea)
hydrochlorothiazide
hydrocortisone
hydroxyprogesterone
hydroxystilbamidine
hydroxyurea
Hylagel Uro viscoelastic gel
Hylutin (hydroxyprogesterone)
hyoscyamine sulfate

medications *(cont.)*
Hypaque contrast medium
Hypaque-Cysto contrast medium
Hypaque-M contrast medium
Hypaque Meglumine contrast medium
Hypaque Sodium contrast medium
Hytrin (terazosin)
Hyzaar (losartan potassium)
Imferon
imipenem
imipramine
imiquimod cream
Imodium
Imodium A-D
Impress Softpatch
Imuran (azathioprine)
Inderal
indomethacin
Infasurf (calfactant) intratracheal suspension
Innofem (estradiol)
insulin glargine
interferon alfa-n3
interleukin-1b
interleukin-2, recombinant (IL-2)
interleukin-3, recombinant (IL-3)
interleukin-6 (IL-6)
IntraDose gel (purified bovine collagen, cisplatin, and epinephrine)
Invicorp (phentolamine mesylate)
Iotrex radiation liquid
I-OXY (intravesical oxybutynin)
iron sucrose
isotretinoin
Jenest-28 oral contraceptive
Kayexalate
K-Dur
Keflex
Kefzol
Kestrone 5
ketoconazole
ketorolac tromethamine
KL4 surfactant
KLH-ImmuneActivator

medications *(cont.)*
Kliovance oral contraceptive
Kontrast U radiopaque medium
K-Y jelly
K-Y Silk-E vaginal moisturizer
K-Y vaginal lubricant
labetalol
Lambda (lanthanum carbonate)
laminaria
Lanoxin
lanthanum carbonate
Lantus (insulin glargine)
Lasix (furosemide)
leflunomide
letrozole
Leukeran (chlorambucil)
Leuprogel (leuprolide)
leuprolide
leuprolide for depot suspension
leuprolide implant
Leuvectin
Levlen oral contraceptive
Levlite (levonorgestrel/ethinyl estradiol)
levobupivacaine
levonorgestrel
levonorgestrel and ethinyl estradiol
levonorgestrel/ethinyl estradiol oral contraceptive
Levora (levonorgestrel/ethinyl estradiol)
levothyroxine sodium
Levoxyl (levothyroxine sodium)
Levulan (5-aminolevulinic acid)
liarozole fumarate
Liazal (liarozole fumarate)
lidocaine
lincomycin
liposomal doxorubicin
liposome encapsulated doxorubicin citrate complex
liposome-encapsulated doxorubicin citrate complex and cyclophosphamide

medications *(cont.)*
- lisinopril
- Loestrin oral contraceptive
- lomefloxacin
- Lo/Ovral oral contraceptive
- Lopid
- Lorabid (loracarbef)
- loracarbef
- losartan potassium
- Low-Ogestrel (norgestrel/ethinyl estradiol) oral contraceptive
- Lubrin vaginal
- Lugol solution
- Lunelle (estradiol cypionate and medroxyprogesterone)
- Lupron
- Lupron Depot (leuprolide)
- Lupron Depot-4 Month
- Lustra
- lutetium texaphryin
- Lutrepulse (gonadorelin)
- Lutrin (lutetium texaphryin)
- lymphocyte immune globulin, antithymocyte
- lyophilized collagenase
- lypressin
- MAb-170 monoclonal antibody
- Macritonin (calcitonin)
- Macrobid (nitrofurantoin)
- macrocyclic lactone
- Macrodantin
- magnesium sulfate
- mannitol
- marimastat
- Marogen (epoetin beta)
- Maxaquin (lomefloxacin)
- Maxipime (cefepime)
- meclizine
- medroxyprogesterone
- mefenamic acid
- Mefoxin
- Megace (megestrol)
- megestrol

medications *(cont.)*
- melphalan (L-phenylalanine mustard)
- Menest
- Menorest (transdermal 17-beta-estradiol)
- menotropin
- Mentax (1% butenafinel)
- Meridia (sibutramine)
- mesalamine
- mesna
- Mesnex (mesna)
- Metamucil
- metformin
- Methergine
- methimazole
- methotrexate
- methylprednisolone
- methysergide
- metolazone
- Metrodin (urofollitropin)
- Metro-Gel Vaginal
- metronidazole
- Mexate (methotrexate)
- Mexitil
- Miacalcin (calcitonin) nasal spray
- miconazole nitrate vaginal cream
- MICRhoGAM
- microbubble contrast agent for color Doppler ultrasound
- Microgestin Fe 1.5/30 oral contraceptive pill
- micronized progesterone
- Micronor oral contraceptive
- Micturin (terodiline)
- Mifegyne (mifepristone)
- mifepristone
- miglitol
- milk of magnesia
- Milli oral contraceptive
- Minesse (gestodene, progestin, and ethinyl estradiol)
- Minovlar oral contraceptive

medications *(cont.)*
Miraluma (technetium ^{99m}Tc sestamibi kit)
Mircette (desogestrel/ethinyl estradiol) oral contraceptive
Mirena (levonorgestrel-releasing intrauterine contraceptive)
Mithracin (plicamycin)
mitomycin
mitoxantrone
MK-906 (finasteride)
MMF (mycophenolate mofetil)
Modicon-28 oral contraceptive
Monistat (miconazole nitrate)
Monistat Dual-Pak
Monistat 1 ointment
Monistat 3 Combo
Monistat 3 vaginal cream
Monistat 7 vaginal cream
Monocid
Monsel paste
Monsel solution
Monurol (fosfomycin tromethamine)
moricizine
morphine
Motrin
MTS1 tumor suppressor gene
MTX (methotrexate)
mutant gene
Multikine (leukocyte; interleukin)
mupirocin ointment
MUSE (medicated urethral system for erection) urethral suppository (alprostadil)
Mutamycin (mitomycin)
MVAC or M-VAC (methotrexate, vincristine, Adriamycin, cisplatin)
MVF (mitoxantrone, vincristine, fluorouracil)
Mycelex (clotrimazole)
Mycelex Twin Pack (clotrimazole)
mycophenolate mofetil
Mycostatin (nystatin)

medications *(cont.)*
Mylocel (hydroxyurea)
Myocet (liposome-encapsulated doxorubicin citrate complex and cyclophosphamide)
M-Zole 3 Combination Pack
M-Zole 7 Combination Pack (miconazole)
M-Zole 7 Dual Pack (miconazole)
nafarelin
nafarelin
naratriptan
Naropin (ropivacaine)
Nashville Rabbit Antithymocyte Serum
Necon 0.5/35 norethindrone/ethinyl estradiol) oral contraceptive
Necon 1/35 norethindrone/ethinyl estradiol) oral contraceptive
Necon 1/50 (norethindrone/ mestranol) oral contraceptive
Necon 10/11 (norethindrone/ethinyl estradiol) oral contraceptive
N.E.E. oral contraceptive
Nelova 10/11 oral contraceptive
Nelulen 1/50 oral contraceptive
Neocon oral contraceptive
Neoral (cyclosporine)
Nephrox (aluminum hyroxide; mineral oil)
Nepro dietary supplement
netilmicin
Nilandron (nilutamide)
nilutamide
nitrofurantoin
Nizoral (ketoconazole)
Nodiol oral contraceptive
Nolvadex (tamoxifen citrate)
nonoxynol-9 spermicidal
Norcept-E oral contraceptive
Nordette oral contraceptive
norethindrone
norethindrone/ethinyl estradiol oral contraceptive

medications *(cont.)*
- norfloxacin
- norgestimate
- norgestrel
- norgestrel/ethinyl estradiol oral contraceptive
- Norimin oral contraceptive
- Norinyl (norethindrone/ethinyl estradiol) oral contraceptive
- Noritate (metronidazole)
- Norlestrin oral contraceptive
- Normodyne (labetalol)
- Noroxin (norfloxacin)
- Norplant (levonorgestrel)
- Nor-QD oral contraceptive
- Nortrel 1/35 (norethindrone and ethinyl estradiol)
- Nortrel-28 (norethindrone and ethinyl estradiol)
- Nortrel 7/7/7 (norethindrone and ethinyl estradiol)
- Novantrone (mitoxantrone)
- Novasome (nonoxynol-9) spermicidal contraceptive
- NuLev (hyoscyamine sulfate)
- NutriMan TNT (*Tribulus terrestris* extract)
- Nutropin (somatropin)
- Nuvera (17-beta estradiol/norethindrone)
- Nyotran
- nystatin
- octoxynol 9
- Oesclim patch
- ofloxacin
- Ogen (estrone)
- OncoScint breast imaging agent
- OncoScint OV103 (ovarian) monoclonal antibody
- One-Alpha (alfacalcidol)
- oral ganciclovir
- Oralgen oral aerosol insulin
- oral phosphate binders
- orBec (beclomethasone)

medications *(cont.)*
- Orlest oral contraceptive
- Ortho-Cept (progesterone desogestrel/ethinyl estradiol)
- Orthoclone OKT3 monoclonal antibody
- Ortho-Cyclen oral contraceptive
- Ortho Dialpak
- Ortho Dienestrol vaginal cream
- Ortho-est (estropipate)
- Ortho-Novum 1/35 oral contraceptive
- Ortho-Novum 1/50 oral contraceptive
- Ortho-Novum 7/7/7 oral contraceptive
- Ortho 1/35 oral contraceptive
- Ortho Personal Pak
- Ortho-Prefest (estradiol/norgestimate)
- Ortho 7/7/7 oral contraceptive
- Ortho Tri-Cyclen (norgestimate/ethinyl estradiol) oral contraceptive
- OvaRex MAb immunotherapy
- O-Vax vaccine
- Ovcon oral contraceptive
- Ovidrel (gonadotropin, chorionic human recombinant)
- Ovral oral contraceptive
- Ovrette oral contraceptive
- Ovysmen 0.5/35 oral contraceptive
- Ovysmen 1/35 oral contraceptive
- Ovysmen oral contraceptive
- oxybutynin chloride syrup
- oxybutynin transdermal patch
- oxytocin
- Oxytrol (oxybutynin transdermal patch)
- Pacis BCG
- paclitaxel
- palladium-103 (^{103}Pd) implantation
- palmetto extract
- Palmettx

medications *(cont.)*
- pamidronate
- paricalcitol
- Parlodel
- Paxene (paclitaxel)
- PC-SPES
- pemtumomab
- Penetrex (enoxacin)
- penicillin
- pentamidine
- pentosan polysulfate sodium
- Percocet
- Pergonal
- Peri-Colace
- Permixon (*Serenoa repens* extract)
- pexiganan
- PharmaSeed iodine-125 seeds
- PharmaSeed palladium-103 seeds
- phenazopyridine
- Phenergan
- phenobarbital
- phenoxybenzamine
- phentermine
- phentolamine mesylate
- phenylpropanolamine
- PhosLo (calcium)
- Photofrin (porfimer sodium)
- pimagedine
- pioglitazone
- piperacillin
- piritrexim
- Pitocin
- Pitressin
- Plan B (levonorgestrel 0.75 mg) postcoital contraceptive pill
- Plaquase (lyophilized collagenase)
- plicamycin
- PMS-Conjugated Estrogens
- podofilox gel
- Podofin (podophyllin)
- podophyllin (podophyllum resin)
- polyantibiotic ointment (neomycin-polymyxin-bacitracin)
- Polycitra-K

medications *(cont.)*
- Ponstel (mefenamic acid)
- poractant alfa
- Potaba
- potassium
- potassium bitartrate
- povidone iodine
- povidine-iodine douche
- Pramet FA prenatal vitamins
- Pramilet FA prenatal vitamins
- pramlintide
- Prandase (acarbose)
- Prandin (repaglinide)
- prazosin
- PreCare Conceive
- Precose (acarbose)
- prednisolone
- prednisone
- Pregnyl (chorionic gonadotropin)
- Prelone (prednisone)
- Premarin
- PremesisRx
- Premphase (conjugated estrogens; medroxyprogesterone)
- Prempro (conjugated estrogens; medroxyprogesterone)
- prenatal vitamins
- Prenavite prenatal vitamins
- Prepidil Gel (dinoprostone cervical gel)
- Preven emergency contraceptive kit
- Pro-Banthine (propantheline)
- probenecid
- Procardia
- Proclim (medroxyprogesterone)
- Procrit (epoetin alfa)
- Profasi (chorionic gonadotropin)
- Progestasert (progesterone) intrauterine device
- progesterone
- Prograf (tacrolimus capsules and injection)
- ProLease encapsulated sustained-release growth hormone

medications *(cont.)*
Proleukin (aldesleukin; IL-2)
Promensil
Prometrium (micronized progesterone)
propantheline
propranolol
propylthiouracil (PTU)
Proscar (finasteride)
prostaglandin E1 (alprostadil)
prostaglandin gel
prostaglandin synthetase inhibitors
ProstaScint (CYT-356 radiolabeled with ^{111}In)
ProstaScint monoclonal antibody imaging agent
ProstaSeed ^{125}I radiation treatment
Prostin (alprostadil)
Protectaid contraceptive sponge with F-5 Gel
Provenge vaccine
Provera (medroxyprogesterone)
Prozac
psyllium hydrocolloid
P-32 chromic phosphate suspension
PTU (propylthiouracil)
Pyridium
Pyridorin (pyridoxamine)
Pyridorin XR (extended release pyridoxamine)
Puregon (follitropin beta)
quinestrol
radioactive seed implants
radiolabeled peptide alpha-M2
raloxifene
ranitidine
Rapamune (sirolimus)
rapamycin
Raplon (rapacuronium bromide)
rasburicase
recombinant human relaxin (ConXn)
recombinant interleukin-2
Regressin
ReLibra (testosterone gel)

medications *(cont.)*
Remifemin
Renacidin
Renagel (sevelamer)
Renografin contrast medium
Renografin-60 contrast medium
Reno-M contrast medium
Reno-M-Dip contrast medium
Reno-M-30 contrast medium
Reno-M-60 contrast medium
Renovist II contrast medium
Renovue-Dip contrast medium
repaglinide
Replens vaginal gel
Repliform
Repronal
Repronex
resiquimod
Rezulin (troglitazone)
Rheomacrodex
Rheumatrex (methotrexate)
RhoGAM
rifampin
risedronate
ritodrine
Rocaltrol (calcitriol)
Rocephin
rofecoxib
rogletimide
ropivacaine
roquinimex
rosiglitazone
RU-486 (mifepristone)
rubitecan (RFS2000)
Salpix contrast medium
Sandimmune (cyclosporine)
SangCya (cyclosporine)
Sarafem (fluoxetine)
SAVVY vaginal microbicide
Seasonale
selenomethionine
SEPA/testosterone gel
Sepracoat coating solution
Sepragel bioresorbable gel

medications *(cont.)*
- Septra
- Septra DS
- Serenoa repens extract
- Serophene
- sevelamer
- 17-beta-estradiol
- sibutramine
- sildenafil citrate
- Silken Secret vaginal moisturizer
- silver nitrate drops
- Simulect (basiliximab)
- sirolimus
- 6-mercaptopurine
- Slow-K
- sodium estrone sulfate
- sodium iothalamate I-125
- sodium polystyrene sulfonate
- sodium propionate
- Solu-Medrol (methylprednisolone)
- somatotropin
- somatropin
- sorbitol
- spectinomycin
- spermicidal contraceptive
- spironolactone
- squalamine
- Stadol
- SteriLyte liquid bicarbonate
- Stuartnatal Plus
- Stuart Prenatal vitamins
- succimer
- sulbactam
- sulfa
- sulfamethoxazole
- sulfisoxazole
- sulodexide
- SU101
- suramin
- Surete contraceptive gel
- Surfak
- Surfaxin (lucinactant)
- Symmetra ^{125}I brachytherapy seed
- Synarel (nafarelin)

medications *(cont.)*
- Synphase oral contraceptive
- Synphasic 28 oral contraceptive
- Synsorb Pk
- synthetic conjugated estrogens
- synthetic vitamin D prohormone
- Synthroid
- tacrolimus
- Talwin
- tamoxifen citrate
- tamsulosin
- Targretin
- taxane
- Taxol (paclitaxel)
- Taxotere (docetaxel)
- teceleukin
- TechneScan MAG3 (^{99m}Tc mertiatide)
- technetium
- Tegretol
- temafloxacin
- TEMP (tamoxifen, etoposide, mitoxantrone, Platinol)
- Tequin (gatifloxacin)
- Terazol 3 (terconazole)
- Terazol 7 (terconazole)
- terazosin
- terbutaline
- terconazole
- terodiline
- Testoderm patch
- Testoderm TTS (testosterone transdermal system) patch
- testolactone
- testosterone gel
- testosterone transdermal patch
- tetracycline
- thalidomide
- TheraCys (BCG live intravesical)
- TheraDerm-MTX
- Theradigm-HPV
- TheraSeed implant
- Therex (monoclonal antibody huHMFG1)

medications *(cont.)*
thiazolidinediones (TZDs)
Thioplex (thiotepa)
thiotepa
Thymoglobulin (antithymocyte globulin, rabbit)
Thyrogyn (thyrotropin alfa)
ticarcillin
Tice BCG
Tigan suppositories
tioconazole
Tobramycin
tocolytic
Tofranil (imipramine)
tolrestat
tolterodine
Topiglan (SEPA/alprostadil) gel
Toradol (ketorolac tromethamine)
toremifene citrate
torsemide
Tostrex (transdermal testosterone gel)
TP-40 chemotherapy drug
transdermal testosterone gel
Trelstar Depot (triptorelin pamoate)
Trelstar LA (triptorelin pamoate)
triamcinolone acetonide cream
triamterene
trichloroacetic acid
Triella oral contraceptive
Tri-Levlen oral contraceptive
trimethoprim
Tri-Norinyl (norethindrone/ethinyl estradiol) oral contraceptive
Trinovin
Trinovum 21 oral contraceptive
Triphasil (levonorgestrel and ethinyl estradiol)
triptolide
triptorelin pamoate
Trivagizole 3 (clotrimazole vaginal cream, 2%)

medications *(cont.)*
Trivora (levonorgestrel/ethinyl estradiol) oral contraceptive
Trivora-21 (ethinyl estradiol/ levonorgestrel)
Trivora-28 (ethinyl estradiol/ levonorgestrel)
troglitazone
trospium
trovafloxacin
Trovan (trovafloxacin)
Trovan/Zithromax Compliance Pak
Trovert
Tru-Scint AD imaging agent
Trysul vaginal cream
TSH-01 transdermal tape with natural estrogen and 17-beta-estradiol
Tylenol Extra Strength
Tylenol No. 3
Tylox
TZDs (thiazolidinediones)
Unasyn
Uprima (apomorphine)
uracil mustard
Urecholine
urethral bulking agent
Urised
Uristat
urofollitropin
Urografin 290 imaging agent
Urografin-76 imaging agent
Urovist Cysto imaging agent
Urovist Meglumine imaging agent
Urovist Sodium imaging agent
UroXatral (alfuzosin)
VAB-6 chemotherapy protocol
Vagifem (17-beta-estradiol)
Vagifem vaginal tablets
vaginal contraceptive film (VCF)
Vagisec Plus vaginal suppositories
Vagistat (tioconazole)
valacyclovir

medications *(cont.)*
- valdecoxib
- Valergen (estradiol)
- Valergen 20 (estradiol)
- Valergen 40 (estradiol)
- Valertest No. 1
- Valium
- valrubicin
- valsartan and hydrochlorothiazide
- Valstar (valrubicin)
- Valtrex (valacyclovir)
- Vantin (cefpodoxime proxetil)
- vardenafil
- Vasodilan
- Vasofem vaginal suppository
- Vasomax (phentolamine mesylate)
- vasopressin tannate in oil
- Velosef
- Venofer (iron sucrose)
- Viadur (leuprolide implant)
- Viagra (sildenafil citrate)
- Vicodin
- vidarabine
- vinblastine
- Vioxx (rofecoxib)
- VIP (VePesid, fosfamide with mesna rescue, and Platinol)
- vitamin C
- vitamin D
- Vivelle (estradiol)
- Vivelle-Dot (estradiol transdermal patch)
- Voltaren (diclofenac)
- Xanax (alprazolam)
- Xatral OD (alfuzosin)
- Xatral SR (alfuzosin)
- Xeloda (capecitabine)
- Xylocaine injectable
- Xylocaine jelly
- Xylocaine ointment
- Xylocaine spray
- Yasmin 28 (dospirenone/ethinyl estradiol) oral contraceptive

medications *(cont.)*
- Yocon (yohimbine)
- yohimbine
- Yohimex (yohimbine)
- Yutopar (ritodrine)
- Yuzpe regimen
- Zantac
- Zaroxolyn
- Zemplar (paricalcitol)
- Zenapax (daclizumab)
- zidovudine
- zinc mesoporphyrin
- zinc oxide
- Zoladex (goserelin)
- zoledronic acid for injection
- Zometa (zoledronic acid for injection)
- Zovia (ethynodiol diacetate/ethinyl estradiol) oral contraceptive
- Zovirax
- Zyloprim (allopurinol)

medicated urethral system for erection (MUSE) urethral suppository

medication-induced allograft dysfunction

medicine (see *medications*)
- maternal-fetal
- neonatal
- perinatal

MediClenze perineal lavage system

Medi-Ject needle-free insulin injection system

Medi-Jector Choice needle-free insulin injection system

Medilas-H holmium laser

Medilas-H pulsed holmium:YAG laser

mediolateral episiotomy

Medisense Pen 2 blood glucose monitor

Mediterranean fever, familial

medium chain acyl-CoA dehydrogenase deficiency (MCAD)

medium, culture

medrogestone

medroxyprogesterone
MEDS (microsurgical extraction
 of ductal sperm)
Medstone STS lithotriptor
Medstone STS shock wave generator
Medstone STS-T transportable
 lithotripsy system
medulla (pl. medullae)
 kidney
 ovarian
 renal
 suprarenal gland
medullary abscess
medullary carcinoma of breast
medullary cyst
medullary cystic disease, adult onset
medullary cystic kidney
medullary interstitium
medullary kidney
medullary necrosis
medullary nephrocalcinosis
medullary osmotic gradient
medullary pyelonephritis
medullary sponge kidney
Medworks urinary incontinence
 surgical device
mefenamic acid
Mefoxin (cefoxitin)
megabase (Mb)
Megace (megestrol)
megacystic-megaureter syndrome
megacystis-microcolon-intestinal
 hypoperistalsis syndrome
megacystic syndrome
megaesophagus
megalencephaly
megalencephaly with hyaline inclusion
megalencephaly with hyaline
 panneuropathy
megalocorneal-mental retardation
 syndrome
megaloblastic marrow change
megalocystis
megaloureter (also megaureter)
megalourethra, congenital
"mega-pocket" augmentation mammoplasty
megaureter
 infected
 primary
 secondary
 sphincteric
megestrol
Meige disease
Meigs syndrome
meiosis
meiotic prophase
melanocyte-stimulating hormone
melanoma
 acral-lentiginous
 Clark classification of vulvar
 malignant
 mucosal
 nodular
 transient neonatal pustular
 vulvar
melanuria
melanuric
MELAS (mitochondrial encephalopathy, lactic acidosis, stroke)
 syndrome
melasma
melasma gravidarum
melena neonatorum
Melkersson syndrome
mellitus
 diabetes
 neonatal diabetes
Melnick-Fraser syndrome
Melnick-Needles osteodysplasty
Melnick-Needles syndrome
melodidymus
melomelia
melphalan
membrane
 anti-glomerular basement
 (anti-GBM)
 artificial rupture of

membrane *(cont.)*
basement
bulging
cellulose
cervical
chorionic
cuprophane
dysmenorrheal
fertilization
fetal
filtering
glomerular basement (GBM)
hemofiltration
high flux
host cell
intact
mucous
peritoneal
placental
polyacrylonitrile
polysulfone
premature rupture of (PROM)
preterm premature rupture of (PPROM)
preterm rupture of
prolonged rupture of
rupture of
semipermeable
Seprafilm bioresorbable
spontaneous rupture of (SROM)
tubular basement (TBM)
urogenital
uterine mucous
membrane attack complex
membrane-based separation
membrane compaction
membrane conditioning
membrane distillation
membrane filter
membranes intact
membrane module
membrane module cell
membrane partition
membrane partition distribution coefficient
membrane permeation and extraction phenomena
membrane physical aging
membrane post-treatment
membrane pretreatment
membrane reactor
membranes ruptured spontaneously
membrane stripping
membrane unit
blood compartment of
clearance characteristics of
hydraulic coefficients of
surface area of
membrane vacuum
membranes were needled
membranes were stripped
membranitis
membranoproliferative glomerulonephritis (MPGN)
membranous dysmenorrhea
membranous endometritis
membranous glomerulonephritis (MGN)
membranous nephritis
membranous nephropathy
membranous part of urethra
membranous pregnancy
membranous urethra
membrum virile
MEN (multiple endocrine neoplasia) syndrome
type 1 (MEN1)
type 2b
menarche
delayed
early
late
normal
onset of
Mendel's first law
Mendel's second law

mendelian disorder
mendelian genetics
mendelian inheritance
Mendelson syndrome
Menest (estrogen)
Menge pessary
Mengert forceps
Mengert index in pelvimetry
Meniere disease
Menkes kinky hair syndrome
meningeal neurosyphilis
meningitis, acute syphilitic
meningocele
meningoencephalitis, syphilitic
meningovascular neurosyphilis
meningovascular syphilis
menometrorrhagia
menopausal bleeding
menopausal estrogen depletion
menopausal menorrhagia
menopausal symptoms
menopausal syndrome
menopause
  artificial
  late
  natural
  premature
  surgical
menopause praecox
Menorest (transdermal 17-beta-estradiol) hormone replacement patch
menorrhagia
  climacteric
  menopausal
  preclimacteric
  pubertal
menorrhagia of hypothyroidism
menorrhalgia
menorrhea
menotropins for injection
menouria
menoxenia
menses
  abnormal
  delayed
  spontaneous
menstrual age
menstrual colic
menstrual cramps
menstrual cycle
menstrual cycle induction
menstrual decidua
menstrual edema
menstrual extraction abortion
menstrual flow
menstrual history
menstrual leukorrhea
menstrual migraine
menstrual molimina
menstrual-ovarian cycle
menstrual period
menstruant
menstruate
menstruating
menstruation
  anovular
  anovulational
  cryoablation reduction of
  delayed
  difficult
  excessive
  frequent
  infrequent
  nonovulational
  painful
  profuse
  regularity of
  regurgitant
  retained
  retrograde
  scanty
  supplementary
  suppressed
  vicarious
mental retardation-osteodystrophy, Ruvalcaba-type

mental retardation with hypoplastic fifth fingernails and toenails
mental retardation with osteocartilaginous anomalies
Mentax (1% butenafinel)
mentoanterior (MA) position
mentoposterior (MP) position
Mentor Alpha 1 inflatable penile prosthesis
Mentor breast implant
mentotransverse position
mentum presentation
meprobamate
mercaptoacetyltriglycine (MAG3)
mercurial diuretic
Meridia (sibutramine)
mermaid syndrome
MERRF (myoclonus epilepsy associated with ragged red fibers) syndrome
Mersilene cerclage strip
Mersilene cerclage tape
Mersilene suture
Mersilene tape
MESA (microsurgical epididymal sperm aspiration)
MESE (microsurgical extraction of sperm from epididymis)
mesangial cell
mesangial cell cytoplasm
mesangial deposit
  C3
  IgA
  IgG
  IgM
mesangial disease
mesangial expansion
mesangial IgA
mesangial IgG deposition
mesangial matrix
mesangial matrix expansion
mesangial nephritis
mesangial phagocytes
mesangial proliferation
mesangial proliferative glomerulonephritis
mesangiocapillary glomerulonephritis (MPGN)
mesangioproliferative glomerulonephritis (MsPGN)
mesangium, renal
mesatipellic pelvis
mesenchymal core cell
mesenchymal tissue
mesenteric pregnancy
mesentery
mesh
  Bard Sperma-Tex preshaped
  Bard Visilex
  Brennen biosynthetic surgical
  Composix
  FortaGen surgical
  Gore-Tex DualMesh Plus
  Gore-Tex MycroMesh Plus
  Herniamesh
  Marlex
  Sepramesh biosurgical composite
  Sperma-Tex preshaped
  Trelex
  Visilex
Mesnex (mesna)
mesoappendix
mesoblastic nephroma
mesocolic hernia
mesoderm, metanephric
mesodermal dysmorphodystrophy
mesoectodermal dysplasia
mesomelic dwarfism
mesoepididymis
mesometric pregnancy
mesometrium
mesonephric adenocarcinoma
mesonephric duct
mesonephric ridge
mesorchium
mesosalpinges
mesosalpinx
mesovarian border of ovary

mesovarium (pl. mesovaria)
messenger RNA (mRNA)
metabolic acidosis, intractable
metabolic acidosis
metabolic alkalosis
metabolic decompensation
metabolic defects
metabolic derangement
metabolic disorders
metabolic disturbance
metabolic process
metabolic waste
metabolism
  acid-base
  nitrogen
metabolized to a more toxic form
metacentric chromosome
metachromatic leukodystrophy
metallic staples
Metamucil (psyllium hydrophilic mucilloid)
metanephric diverticulum
metanephric duct
metanephric mesoderm
metanephric tubule
metaphase
metaphase banding
metaphase stage of mitosis
metaphyseal chondrodysplasia, Schmidt- and McKusick-type
metaphyseal lesion in abused infants
metaphysis, apocrine
metaplasia
  apocrine
  coelomic
  squamous
metastasis (pl. metastases)
  advanced
  breast skin satellite
  calcareous
  distant
  nonskeletal
  retrograde
  skeletal
  skin
metastatic abscess
metastatic breast cancer
metastatic calcification
metastatic cascade
metastatic disease
metastatic mumps involving testis, breast, or pancreas
metastatic ovarian cancer
metastatic seeding
metastatic trophoblastic disease (MTD)
metasyphilis
metasyphilitic
metatarsus varus
metatropic dysplasia
metformin
methanol
methemoglobinuria
Methergine (methylorgonovine maleate)
methicillin-resistant *Staphylococcus aureus* (MRSA, pronounced "mer-sah")
methimazole
method
  Edwards-Steptoe in vitro fertilization
  Grantly Dick-Reed
  Krivitski
  Slow-Stop Flow Recirculation
  transvaginal ultrasound-guided drainage with trocar
  Yuzpe contraceptive
methotrexate
methyldopa
methylated X-chromosome
methylation analysis
methylene blue dye
methyl groups
methylmalonic acidemia (MMA)
methylprednisolone
methysergide
meticulous dissection
meticulous hemostasis
metoidioplasty
metolazone
metoprolol and propranolol

MetraGrasp ligament grasper
MetraPass suture passer
MetraTie knot pusher
metratonia
Metrodin (urofollitropin)
metrodynia
Metro-Gel Vaginal
metronidazole
MetraPS kit
metropathia hemorrhagica
metropathic
metropathy
metroperitonitis
metrophlebitis
metroplasty
metrorrhagia, metrorrhexis
metrorrhea
metrorrhexis metrorrhagia
metrosalpingitis
metrosalpingography
metrostaxis
metrostenosis
metrotomy
"mets" (slang for metastases)
metyrapone test
metyrosine
"Metz" (slang for Metzenbaum scissors)
Metzenbaum scissors
Mexate (methotrexate)
Mg (magnesium)
MG (myasthenia gravis)
MGN (membranous glomerulonephritis)
$MgSO_4$ (magnesium sulfate)
MHA-TP (microhemagglutination assay for antibodies to *T. pallidum*)
MHC (myosin heavy chain)
Miacalcin (calcitonin) nasal spray
MIBB breast biopsy system
Michaelis-Gutmann bodies
miconazole nitrate
Micral chemstrip urine test
Micral urine dipstick test
MICRhoGAM
micrencephaly
microadhesiolysis
microalbuminuria
microangiopathic hemolytic anemia
microarray technology
microbial genetics
microbubble contrast agent
microcalcifications
  breast
  clustered
microcephaly
microcoil
  Intercept prostate
  Intercept urethra
microcystic disease of renal medulla
microcystic dysplasia
microcytic anemia
microdeletion
microdeletion syndrome
microdialysis
microepididymal sperm aspiration (MESA)
micro-F (microimmunofluorescence)
microfiltration
microflora, vaginal
microfocal spot mammography
microgamete
microgametocyte
microgenitalism
Microgestin Fe 1.5/30 oral contraceptive pill
micrognathia
Microgyn resectoscope safety sheath
microgyria
Micro-H hysteroscope
microhemagglutination assay for antibodies to *T. pallidum* (MHA-TP)
microinjection of a single sperm
microimmunofluorescence (micro-F) test
microinvasion
MicroLap and Microlap Gold microlaparoscopy systems

microlaparoscope (see *also endoscope; laparoscope*)
  MicroLap
  MicroLap Gold
  VerreScope
Microlens
Microlet Vaculance finger stick device
microlithiasis, testicular
micromanipulating and cloning embryos
micromanipulation
micromanipulation of sperm and egg
micromazia
micromelia
micrometastatic disease
micrometastatic involvement of pelvic lymph nodes
micromoles per liter (μmol/L)
micronized progesterone
micropenis
microphthalmia
microsalpingoplasty
microsatellite
microsatellite instability (MSI)
microscope
  dark-field
  electron
  light
  phase-contrast
microscopic fern pattern of amniotic fluid
microscopic hematuria
microscopic polyarteritis
microscopic tubal ligation reversal
microscopic vasectomy reversal
microscopy
  electron
  immunofluorescence
  immunofluorescent
  light
  polarized light
  scanning electron
microsomal autoantibodies (MSA)
microsomia
MicroSpan microhysteroscopy system
MicroSpan minihysteroscopy system
MicroSpan sheath
Microspike approximator clamp
Microsulis microwave endometrial ablation system
microsurgery
microsurgical denervation of spermatic cord
microsurgical epididymal sperm aspiration (MESA)
microsurgical epididymovasostomy (MSEV)
microsurgical extraction of ductal sperm (MEDS)
microsurgical free tissue transfer
microsurgical inguinal varicocele repair
microsurgical reconstruction of the seminal tract
microsurgical technique
microsurgical tubal reanastomosis (MTR)
microthelia
microthrombosis
microtubular glomerulopathy
microtia
microvascular technique
microvillus inclusion disease
microwave endometrial ablation (MEA)
microwave nonsurgical treatment for benign prostatic hypertrophy
microwave thermotherapy
  Prostatron
  Urowave
microwave thermotherapy of prostate
micturate
micturating cystourethrogram
Micturin (terodiline)
micturition, frequent
micturition reflex
micturition syncope
Miculicz peritoneal clamp
midback, right
middle fetal death

middle kidney
middle lobe hyperplasia
middle molecules
middle suprarenal artery
midface, fetal
midforceps delivery
midgestational sciatic nerve transection
midgut volvulus
mid-isthmus
midline episiotomy
midline incision
midmenstrual
midpelvis
midportion of fallopian tube
midposition uterus
midshaft of penis
midstream
midstream urine (MSU)
midtubal in the ampulla
midway between symphysis pubis and umbilicus
midwife
migration
migration pattern
Mifegyne (mifepristone)
mifepristone (RU 486)
migraine, menstrual
migration of ovum
mild fetal bradycardia
mild hydronephrosis
mild hyperemesis gravidarum
mild pre-eclampsia
mild urge incontinence
milestones, developmental
miliaria
milk-alkali syndrome
milk anemia
milk duct
milk, inspissated
milk let-down reflex
milk of magnesia (MOM)
milky nipple discharge
milky urine
Millen retropubic prostatectomy
Millennium MLC-120
Miller-Dieker syndrome
Miller syndrome
millimoles per liter (mmol/L)
Millin bladder neck spreader
Millin-Read urethrovesical suspension
Milli oral contraceptive
Millon reagent
Milne-Murray axis traction
Milroy disease
Miltex IUD extractor
Miltex-Kogan endocervical speculum
mimetic labor
mimic gene
mineralocorticoid replacement therapy
Minesse (gestodene, progestin, and ethinyl estradiol)
mini-colpostat tandem and ovoids system
Miniguard urinary incontinence device
minilap (minilaparotomy)
minilaparotomy
minilaparotomy incision
minilaparotomy pelvic lymph node dissection
minilaparotomy staging pelvic lymphadenectomy
minimal cervical dysplasia
minimal change disease (MCD)
minimal change glomerulonephritis (MCGN)
minimal change glomerulopathy
minimal change nephropathy
minimal change nephrotic syndrome
minimally invasive fetal surgery
minimally invasive kidney donation
minimally invasive surgery
miniretractor, laparoscopic
minisatellite
MiniSite laparoscope
mini Tischler delicate biopsy punch
minor calices
minora, labia
minor, emancipated

Minovlar oral contraceptive
minus, labium
Miralene suture
Miraluma (technetium ^{99m}Tc sestamibi kit)
Miraluma nuclear breast imaging
Mircette (desogestrel/ethinyl estradiol) oral contraceptive
Mirena (levonorgestrel-releasing intrauterine contraceptive)
mirror image breast biopsy
mirror imaging
MIS (müllerian inhibiting substance)
miscarriage
miscegenation
mismatch repair mechanism
mispairing
missed abortion
missed delivery
missed labor
missense mutation
missing chromosomes
Mitchell epispadias repair
Mitek suture anchor
Mithracin (plicamycin)
mitochondria
mitochondrial chromosome
mitochondrial dysfunction
mitochondrial DNA (mtDNA)
mitochondrial encephalopathy (MELAS)
mitochondrial gene
mitochondrial inheritance
mitochondrial myopathy
mitochondrial myopathy, encephalopathy, lactic acidosis, and strokelike episodes
mitomycin, mitomycin-C
mitosis (pl. mitoses)
mitoxantrone
mitral valve prolapse (MVP)
Mitrofanoff appendicovesicotomy
Mitrofanoff continent urinary diversion
Mitrofanoff neourethra procedure
Mitrofanoff principle
mittelschmerz
Mityvac cup
Mityvac vacuum delivery system
mixed apnea
mixed connective tissue disease (MCTD)
mixed cryoglobulinemia
mixed hemorrhoids
mixed hyperlipidemia
mixed genital flora
mixed membranous and proliferative glomerulonephritis
mixed mesodermal tumor
mixed-type incontinence
Miyazaki-Bonney test for stress urinary incontinence
ML4 (mucolipidosis, type 4)
MLL gene
MMA (methylmalonic acidemia)
MMF (mycophenolate mofetil)
MMK (Marshall-Marchetti-Krantz) procedure
MMMK (modified Marshall-Marchetti-Krantz) procedure
MMP21-22
μmol/L (millimoles per liter)
MMPI (matrix metalloproteinase inhibitor)
MMR (measles-mumps-rubella) vaccine
MoAb monoclonal antibody
Mobetron electron accelerator
mobile carrier
mobile kidney
mobile uterus
mobilization
  breast
  cecum
  rib
  uterine
Möbius syndrome (also Moebius)

model
  Claus breast cancer
  Gail breast cancer
  Markov simulation
modeling
  fetal skull
  kinetic
mode of inheritance
moderate ductal hyperplasia
moderate hydronephrosis
moderately dilated ureter
moderate postvoid residual
modern genetics
Modicon-28 oral contraceptive
modified Benelli round block mastopexy
modified bulbar urethral sling
modified citrus pectin
modified dorsal lithotomy position
modified Kun colocolponeopoiesis
modified Kun colocolpopoiesis
modified Marshall-Marchetti-Krantz (MMMK) procedure
modified mastopexy
modified Pereyra bladder neck suspension
modified Pomeroy technique
modified Prague maneuver
modified radical hysterectomy
modified radical mastectomy
modified Thayer-Martin medium (MTM)
modified vulvectomy
modified Wertheim procedure for microinvasive carcinoma
modifier gene
MODM (maturity onset diabetes mellitus)
MODS (multiple organ dysfunction syndrome)
Modulap coagulation probe
modular clip application system (MCAS)
Modulith SL 20 lithotriptor
MODY (maturity onset diabetes of the young)
Moebius syndrome (also Möbius)
MOF (multiple organ failure)
Mogen circumcision clamp
Mohr syndrome
moist sponge on ring forceps
molar
  hutchinsonian
  mulberry
molar pregnancy
molding and caput of fetal vertex
molding of fetal head by birth canal
molding of head
mold nephrosis
mole
  carneous
  cystic
  fleshy
  hydatid
  hydatidiform
  invasive
  malignant hydatidiform
  stone
  vesicular
molecular genetics
molecular genetic testing
molecular heterogeneity
molecular technique
molecular-weight cutoff
molecule
  antibody
  filtered
  middle
  secreted
mole fractions
molimen, menstrual
molimina
  menstrual
  premenstrual
MOLLY bipolar forceps
Molnar disk
MoM (multiples of the median)
Mondor disease

mongolian spots
mongolism
monilethrix
monilia infection
monilial cystitis
monilial prostatitis
monilial vulvovaginitis
moniliasis, neonatal
Monistat (miconazole nitrate)
Monistat Dual-Pak
Monistat 1 ointment
Monistat 3 Combo
Monistat 3 vaginal cream
Monistat 7 vaginal cream
monitor (also monitoring)
  actocardiotocograph
  Bear NUM-1 tidal volume
  CALM II (computer-assisted labor)
  ClearPlan fertility
  Colormate TLc.BiliTest bilirubinometer
  Corometrics maternal/fetal
  Doppler ultrasonic fetal heart
  DRx quantitative hCG patient
  EFM (electronic fetal)
  electronic fetal heart (EFM)
  end-tidal carbon dioxide
  external fetal
  fetal
  fetal scalp
  Flo-Stat
  Glucochek Pocketlab II blood glucose
  Glucometer DEX
  Gluco-Protein OTC self-test
  Healthdyne apnea
  internal fetal
  OLC (On Line Clearance)
  On Line Clearance (OLC) dialysis
  One Touch Basic blood glucose
  One Touch FastTake blood glucose
  One Touch II hospital blood glucose
  OxiFirst fetal
  Propaq Encore neonatal vital signs

monitor *(cont.)*
  PSC Fertility
  Select GT blood glucose
  Sof-Tact glucose
  Supreme II blood glucose
  SureStep blood glucose
  TD Glucose
  television
monoamine oxidase (MAO) inhibitors
monoaminuria
monoamnionic
monoamniotic sac
monoamniotic twins
monochorial twins
monochorionic diamnionic placenta
monochorionic diamniotic placenta
monochorionic monoamnionic placenta
monochorionic monoamniotic placenta
monochorionic twins
Monocid (cefonicid sodium)
monoclonal antibody
  anti-HER2
  anti-HER2 humanized
  basiliximab
  Campath
  dacliximab
  daclizumab
  Ha1A
  Herceptin (trastuzumab) anti-HER2
  IgG 2A (Immurait)
  Immurait (IgG 2A)
  MAb
  MAb-170
  MoAb
  Muromonab-CD3
  Orthoclone OKT3
  satumomab pendetide
  Simulect (basiliximab)
  trastuzumab
Monocryl suture
monocyte
monocyte/macrophage
monoecious
monofilament nylon sutures

monogamous sexual relationship
monogenic
monogenous
monohybrid cross
Monojector finger stick device
monolayers of surface-active component
monomodal visual amnesia
mononuclear interstitial infiltrate
mono-ovular twins
monopolar cautery or electrocautery
monopolar plug
monorchia
monorchid
monorchidism
monorchism
monorhinic
monosomia
monosomy (see also *syndrome*)
monosomy 1p36
monosomy 2q37.3
monosomy 10
monosomy 15q
monosomy 21q
monosomy 22
monosomy 22q11
monosomy X
monosomy X with gonadal streak
monospermy
monosyphilide
monotherapy
monozygosity
monozygotic twins
mons (pl. montes)
mons pubis
mons ureteris
mons veneris
Monsel hemostatic solution
Monsel paste
Monsel' solution
Montevideo units
Monurol (fosfomycin tromethamine)
Moolgaoker forceps
moon face or facies
Moore Graves vaginal speculum
Moore ovum forceps
Moravcsik-Marinesco-Sjögren syndrome
morbidity
  maternal
  puerperal
morbidity following biopsy
morcellated nephrectomy
morcellation
  tissue
  uterine
morcellation vaginal hysterectomy
morcellator
  Cook tissue
  Diva laparoscopic
Morgagni cyst
Morgagni hydatid
Morganstern continuous-flow operating cystoscope
moricizine
morning after pill
morning erection
morning sickness
morning urine
morning vomiting
Moro reflex
morphine
morphological proportions
morphologic data
morphology
Morquio syndrome
Morris syndrome
mortality
  fetal
  maternal
  perinatal
mortar kidney
Morvan disease
mosaic chromosome complement
mosaic 5p tetrasomy
mosaicism
  chromosomal
  germinal
  gonadal

mosaic state
mosaic tetrasomy
Moschcowitz culdoplasty
mosquito clamp
moth-eaten alopecia of secondary
  syphilis
"moth-eaten" appearance on imaging
mother and baby endoscope
mother-infant bonding
motherscope
mother surrogate
Mother2Be skin and body care products
motif
motile organism
motile sperm per high power field (hpf)
motility
motion, fetal
motor impulse of bladder
motor neuron disease
motor paralytic bladder
moulage for custom breast implant
mouse model
mouth, pursestring
movable kidney
movable testis
movement
  fetal
  spontaneous fetal
moyamoya disease
MP (mentoposterior) position
MPGN (membranoproliferative
  glomerulonephritis)
MPIF-1 (myeloid progenitor inhibitory
  factor-1)
MPO (myeloperoxidase)
MPS (mucopolysaccharidosis)
MPS I-H Hurler
MPS I-H/S Hurler/Scheie
MPS I-S Scheie
MPS II Hunter
MPS IIIA Sanfilippo
MPS IVA Morquio
MPS VI Maroteaux-Lamy
MPS VII Sly
MQSA (Mammography Quality
  Standards Act)
MRI (magnetic resonance imaging)
MRI-guided breast biopsy
MRI procedures
  3-D gadolinium-enhanced MR
    angiography
  magnetic resonance mammography
  magnetic resonance urography
  proton magnetic resonance
    spectroscopy
MRM (magnetic resonance mammog-
  raphy)
mRNA (messenger RNA)
MRSA (methicillin-resistant
  Staphylococcus aureus)
MR-915 pediatric cystoscope
MRO-6 operating ureteroscope
MRO-2004 rigid percutaneous
  nephroscope
MRO-2005 rigid percutaneous
  nephroscope
MRU (magnetic resonance urography)
MS (multiple sclerosis)
MSA (microsomal autoantibodies)
MSAFP (maternal serum alpha-
  fetoprotein)
MSEV (microsurgical epididymo-
  vasostomy)
MSI (microsatellite instability)
MSOF (multisystem organ failure)
MsPGN (mesangioproliferative
  glomerulonephritis)
MSU (midstream urine)
MSUD (maple sugar urine disease)
mtDNA (mitochondrial DNA)
M3G telescope
MTM (modified Thayer-Martin
  [culture] medium)
MTM (myotubular myopathy)
MTR (microsurgical tubal
  reanastomosis)
MTS1 tumor suppressor gene
MTX (methotrexate)

mucinous carcinoma
mucinous cyst
mucinous cystadenocarcinoma
mucocutaneous lesion
mucocutaneous relapse
mucoid material
mucolipidosis types 1-4
mucopolysaccharide
mucopolysaccharidosis (MPS)
mucoprotein, Tamm-Horsfall
mucopurulent discharge
mucormycosis
mucorrhea
mucosa
  appendiceal
  bladder
  cervix uteri
  endocervical
  intussuscepted appendiceal
  necrosis of bladder
  prolapsed urethral
  renal pelvis
  seminal gland
  ureteral
  urethral
  urinary
  uterine tube
  vaginal
mucosal dissection
mucosal fold
mucosal melanoma
mucosal neuroma syndrome
mucosal surface
mucosal ulceration
mucosanguineous discharge
mucosulfatidosis
mucous (adj.)
mucous membrane
mucous plug
mucous polyp of cervix
mucoviscidosis
MUCP (maximum urethral closure pressure)
mucus aspiration bulb for infant suctioning
mucus, cervical
mucus receptivity
mucus secretion
Mueller-Hillis maneuver
mulberry calculus
mulberry molar
mulberry ovary
mulibrey nanism syndrome
Müller duct
mullerian agenesis
mullerian cyst
mullerian duct
mullerian duct abnormality
mullerian duct anomaly
mullerian dysgenesis
mullerian inhibiting substance (MIS)
MultAport cannula
MultApplier clip applier
MultApump disposable pump
MultAvalue laparoscopic system
multiagent therapy
multicentric cancerous lesions
multicentric lesion
multichannel implantable urinary prosthesis
multicolor banding (MCB) studies
multicystic dysplastic kidney
multicystic ovaries with thickened capsules
multidrug systemic chemotherapy
multifactorial disorder
multifactorial inheritance
multifetal pregnancy
multifetal pregnancy reduction
Multifire Endo GIA stapler
Multifire GIA stapler
Multifire VersaTack
Multi-Flex urologic stent
multigenic disorder
multigravida
Multikine (leukocyte; interleukin)

multilamination of lamina densa
multilocal genetics
multilocular cyst
multiloculated cyst
multinodular goiter
multiorgan dysfunction syndrome (MODS)
multipara
multiparity, grand
multiparous cervix
multiparous uterus
multiple abscess formation
multiple allelism
multiple angiomas and enchondromas
multiple arbitrary amplicon profiling (MAAP)
multiple birth
multiple cartilaginous exostoses
multiple colloid adenomatous goiter (MCAG)
multiple congenital anomaly (MCA) syndrome
multiple endocrine adenomatosis (MEA), types 1-3
multiple endocrine deficiency syndrome type II, Schmidt-type
multiple endocrine neoplasia (MEN)
multiple epiphyseal dysplasias
multiple fetuses
multiple gestation
multiple hereditary exostoses
multiple lentigines syndrome
multiple myeloma
multiple organ dysfunction syndrome (MODS)
multiple organ failure (MOF)
multiple organ involvement
multiple organ system failure
multiple polyposis
multiple pregnancies
multiple pterygium syndrome
multiple renal calculi
multiple sclerosis (MS)
multiple sexual partners
multiple-site perineal applicator (MUPIT)
multiple sulfatase deficiency
multiples of the median (MoM)
multiplexing
multiprong administration manifold and drainage bag
MultiPulse laser
Multispatula cervical sampling device
multisynostotic osteodysgenesis
multisystem disease
multisystem organ failure (MSOF)
MultiVysion PB assay for identification of chromosomal abnormalities
Mulvihill-Smith syndrome
mummified fetus
mumps, metastatic
mumps orchitis
Munro and Parker LAVH procedure
Munro-Kerr cesarean section
mupirocin ointment
MUPIT (multiple-site perineal applicator)
mural kidney
mural pregnancy
MURCS association
Murdoch intraoperative laparoscopic lens cleaner
Murless fetal head extractor
murmur
  functional
  innocent
  machinery
muromonab-CD3 monoclonal antibody
muscle
  artificial sphincter
  bulbocavernosus
  bulbospongiosus
  coccygeus
  detrusor
  gracilis
  Houston
  internal oblique
  ischiocavernous

muscle *(cont.)*
- ischiospongiosus
- latissimus dorsi
- levator ani
- pectoral
- pectoralis
- pectoralis major
- pectoralis minor
- pelvic
- pelvic floor
- psoas
- pubococcygeal
- rectouterine
- rectovesicalis
- rectovesicle
- rectus urethralis
- serratus anterior
- sphincter
- superficial transverse perineal
- teres major
- ureteral smooth
- urinary sphincter

muscle clonus
muscle core disease
muscle-eye-brain disorder
muscle guarding
muscle layer
- female urethra
- male urethra
- renal pelvis
- seminal gland
- spongy urethra
- ureter
- urinary bladder
- uterine tube
- vaginal

muscle pedicle
muscle phosphofructokinase deficiency
muscle phosphorylase deficiency
muscle-splitting incision
muscular atony
muscular dystrophy (MD)
- Duchenne
- Landouzy-Dejerine

muscularis
musculofascial sling
musculoglandular organ
musculomucoid intimal hyperplasia
MUSE (medicated urethral system for erection) urethral suppository
Mutamycin (mitomycin)
mutant allele
mutant gene PKD1 in diagnosis of ADPKD
mutation
- BRCA
- gene
- p53

mutational event
mutation analysis
mutation, disease-causing
mutation scanning
mutation variability
mutator mutation
mutilation, female genital
mutism, elective or selective
MVAC (methotrexate, vincristine, Adriamycin, cisplatin) chemotherapy protocol
MVAC or M-VAC (methotrexate, vincristine, Adriamycin, cisplatin)
MVF (mitoxantrone, vincristine, fluorouracil) chemotherapy protocol
MVP (mitral valve prolapse)
myalgia
myasthenia gravis (MG), neonatal
myasthenic syndrome of Lambert-Eaton
Mycelex (clotrimazole)
Mycelex Twin Pack (clotrimazole)
mycobacteria
Mycobacterium tuberculosis
mycophenolate mofetil (MMF)
Mycoplasma
mycosis
Mycostatin (nystatin)
mycotic nephrosis
mycotic penile disease
myelin kidney

myelinoclastic diffuse sclerosis
myelodysplasia
myeloid progenitor inhibitory factor-1 (MPIF-1)
myeloma
  kidney
  multiple
myeloma protein
myelomeningocele closure in utero
myelomeningocele, fetal
myelomonocytic leukemia
myeloperoxidase (MPO)
myeloschisis
myelosuppression
myelosyphilis
myelosyringosis
Myhre syndrome
Mylocel (hydroxyurea)
myoadenylate deaminase deficiency
Myocet (liposome-encapsulated doxorubicin citrate complex and cyclophosphamide)
myoclonic encephalopathy of infants
myoclonic epilepsy associated with ragged red fibers (MERRF)
myoclonus
myocolpitis
myocutaneous flap
myoencephalopathy ragged red fiber disease
myofibromatosis
  infantile
  juvenile
myoglobinuria
myoglobulinuria
myoma (pl. myomata)
  pedunculated uterine
  prostatic
  uterine
myoma screw
  hysteroscopic
  laparoscopic
myomatous uterus
myomectomy
  abdominal
  uterine
  vaginal
myometrial activity
myometrial endometriosis
myometritis
myometrium
  endometriosis of
  hypotonic
  intervening
myometrium of corpus of uterus
myoneurogenic disorder
myopathy
  congenital, Batten-Turner-type
  desmin storage
  distal
  lipid
  metabolic
  mitochondrial
  myotubular
  scapuloperoneal
  steroid
  uremic
myophosphorylase deficiency
myopia
myosalpingitis
myosalpinx
myosin heavy chain (MHC)
myositis, inclusion body (IBM)
myotonia congenita
myotonic dystrophy (MD)
myotubular myopathy (MTM)
myouterine flap
myxedema coma
myxedema madness
myxedema, pretibial
myxedematous infantilism
M-Zole 3 Combination Pack
M-Zole 7 Combination Pack
M-Zole 7 Dual Pack

N, n

N (nitrogen)
Na (sodium)
nabothian cyst
nabothian follicle
N-acetyl glutamate synthetase (NAGS) deficiency
NaCl (sodium chloride)
NACS (Neurologic and Adaptive Capacity Score)
nafarelin
Nägele rule for calculation of EDC
Nager syndrome
nail-patella syndrome
nails, half-and-half
NALS (neonatal adjuvant life support)
nanocephaly
nanofiltration
nanogram (millimicrogram)
naratriptan
narcolepsy
Naropin (ropivacaine)
narrow lateral Heaney retractor
narrowness of the vagina
NAS (neonatal abstinence syndrome)
nasal cannula
nasal flaring
nasalfrontofacial dysplasia
Nashville Rabbit Antithymocyte Serum
nasogastric (NG) tube
nasolabial
nasolacrimal embryonic groove
nasomaxillary hypoplasia
NASS (Neonatal Abstinence Scoring System)
National CAPD Registry
National Diabetes Data Group
National Institute of Diabetes and Digestive and Kidney Diseases (NIDDK)
National Kidney Foundation
National Organization of Circumcision Information Resource Centers (NOCIRC)
native C3
native dilated ureter
native kidney
native vasculature
natriuresis
natural childbirth
natural cleavage of placenta
natural family planning methods
natural father
natural fertility signs

natural hormone replacement therapy (NHRT)
natural selection
naturopath (NP)
nausea and vomiting (N/V)
nausea gravidarum
nausea, pregnancy-related
navel cord infection
navel string
navicular fossa of the urethra
Navratil retractor
NB/70K ovarian cancer test
NBS1 gene
NDI (nephrogenic diabetes insipidus)
near-fatal hemorrhage of kidney
Nearly Me breast implant
Nearly Me breast prosthesis
near-syncopal episode
near-syncope necrotic tumor
nebulous urine
NEC (necrotizing enterocolitis)
necessary cause
neck
  bladder
  cord around
  cord tightly around
  cord wrapped around
  urinary bladder
  uterine
  vesical
  womb
Necon 0.5/35 norethindrone/ethinyl estradiol) oral contraceptive
Necon 1/35 norethindrone/ethinyl estradiol) oral contraceptive
Necon 1/50 (norethindrone/mestranol) oral contraceptive
Necon 10/11 (norethindrone/ethinyl estradiol) oral contraceptive
necrosadism
necrosis
  acute tubular (ATN)
  bladder epithelium
  bladder mucosa

necrosis *(cont.)*
  blood vessel
  cortical
  endometrial
  fat
  focal
  glomerular fibrinoid
  gummatous
  ischemic
  medullary
  papillary
  papillary tissue
  penile
  radiation
  renal artery
  renal cortical
  renal medullary
  segmental
  soft tissue
  tubular
  tumor
  vascular
necrospermia
necrotic fibroid
necrotizing arteriolitis in kidney
necrotizing enterocolitis (NEC)
necrotizing enterocolitis in newborn
necrotizing fasciitis
necrotizing glomerulitis
necrotizing glomerulonephritis
necrotizing nephrosis
necrotizing renal papillitis
needle
  Accucore II
  Baker amniocentesis
  Biopty cut
  Chiba biopsy
  Cobb-Ragde
  colposuspension
  Core aspiration/injection
  core biopsy
  Core aspiration/injection
  Core CO_2 insufflation
  Craft aspiration

needle *(cont.)*
DiaCan fistula
dialysis fistula
Dominion aspiration
Echo-Coat ultrasound biopsy
Echotip amniocentesis
Echotip culdocentesis
Echotip Dominion aspiration
Echotip Foothills
Echotip Kato-Asch coaxial
Echotip LANCET
Echotip Mannuti sampling
Echotip Norfolk aspiration
Echotip percutaneous entry
Echotip Pivet-Cook double lumen
electrode
Endoknot suture
Endopath Ultra Veress
Fettouh bladder suspension
Foothills
Franseen biopsy
GraNee
Gynepath biopsy
Gynex extended-reach
Hawkins breast localization
Kopans breast lesion localization
LANCET
laparoscopic port closure
Lee-Ray aspiration biopsy
Maciol laparoscopic suture
Madayag biopsy
Mannuti
Martin cutting
Mayo
Mayo noncutting
Neuro-Trace
Norfolk aspiration
Nottingham colposuspension
PCB (paracervical block)
paracervical block (PCB)
P.D. Access
pencil-point suprapubic access
Pivet-Cook double lumen

needle *(cont.)*
pneumoperitoneum
Pneu-Stick
Quick-Core II biopsy
Quintero amniocentesis
Riza-Ribe grasper
Rutner biopsy
Safety AV fistula
silicon
Silverman
spinal
Stamey
Sutureloop needle/suture
Terry-Mayo
Touhy
transluminal angioplasty
Turner biopsy
ultrasound biopsy
Unimar J-Needle
Veress (not Verres)
Visi-Black surgical
Voorhees

needle aspiration
needle aspiration of cystic structure
needle biopsy
needle decompression of corpora
needle driver
endoscopic curved
Talon curved
needle electrode, BiLAP bipolar
needle guide, Iowa trumpet
needle holder
Bihrle
Dubecq-Princeteau angulating
Nolan
needle inserted under fluoroscopic control
needle localization, mammographically guided
needle localization of breast lesion
needle-nose forceps
needlepoint electrocautery
needle-tip electrocautery

needle urethropexy incontinence
procedure
needling of hydrocephalic head
needling of membranes
N.E.E. oral contraceptive
negative antibody screen
negative breast biopsy
negative cytology
negative interference
negative predictive value
negative serology
negative stroke margin on breast biopsy
negative, Rh
neighboring alleles
neighboring loci
Neisseria gonorrhoeae, chromosomally
mediated resistant
Nellcor oximetry
Nelova 10/11 oral contraceptive
Nelson tissue forceps
Nelulen 1/50 oral contraceptive
nemaline myopathy (NM)
neoadjuvant hormonal therapy (NHT)
neobladder
ileal
orthotopic
W-stapled ileal
neobladder construction following total
cystectomy
Neo-Calglucon
Neocate infant formula
neocentromerization
neoclitoris
Neocon oral contraceptive
NeoControl pelvic floor therapy system
NeoControl urinary incontinence
control device
NeoCure Cryoablation System
neodarwinism
neodymium:yttrium-aluminum-garnet
(Nd:YAG) laser
neofetal
neofetus
Neoflex bendable knife electrocautery
NeoKnife electrosurgical instrument
neomycin
Neonatal Abstinence Scoring System
(NASS)
neonatal abstinence syndrome (NAS)
neonatal adjuvant life support (NALS)
neonatal acne
neonatal adrenal ultrasound
neonatal adrenoleukodystrophy
neonatal anemia
neonatal apoplexy
neonatal *Candida* infection
neonatal candidiasis
neonatal conjunctivitis
neonatal cystic pulmonary emphysema
neonatal dacryocystitis
neonatal death, early
neonatal dehydration
neonatal diabetes mellitus
neonatal diagnosis
Neonatal Facial Coding System
neonatal fellow
neonatal hepatic conjugating enzymes
neonatal hepatitis
neonatal hyperammonemic encephalopathy
neonatal hyperbilirubinemia
neonatal hyperthyroidism
neonatal hypocalcemic tetany
neonatal hypoglycemia
neonatal hypoparathyroidism
Neonatal Infant Pain Scale (NIPS)
neonatal infective mastitis
neonatal intensive care unit (NICU)
neonatal intracranial hemorrhage
neonatal jaundice
neonatal line
neonatal lupus
neonatal lupus erythematosus
neonatal medicine
neonatal moniliasis
neonatal mortality rate
neonatal mortality risk (NMR)
neonatal myasthenia gravis

neonatal neutropenia
neonatal nurse practitioner
neonatal resuscitation team
neonatal sepsis
neonatal survival and neurological morbidity
neonatal tetanus
neonatal tetany
neonatal thrombocytopenia
neonatal thyrotoxicosis
neonatal urinary tract infection
neonate
neonatologist
neonatology
neonatorum
  acne
  anoxia
  edema
  erythroblastosis
  icterus
  icterus gravis
  impetigo
  keratolysis
  ophthalmia
  pemphigus
  polycythemia
  sclerema
  tetanus
  urticaria
neopenis
neophalloplasties
neophalloplasty
neoplasia
  cervical
  cervical intraepithelial (CIN)
  endometrial intraepithelial
  gestational trophoblastic (GTN)
  preinvasive urothelial
  tubal
  urinary tract
  urinary tract epithelial
  vaginal intraepithelial
  vulvar intraepithelial
neoplasm
  androgen-producing
  benign
  breast
  cystic
  encapsulated
  estrogen-producing
  firm
  functioning
  germ cell ovarian
  gonadal
  lethal
  low grade
  ovarian
  primary
  spherical
  well-circumscribed
neoplasms producing androgens
neoplasms producing estrogens
neoplasms producing hCG
neoplastic cyst of ovary
neoplastic extension
neoplastic lesion
neoplastic ovarian cyst
Neoprobe 1000 gamma-detection probe
Neoral (cyclosporine)
neosalpingostomy, CO_2 laser surgery
Neosar (cyclophosphamide)
neoscrotum
Neo-Sert umbilical vessel catheter insertion set
Neostar hemodialysis catheter
Neosure infant formula
NeoTect disease-specific imaging agent
Neotrend system
neourethra, unobstructed
neovagina, rectal
neovascularization in human breast cancer
NephrAmine amino acid preparation
nephrectomy
  abdominal
  laparoscopic
  lumbar

nephrectomy *(cont.)*
  morcellated
  paraperitoneal
  partial
  posterior
  radical
  transabdominal radical
nephredema
nephrelcosis
nephric
nephritic calculus
nephritic colic
nephritic factor, C3
nephritic syndrome
nephritis (pl. nephritides)
  acute
  acute interstitial
  acute noninfective tubulointerstitial
  allergic interstitial
  analgesic
  anti-glomerular basement membrane
  anti-kidney serum
  arteriosclerotic
  azotemic
  bacterial
  Balkan
  capsular
  caseous
  cheesy
  chloroazotemic
  chronic
  congenital
  diffuse
  diffuse membranous lupus
  dropsical
  epimembranous
  exudative
  fibrolipomatous
  fibrous
  focal
  focal mesangial lupus
  glomerular
  glomerulocapsular
  hemorrhagic

nephritis *(cont.)*
  Henoch-Schönlein
  hereditary
  Heymann
  immune complex
  indurative
  interstitial
  Lancereaux
  lupus
  Masugi
  membranous
  mesangial
  nephrotoxic serum
  parenchymatous
  pneumococcus
  potassium losing
  salt-losing
  saturnine
  scarlatinal
  serum
  subacute
  suppurative
  syphilitic
  toxic
  transfusion
  tubal
  tubular
  tuberculous
  tubulointerstitial
  vascular
nephritis caseosa
nephritis dolorosa
nephritis gravidarum
nephritis of pregnancy
nephritis repens
nephritogenic
nephroangiosclerosis
  benign
  malignant
nephroblastoma
nephrocalcinosis, medullary
nephrocardiac
nephrocele
nephrocyst anastomosis

nephrocystosis
nephrogenetic
nephrogenic adenoma
nephrogenic ascites
nephrogenic diabetes insipidus (NDI)
nephrogenous
nephrogram effect
nephrographic phase (NP)
nephrography
nephrohypertrophy
nephroid
nephrolith
nephrolithiasis
  calcium
  urate
  uric acid
nephrolithotomy, percutaneous (PCNL)
nephrolithotripsy, percutaneous
nephrologist, pediatric
nephrology
nephrolysin
nephrolysis
nephrolytic
nephromalacia
nephroma, mesoblastic
nephromegaly
nephron
  distal
  residual
nephron function
nephron involvement
nephron solute exchange
nephronophthisis
  familiar juvenile
  juvenile
nephronophthisis-uremic medullary
  cystic disease (UMCD)
nephropathic
nephropathy
  acute
  analgesic
  Balkan
  benign reflux
  bilateral reflux

nephropathy *(cont.)*
  chronic
  Danubian endemic familial
  diabetic (DN)
  gouty
  hereditary
  HIV-associated
  hypazoturic
  hypercalcemic
  hypocalcemic
  hypokalemic
  hypomagnesemic
  idiopathic membranous
  IgA (immunoglobulin A)
  IgM (immunoglobulin M)
  ischemic
  light chain
  malignancy-associated
  membranous
  minimal change
  mycotoxic
  obstructive
  potassium depletion
  potassium losing
  reflux
  sickle cell
  silicon
  thin basement membrane
  toxic
  urate
  uric acid
  vasomotor
nephropathy in pregnancy
nephropexy, laparoscopic
nephrophthisis, familial juvenile
nephroptosis
nephropyeloureterostomy
nephropyosis
nephrorrhaphy
nephros
nephrosclerosis
  arterial
  arteriolar
  arteriosclerotic

nephrosclerosis *(cont.)*
- benign
- benign arteriolar
- hypertensive
- malignant
- senile

nephrosclerotic
nephroscope (see also *endoscope*)
- ACMI
- Elite
- MRO-20
- MRO-2004
- MRO-2005
- Olympus CHF-P10
- Pentax ECN-1530 choledocho-nephroscope
- percutaneous
- rigid

nephroscopy
nephrosis
- acute
- acute lobar
- amyloid
- cholemic
- chronic
- Epstein
- familial
- functional
- glycogen
- hemoglobinuric
- hydropic
- hypokalemic
- hypoxic
- infectious avian
- lavral
- lipid
- lipoid
- lower nephron
- mold
- mycotic
- necrotizing
- osmotic
- toxic
- vacuolar

nephrostogram, postprocedure
nephrostolithotomy, percutaneous (PCNL)
nephrostoma
nephrostome
nephrostomy
- cutaneous intubated
- percutaneous

nephrostomy balloon catheter
nephrostomy drainage
nephrostomy tube
nephrostomy-type catheter
nephrotic edema
nephrotic-range hematuria
nephrotic-range proteinuria
nephrotic syndrome with hematuria
nephrotome
nephrotomic
nephrotomogram
nephrotomography
nephrotomy, anatrophic
nephrotoxic agent
nephrotoxic aminoglycoside
nephrotoxic antibiotics
nephrotoxic contrast medium
nephrotoxic drug
nephrotoxic reaction
nephrotoxic serum nephritis
nephrotoxicity
- acute cyclosporine
- drug-induced
- solvent

nephrotoxin
nephrotropic MR imaging contrast
nephrotuberculosis
nephroureterectasis
nephroureterectomy, radical
nephroureterocystectomy
Nephrox (aluminum hyroxide; mineral oil)
Nepro dietary supplement
Nepro nutritional formula
nerve
- genitofemoral
- ilioinguinal

nerve *(cont.)*
  intercostal
  long thoracic
  obturator
  splanchnic
  thoracodorsal
  vaginal
nerve block infusion kit
nerve impulse propagation
nerve-sparing radical cystoprostatectomy
nerve-sparing radical prostatectomy
nerve-sparing technique
nervous pregnancy
Nesacaine (chloroprocaine)
Nesbit-Kelami technique for correction of congenital penile curvature
Nesbit operation for Peyronie disease
Nesbit resectoscope
nesidioblastosis
NESP (Novel erythropoiesis-stimulating protein)
nests, Brunn
Netherton syndrome
Neu-Laxova syndrome
Neupogen-mobilized PBPC transplantation
Neupogen (filgrastim) recombinant G-CSF
neural tube
neural tube defect (NTD)
neural tube disorder
neuralgia, mammary
neurectomy
  presacral
  sacrouterine
neurinoma
neuritis (pl. neuritides), fallopian
neuroacanthocytosis
neurobehavioral abnormality
neurocutaneous disease
neurocutaneous melanosis
neuroendocrine regulation of menstrual cycle
neurofibroma, multiple (NF)
neurofibromatosis (NF)
  bilateral acoustic
  central
  peripheral
  type 1 (NF1)
  type 2 (NF2)
neurogenic bladder
  contracted
  flaccid
  hypotonic
  spastic
neurogenic bladder dysfunction
neurogenic dysfunction of bladder
neurogram, pudendal
neurohypophysis
Neurologic and Adaptive Capacity Score (NACS)
neurologic bladder lesion
neurologic morbidity
neuromodulation for overactive bladder
neuromuscular diseases
neuromuscular transmission, impairment of
neuronal ceroid lipofuscinosis
neuronephric
neuron-specific aldolase
neuropathic bladder
neuropathic cystinosis
neuropathic GU tract lesion
neuropathy
  congenital hypomyelination
  diabetic
  giant axonal
  hereditary sensory, type 1
  hereditary sensory, type 2
  peripheral
  uremic
neuroretinopathy
NeuroSector ultrasound
neurosyphilis
  asymptomatic
  meningeal
  meningovascular

neurosyphilis *(cont.)*
  parenchymatous
  paretic
  symptomatic
  tabetic
Neuro-Trace insulated needle
Neuro-Trace needle
Neuro-Trace II nerve locator
neurovascular bundle
neutral lipid storage disease
neutropenia
  congenital
  isoimmune
  maternal transfer
  transient neonatal
neutrophil granules
  azurophilic
  primary
Neville-Barnes forceps
nevoid basal cell carcinoma syndrome
nevus
nevus comedinecus
nevus flammeus
newborn (see also *baby; infant*)
  ABO hemolytic disease of
  aseptic myocarditis of
  breast engorgement in
  bullous impetigo of
  cerebral irritability in
  chloramphenicol administration in
  cold injury syndrome of
  congenital epulis of
  congenital pneumonia in
  dehydration fever
  diabetes mellitus syndrome in
  disseminated intravascular coagulation in
  extreme immaturity of
  fits in
  hemolytic anemia of
  hemolytic disease of
  hyaline membrane disease of
  hyperthermia in
  hypocalcemia of

newborn *(cont.)*
  hypomagnesemia of
  jaundice of
  late metabolic acidosis of
  leukocytosis of
  necrotizing enterocolitis
  noninfective mastitis of
  omphalitis of
  plethora of
  regurgitation of food in
  seizures in
  spontaneous gangrene of
  superficial hematoma of
  thrush in
  transient tachypnea of
  transitory fever of
  transitory ileus of
  vitamin K deficiency of
newborn drug withdrawal syndrome
newborn nursery
newborn pediatrics
newborn screening
newly constructed introitus
new mutation
Newport lateral vaginal retractor
new sigmoid reconfiguration technique
New York Heart Association Classification of Heart Disease (1-4)
Nezhat-Dorsey trumpet valve
NF (neurofibromatosis)
NF1 (neurofibromatosis, type 1)
NF2 (neurofibromatosis, type 2)
NFkB-dependent gene activation
NG (nasogastric) tube
NGU (nongonococcal urethritis)
NHRT (natural hormone replacement therapy)
NHT (neoadjuvant hormonal therapy)
Niagara high flow pump
Niagara temporary dialysis catheter
Nibbler
Nibblit laparoscopic device
Nichol vaginal suspension procedure
nick

nicked-free beta subunit
nicked dimer
nicking (of fascia)
nick translation
"nick-u" (NICU)
Nicoladoni-Branham sign
NICU staff nurse
NIDDK (National Institute of Diabetes and Digestive and Kidney Diseases)
NIDDM (non-insulin-dependent diabetes mellitus)
nidus, uric acid
Niemann-Pick disease, type C (NPC)
night cycler method
night sweats
night sweats, chills, and fever
Niikawa-Kuroki syndrome
nil disease
Nilandron (nilutamide)
nilutamide
9 duplication
90° angle to the needle driver shaft
19 duplication
nipple
  accessory
  aortic
  bleeding from
  cracked
  discharge from
  everted
  fissure of
  inverted
  level of
  retracted
  retraction of
  slough of
  supernumerary
  ulcer of
nipple abscess
nipple-areola complex
nipple change
nipple discharge
  bloody
  guaiac-positive
nipple *(cont.)*
  milky
  persistent
  spontaneous
nipple eversion
nipple exploration with excision
nipple-flap duct resection
nipple infection
nipple inversion
nipple lesion
nipple level
nipple marker
nipple rash
nipple reconstruction
nipple retraction
nipple stimulation test
nipple valve
nippled stoma
NIPS (Neonatal Infant Pain Scale)
Nissen fundoplication
nitrate
Nitrazine paper
Nitrazine-positive
Nitrazine test
nitrite
nitrite testing
nitrituria
nitrofuran delivery catheter
nitrofurantoin
nitrogen (N)
nitrogen metabolism
nitrogenous base
nitrogenous solutes
nitrogenous waste
nitrogen retention
nits
Nizoral (ketoconazole)
NKHHC (nonketotic hyperglycemic-hyperosmolar coma)
NM (nemaline myopathy)
NMP22 test for early detection of transitional cell CA of bladder
NMR (neonatal mortality risk)
NOA (nonobstructive asoospermia)

NOA implanted urinary prosthesis
no clonus
Noble position
NOCIRC (National Organization of Circumcision Information Resource Centers)
nocturia times 3 (nocturia x 3)
nocturia x 3 (nocturia times 3)
nocturnal automated-cycler IPD
nocturnal enuresis
nocturnal myoclonus
nocturnal penile tumescence
nodal involvement
nodal metastases/metastasis
nodal status
nodal tissue
node
  axillary lymph
  common iliac
  external iliac
  iliac
  inguinal
  internal iliac
  internal mammary lymph
  intramammary
  intramammary lymph
  ipsilateral internal mammary lymph
  lymph
  para-aortic
  paramammary lymph
  parauterine lymph
  paravaginal lymph
  periaortic
  rectovaginal
  Sister Mary Joseph
  syphilitic
  Troisier
node-negative breast cancer
node-negative patient
node-positive patient
node sampling
nodes of Cloquet
Nodiol oral contraceptive
nodosa, isthmica
nodosum, amnion
nodular glomerulosclerosis
nodular glomerulonephritis
nodular goiter
nodularity of uterosacral ligaments
nodular mass
nodular prostate
nodule
  adenomyotic
  Albini
  axillary
  Bohn
  breast
  endometriotic
  fibroadenomatous
  Jeanselme
  juxta-articular
  Lutz-Jeanselme
  lymphatic
  prostatic
  satellite
  Sister Mary Joseph
  testicular
Nolan needle holder
Nolvadex (tamoxifen citrate) tablets
nomogram
nonarteriosclerotic cerebral calcification
nonbacterial epididymitis
nonbacterial epididymo-orchitis
nonbacterial prostatitis
nonbarrier contraceptives
nonbiodegradable suture
noncalcified stone
noncoding DNA
noncoding sequences
noncollagenous domain
noncommunicating hydrocele
noncommunicating hydrocephalus
noncommunicating uterine horn
noncontraceptively sterile
non-contrast-enhanced CT scan
nondeciduate placenta
nondeciduous placenta
nondiabetic glycosuria

nondialytic management of ARF
nondialytic management of CRF
nondirectiveness
nonemptying bladder
nonestrogenic progesterone derivatives
nonexcretory portions of kidney
nonfenestrated forceps
nonfunctional genes
nonfunctioning fallopian tube
nonfunctioning kidney
nongonococcal cervicitis
nongonococcal mucopurulent cervicitis
nongonococcal urethritis (NGU)
nonhomologous chromosomes
nonhyperglycemic glycosuria
nonidentical morphology
nonimmune fetal hydrops
nonimmunological fetal hydrops
nonimplantation
noninfective mastitis of newborn
noninfiltrating lobular carcinoma
non-insulin-dependent diabetes mellitus (NIDDM)
noninvasive carcinoma
nonisolated proteinuria
nonketotic hyperglycemic-hyperosmolar coma (NKHHC)
nonketotic hyperglycemia
nonlethal fetal malformations
nonlinkage
nonmorular solid growth pattern
non-neoplastic ovarian cyst
Nonne syndrome
non-neurogenic bladder
non-nodular prostate
non-nutritive sucking
nonobstructed anastomosis
nonobstructive azoospermia
nonoliguric renal failure
nonopaque calculi
nonopaque stone
nonovulational menstruation
nonoxynol 9 spermaticide
nonpalpable mass on mammogram
nonpapillary renal cell carcinoma (RCC)
nonpapillary transitional cell carcinoma
nonpathologic endogenous microflora
nonpedunculated hydatid
nonpermeating stream
nonpitting edema
nonprogressive congenital myopathy
nonpuerperal abscess of breast
nonpurulent mastitis
nonrandom or skewed X-inactivation
nonreduced twin gestation
nonreducible mass
nonrenal antigen
nonrenal azotemia
nonrenal hematuria
nonretractable foreskin
nonrigid technique reduction mammoplasty
nonrubella immunity
nonseminomatous germ cell tumor
nonsense mutation
nonsexual generation
nonskeletal metastases
nonsolvent bath
nonspecific urethritis (NSU)
nonspecific vaginitis (NSV)
nonsquamous solid growth pattern
nonstaining area of cervix
nonsteroidal anti-inflammatory drug (NSAID)
nonstreptococcal acute glomerulo-nephritis
nonstress test (NST)
nonstress test/contraction stress test (NST/CST)
nonsurgical sperm retrieval
nonsymptomatic urethritis
nontoxic diffuse goiter
nontoxic nodular goiter
nontraditional surrogacy arrangement
nontraumatic rupture of bladder
nontraumatic rupture of urethra
nonuterotropic

nonvenereal syphilis
nonviable fetus
nonviable infant
nonviable intrauterine pregnancy
Noonan syndrome
Norcept-E oral contraceptive
Nordette oral contraceptive
norethindrone
norethindrone/ethinyl estradiol oral contraceptive
norfloxacin
Norfolk aspiration needle
Norfolk intrauterine catheter
norgestimate
norgestrel
norgestrel/ethinyl estradiol oral contraceptive
Norimin oral contraceptive
Norinyl (norethindrone/ethinyl estradiol) oral contraceptive
Noritate (metronidazole)
Norlestrin oral contraceptive
normal allele
normal-appearing endometrium
normal blood pressure
normal collecting system
normal female genitalia
normal flora
normal fundus
normal gigantism
normal hemodynamic gradient
normal in position and contour
normal male genitalia
normal menarche
normal menstrual cycles
normal saline
normal-size uterus
normal spontaneous vaginal delivery (NSVD)
normal vaginal flora (NVF)
Norman-Roberts syndrome
normocephalic
normochromic-normocytic anemia
Normodyne (labetalol)
normoglycemia, absolute
normoglycemic glycosuria
normogonadotropic pattern
normospermatogenic sterility
normosthenuria
Noroxin (norfloxacin)
Norplant (levonorgestrel) implantable contraceptive system
Nor-QD oral contraceptive
Norrie disease
Northern blot
Northern blotting
Nortrel 1/35 (norethindrone/ethinyl estradiol)
Nortrel 7/7/7 (norethindrone/ethinyl estradiol)
Nortrel-28 (norethindrone/ethinyl estradiol)
notching, ureteral
notch, suprasternal
Nottingham colposuspension needle
NovaGold breast implant
Novak endometrial suction biopsy curette
Novantrone (mitoxantrone)
NovaSaline inflatable saline breast implant
NovaSaline pre-filled breast implant
Novasome (nonoxynol-9) spermicidal contraceptive
NovaSure endometrial ablation system
Novel erythropoiesis-stimulating protein (NESP)
Novofem disposable douche
Novolin Pen insulin device
NovoNorm (repaglinide)
Novy cornual cannulation catheter
NP (naturopathic physician)
NP (nephrographic phase)
NPC (Niemann-Pick disease, type C)
NSAID (nonsteroidal anti-inflammatory drug)
NST (nonstress test)
NSU (nonspecific urethritis)

NSV (nonspecific vaginitis)
NSVD (normal spontaneous vaginal delivery)
NTD (neural tube defect)
NTx Assay
nubain
nuchal cord
nuchal translucency
Nuck, canal of
nuclear atypia
nuclear/cytoplasmic ratio
nuclear density
nuclear matrix-based chemotherapy
nuclear matrix protein
nuclear medicine
nuclear steroid receptor
nuclease
nucleated cell
nucleic acid
nucleolar chromosome
nucleolar organizing region (NOR) chromosome staining method
nucleolus (pl. nucleoli)
nucleoside
nucleosome
nucleotide deletion
nucleotide substitution
nucleus
NuLev (hyoscyamine sulfate)
nulliparous cervix
null alleles
nulligravida
nullipara
nulliparous
null mutations
number of different sexual partners
nurse cell
Nursoy infant formula
nutcracker syndrome/phenomenon
Nutramigen infant formula
NutriMan TNT (*Tribulus terrestris* extract)
nutritional amenorrhea
nutritional deficiency
nutritional edema
nutritional gynecomastia
nutritional product
nutritional supplement
nutritionally deficient infant
nutritive sucking
Nutropin (somatropin)
NuvaRing (etonogestrel/ethinyl estradiol) contraceptive vaginal ring
Nuvera (17-beta estradiol/norethindrone)
N/V (nausea and vomiting)
NVF (normal vaginal flora)
Nyhan disease
nymphectomy
nympholabial
nymphomania
nymphomaniac
nymphomaniacal
Nyotran
nystatin

O, o

OA (occipitoanterior) position
OAC (optical aspirating curette)
O&P (ova and parasites)
Oasis thrombectomy system
oasthouse urine disease
OB (obstetrics)
obesity
  abdominal
  android
  gynecoid
  hypothalamic
obligate bicarbonate loss
obligate carrier
obligate heterozygote
oblique films
oblique incision
oblique lie
oblique presentation
obliterans, *Balanitis xerotica*
obliteration of caliceal diverticulum
obliteration of vagina
obliterative diabetic glomerulosclerosis
O'Brien suprapubic peel-away access set
Obrinsky syndrome
observable phenotype
observation
obstetrical air embolism
obstetric and perinatal risk
obstetrical binder
obstetrical blood clot embolism
obstetrical forceps
obstetrical history
obstetrical injury
obstetrical sonography
obstetrical symphysiotomy
obstetrical trauma
obstetric canal
obstetric conjugate
obstetric conjugate diameter
obstetric conjugate of pelvic inlet
obstetric conjugate of pelvic outlet
obstetric dates
obstetrician
obstetrician-gynecologist (OB-GYN)
obstetric palsy
obstetric perineal laceration
obstetric position
obstetrics (OB)
obstetrics and gynecology (Ob-Gyn, OB-GYN)
obstetric shock
obstetrics, perioperative
obstetric tamponade
obstetric ultrasound
obstetric yellow atrophy

obstructed calix
obstructed labor
obstructing periureteral fibrosis
obstruction
  Bartholin gland
  bladder neck
  bladder outlet
  cornual
  duct
  efferent duct
  extrinsic malignant ureteral
  functional ureteral
  hollow viscus
  hydronephrosis due to ureteral
  infravesical
  intravesical
  lower tract
  mammary duct
  meconium
  outflow
  partial ureteral
  prostatic
  recurrent bladder neck
  renal
  renal artery
  secretory duct of Bartholin gland
  supravesical
  tubal
  tubular
  upper tract
  ureteral
  ureteric
  ureteropelvic junction (UPJ)
  ureterovesical
  urethral
  urinary
  urinary tract (UTI)
  vesical outlet
obstructive anuria
obstructive apnea
obstructive azoospermia
obstructive azotemia
obstructive dysmenorrhea
obstructive hydrocephalus
obstructive nephropathy
obstructive prostate
obstructive prostatism
obstructive renal dysplasia
obstructive renal failure
obstructive symptoms
obstructive uropathy
obstructive voiding symptoms
obtundation
obtunded
obturator
  LaparoSac single-use
  malleable
  stiffening
  Syed
  Timberlake
obturator and cannula
obturator fossa
obturator nerve
obturator nodes
OC (oral contraceptive)
occasional bacteria
occipital fontanelle
occipital osteodiastasis
occipital prominence of fetus
occipitoanterior (OA) position
occipitofrontal circumference (OFC)
occipitoposterior (OP)
occipitotransverse (OT)
occiput
occiput-anterior (OA) presentation of fetus
occiput-posterior (OP) presentation of fetus
occludens, zonula
occlusion
  breast duct
  cervical
  fallopian tube
  fimbria
  renal arterial
  renal artery
  renal venous
  testicular blood flow

occlusion *(cont.)*
tubal
tubal mucosa
ureteral
ureteral orifice
occulta, spina bifida
occult blood
occult blood in urine
occult cervical cancer
occult renal disease
occult tumor cell deposit
occult urinary tract infection
occupational therapist
ochiotomy
Ochoa syndrome
o'clock position (e.g., 9 o'clock position)
O'Connor-O'Sullivan retractor
O'Connor sheath
OCN (over-the-needle) catheter
OCP (oral contraceptive pill)
OCT (oxytocin challenge test)
octocephaly
octoxynol 9
octuplet pregnancy
ocular hypertelorism
ocular hypotelorism
oculoauriculovertebral syndrome
oculocerebral syndrome with hypopigmentation
oculocerebrocutaneous syndrome
oculocerebrorenal
oculocraniosomatic neuromuscular disease
oculodentodigital dysplasia
oculogenitolaryngeal syndrome
oculomandibulodyscephaly
oculomandibulofacial syndrome
odd chromosome
O_2 (oxygen) debt in resuscitation of newborn
Oesclim patch
OFC (occipitofrontal circumference)
OFD (orofaciodigital) syndrome
offspring
ofloxacin
OG (orogastric tube)
Ogden soft tissue anchor
Ogen (estrone)
OHCS (17-hydroxycorticosteroid)
Ohdo syndrome
Ohio infant warmer
OHSS (ovarian hyperstimulation syndrome)
OI (osteogenesis imperfecta)
ointment
antifungal vaginal
mupirocin
zinc oxide
OKT3 (orthoclone K T-cell receptor 3) antibody)
olfactory ganglion
oligoanuric renal failure
oligohydramnios sequence or tetrad
oligohypermenorrhea
oligohypomenorrhea
oligomeganephronia
oligomenorrhea
Oligon Foley catheter
oligonucleotide
oligonucleotide primers
oligo-ovulation
oligo-ovulatory
oligosaccharide
oligospermia
oligoteratoasthenozoospermia syndrome
oligozoospermia
oliguria
oliguric acute renal failure (ARF)
oliguric phase of ARF
olive catheter tip
olive-tipped catheter
Olivier retractor
olivopontocerebellar atrophy (OPCA)
Ollier disease
Olympus A2010 0° 4 mm cystoscope

Olympus CHF-P10
Olympus CYF-3 OES cystofiberscope (also cystofibroscope)
Olympus 35 mm laparoscope camera
Ombrédanne transseptal orchiopexy
omental hernia
omental wrapping
omentectomy
 complete
 partial
omentum
omentumectomy
Omni-Lift retractor
OmniPulse-MAX holmium laser
Omni retractor
Omni-Tract retractor
omphalectomy
omphalelcosis
omphalic
omphalitis of the newborn
omphalitis, tetanus
omphaloangiopagus
omphalocele
omphaloenteric
omphalomesenteric cyst
omphalomesenteric duct
omphalopagus
omphalophlebitis
omphalorrhagia
omphalorrhea
omphalorrhexis
omphalosite
omphalotomy
omphalotripsy
omphalovesical
onanism
oncofetal antigen
oncofetal marker
oncogene
 Bc1-2
 c-erb B-2
 c-fos
 germline RET proto-oncogene point mutations

oncogene *(cont.)*
 HER-2-neu oncogene marker for breast cancer
 HER2/neu
 RET proto-oncogene
oncogenesis
oncogenic human papillomavirus
oncogenic virus
oncologist, gynecologic
On-Command catheter
oncovirus
On Line Clearance (OLC) dialysis monitor
OncoScint breast imaging agent
OncoScint OV103 (ovarian) monoclonal antibody
Oncoseed I-125 prostate brachytherapy seeds
oncosuppressor gene
Oncotech Extreme Drug Resistance Assay
OnCyte newborn sepsis detection system
One-Alpha (alfacalcidol)
one-horned uterus
one-hour glucose tolerance test
100° series endoscopic grasping forceps
1p21-22 deletion syndrome
1p22-p36.2 deletion syndrome
1p36 deletion syndrome
1p36.3 deletion syndrome
1q deletion syndrome
1q41 deletion syndrome
One Touch Basic glucose monitor
One Touch blood glucose monitor
One Touch FastTake blood glucose monitor
One Touch Profile glucose monitor
One Touch II hospital blood glucose monitor
onion bulb neuropathy
onset of menarche
onset of menses
ontogeny

onycho-osteodysplasia, hereditary
oocyesis
oocyte
  primary
  secondary
  trapped
oocyte donation
oocyte retrieval
oocyte transfer
oogenesis
oogenetic
oogonia
ookinesia
ookinesis
oophoralgia
oophorectomy
  bilateral
  unilateral
oophoritis
oophorocystectomy
oophorocystosis
oophorohysterectomy
oophoron
oophoropathy
oophoropeliopexy
oophoropexy
oophoroplasty
oophororrhaphy
oophorosalpingectomy
oophorosalpingitis
oophorotomy
oophorrhagia
ooplasm
oosome
oospore
ootid
ootype
oozing
  capillary
  venous
opacification
  complete
  extravesical
  incomplete
  poor
Opal R.F. tissue ablation device
opaque calculi
OPCA (olivopontocerebellar atrophy)
Opdima digital mammography system
open abdominal suturing
open biopsy
open cervix
open channel
open crib
open-end ureteral catheter
open fetal approach to spina bifida repair
open hydronephrosis
opening
  gland
  urethral
  ureteral
  uterine
  utricular
open laparotomy
open periprosthetic capsulotomy
open pyeloplasty
open radiant infant warmer
open reading frame (ORF)
open renal biopsy
open resection of bladder diverticulum
open-wound fetal surgery
OPERA (outpatient endometrial resection/ablation) procedure
OPERA STAR SL (outpatient endometrial resection/ablation; specialized tissue aspirating resectoscope) hysteroscope
operating laparoscope
operating microscope
operating room (OR)
operation or procedure (including diagnostic procedures, invasive and noninvasive studies, and surgical procedures, approaches, maneuvers, methods, and techniques)
  A&P (anterior and posterior) repair
  Abbe-McIndoe vaginal construction
  abdominal hysterectomy

operation *(cont.)*
abdominal hysterotomy
abdominal laparotomy
abdominal myomectomy
abdominal nephrectomy
abdominopelvic procedure
abdominal-sacral colopoperineopexy
abdominal sacrocolpopexy
abdominouterotomy
abdominovaginal hysterectomy
ablation
ablation of condylomata accumulata
Acucise endopyelotomy
adhesiotomy
adnexectomy
adrenalectomy
Aldridge-Studdiford
Altemeier perineal rectosigmoidectomy
ambulatory
anatrophic nephrolithotomy
anatrophic nephrotomy
AngioJet rapid thrombectomy
AngioJet Rheolytic thrombectomy
anorectovaginoplasty
antegrade endopyelotomy
antegrade scrotal sclerotherapy
antepartum tamponade
anterior and posterior (A&P) repair
anterior colporrhaphy
anterior urethropexy
anterior vesicourethropexy
appendicovesicostomy
appendicovesicotomy
Aries-Pitanguy correction of mammary ptosis
aspiration curettage
atrioseptoplasty
Auchincloss modified radical mastectomy
augmentation cystoplasty
augmentation mammoplasty
augmentation of bladder
autoaugmentation of bladder

operation *(cont.)*
autocystoplasty
autologous bone marrow transplantation
axillary dissection
axillary node dissection mastectomy
Bacon-Babcock correction of rectovaginal fistula
balanoplasty
Baldy-Webster correction of uterine retrodisplacement
balloon dilation of prostatic urethra
balloon tuboplasty
Ball pruritus ani treatment
BAMBI (breast augmentation mammoplasty by injection)
Barcat hypospadias repair
Bartholin cystectomy
Basset en-bloc radical vulvectomy
Bassini hernia repair
Bell-Buettner hysterectomy
"belly button" augmentation mammoplasty
Benelli mastopexy
Benelli pursestring mastopexy
Benenenti rotation of bulbous urethra
bilateral inguinofemoral lymphadenectomy
bilateral mastectomy
bilateral oophorectomy
bilateral orchiectomy
bilateral salpingectomy
bilateral tubal ligation
bilateral vasectomy
bisection of ovary
bladder neck elevation
bladder neck suspension
bladder suspension
Bonney abdominal hysterectomy
bottle repair of hydrocele
Bozeman uterovaginal fistula
breast-conserving therapy (BCT)

operation *(cont.)*
breast open periprosthetic capsulotomy
breast reconstruction during mastectomy
breast-sparing mastectomy
Bricker ureteroileostomy
Brunschwig total pelvic exenteration
bulbourethral sling
Burch bladder neck suspension
Burch colposuspension for stress incontinence
Burch iliopectineal ligament urethrovesical suspension
Burch laparoscopic bladder neck suspension
Burch retropubic urethropexy
burying of fimbriae in uterine wall
calicectomy
calicoplasty
calicotomy
calioplasty
Camey ileocystoplasty
Campbell radical retropubic prostatectomy
capsular flap pyeloplasty
capsulectomy of breast
CARMEN (cryoablation reduction of menstruation)
CASH (classic abdominal Semm hysterectomy)
cavernosography
cavernosometry
cavernosphenous shunt
cavernosal dilation
Cecil urethroplasty
central cone technique reduction mammoplasty
cephalotomy
cerclage of isthmus uteri
cervicectomy
cervicoplasty
cervicosigmoid fistulectomy
cervicotomy

operation *(cont.)*
cesarean
cesarean hysterectomy
cesarean section
circumcision
Clark perineorrhaphy
clavicotomy of fetus
cleavoplasty augmentation mammoplasty
clitoridectomy
clitoridotomy
clitoroplasty
coagulum pyelolithotomy
Coffey ureterointestinal anastomosis
cold cup bladder biopsy
colliculectomy
colocolponeopoiesis
colpocystotomy
colpocystourethropexy
colpohysterectomy
colpohysterotomy
colpomyomectomy
colpoperineopexy
colpoperineoplasty
colpoplasty
colpostenotomy
colposuspension
colpoureterotomy
complete mastectomy
complete omentectomy
complete penectomy
complete vaginectomy
conization of cervix
construction of ileal conduit
continent supravesical bowel urinary diversion
conventional abdominal hysterectomy
corpora cavernosa-corpus spongiosum shunt
corporotomy
Costello laser ablation of prostate
"crash" cesarean section

operation *(cont.)*
- Credé method of expressing placenta from uterus
- "cross-the-heart" augmentation mammoplasty
- cryoablation reduction of menstruation (CARMEN)
- cryoablation for prostate cancer
- cryoconization of cervix
- cryoprostatectomy
- cryosurgery
- C-section (cesarean section)
- culdocentesis
- culdolaparoscopy
- culdoplasty
- culdotomy
- Culp pyeloplasty
- culpoperineorrhaphy
- cutaneous intubated nephrostomy
- cutaneous intubated ureterostomy
- cutaneous vesicostomy
- Cyclops procedure
- cystectomy with urinary diversion
- cystocolic anastomosis
- cystolithalopaxy
- cystolithotomy
- cysto-ophorectomy
- cystoprostatectomy
- cystoscopy through artificial stoma
- cystostomy
- cystourethroplasty
- D&C (dilation and curettage)
- D&E (dilation and evacuation)
- D&X (partial birth abortion)
- Davydov vagina construction
- decapsulation of kidney
- decortication of kidney
- defatting of pannus
- degloving of penis
- destruction of fetus
- detorsion of testicle
- detorsion of testis
- dilation and curettage (D&C)
- dilation and evacuation (D&E)

operation *(cont.)*
- direct-vision internal urethrotomy (DVIU)
- disjoined pyeloplasty
- dismembered pyeloplasty
- diverticulectomy
- division of sacrouterine ligaments
- Döderlcin (Doederlein) laparoscopic hysterectomy
- dorsal onlay graft urethroplasty
- dorsal slit of prepuce
- douglasectomy
- Doyle paracervical uterine denervation
- drainage of bulbourethral gland
- drainage of ovarian cyst
- Duhrssen incision of cervix
- elective bilateral vasectomy
- embolectomy
- embryotomy
- emergency laparotomy
- en bloc augmentation mammoplasty
- endocervical biopsy
- endocervical curettage
- endometrectomy of bladder
- endometrial resection
- endopyelotomy
- endoscopic bladder neck suspension
- endoscopic destruction of fallopian tubes
- endoscopic fetal surgery
- endoscopic needle bladder neck suspension
- endoscopic needle suspension of bladder
- endoscopic needle suspension of vesical neck
- endoscopic strip craniectomy
- endoscopic suspension of vesical neck
- endoscopic transaxillary augmentation mammoplasty
- endoscopic-assisted transumbilical augmentation mammoplasty

operation *(cont.)*
- enterocele repair
- enterocystoplasty method of bladder augmentation
- epididymectomy
- epididymoplasty
- epididymostomy
- epididymotomy
- epididymovasectomy
- episioplasty
- episioproctotomy
- episiorrhaphy
- episiotomy repair
- Estes sterility
- excision of appendix testis
- excision of bladder dome
- excision of cyst of Morgagni
- excision of fistulous tract
- excision of median bar of prostate
- excisional biopsy
- exenterative surgery for pelvic cancer
- explantation of breast implants
- exploration of scrotum
- exploratory laparotomy
- exploratory pelvic laparotomy
- extended radical mastectomy
- external ureteral ileostomy
- extirpation of uterus and adnexa
- extracervical
- extrafascial total abdominal hysterectomy with wide vaginal cuff
- extraperitoneal pelvioscopy
- ex utero fetal surgery
- ex vivo extracorporeal kidney surgery
- fallopian tube prosthesis insertion
- female castration
- fetal endoscopic clip procedure
- fibroidectomy
- fibromectomy
- filtration
- fimbriectomy
- fimbrioplasty

operation *(cont.)*
- fistulectomy of bladder
- fistulotomy
- Foley Y-plasty pyeloplasty
- formation of open ileal bladder
- Fowler-Stephens orchiopexy
- fractional dilation and curettage (D&C)
- Frank and McIndoe vagina construction
- free nipple transposition reduction mammoplasty
- frenulectomy
- frenuloplasty
- Freund total abdominal hysterectomy for uterine cancer
- fundectomy
- gamete intrafallopian tube transfer (GIFT)
- gastric neobladder procedure
- gastrocystoplasty
- Gilliam uterine suspension
- Gittes urethral suspension
- Goebel-Frangenheim-Stoeckel urethrovesical suspension
- gonadectomy
- Goulian mammoplasty
- gracilis muscle transplant
- groin dissection
- Halsted radical mastectomy
- hand-assisted laparoscopic surgery (HALS)
- Heaney vaginal hysterectomy
- heminephrectomy
- hemivulvectomy
- hemodialysis
- hemofiltration
- Higgins ureterointestinal anastomosis
- high ligation of spermatic vein
- high McCall vaginal vault suspension
- high vasal ligation
- hydrocelectomy

operation *(cont.)*
- hymenectomy
- hymenotomy
- hypocystotomy
- hypophysectomy
- hysterectomy
- hysteromyomectomy
- hysteromyotomy
- hystero-oophorectomy
- hysteroplasty
- hysteroscopy
- hysterosalpingectomy
- hysterosalpingography
- hysteroscopic myomectomy
- hysterotomy
- hysterotrachelectomy
- hysterotrachelotomy
- ileal loop urinary conduit diversion
- ileocecocystoplasty
- ileocystoplasty
- implantation of inflatable cylinders
- incidental appendectomy
- Indiana pouch
- inferior pedicle technique reduction mammoplasty
- inframammary approach in augmentation mammoplasty
- inguinal exploration
- inguinal lymphadenectomy
- inguinal orchiectomy
- insertion of penile prosthesis
- insertion of ureteral catheter
- interstitial laser coagulation
- internal urethral meatotomy
- internal urethrotomy
- internal urinary diversion
- intra-abdominal endoscopic procedure
- intraperitoneal transplantation of ureters
- intrauterine myelomeningocele repair
- intrauterine pressure determination

operation *(cont.)*
- intravesical crushing and irrigation
- intravesical crushing of bladder calculi
- in utero fetal surgery
- in utero repair of congenital myelomeningocele
- in utero repair of neural tube defects
- InVance male sling procedure
- in vitro fertilization (IVF)
- irrigation of urinary tract
- Irving tubal ligation
- Kelly correction of retroversion of uterus
- Kelly correction of urinary stress incontinence
- Kelly-Kennedy urethral
- Kelly-Stoeckel urethral plication
- Kiricuta reconstructive breast
- Kock ("coke") ileostomy
- Kock pouch
- Kropp bladder neck reconstruction
- Kun colocolponeopoiesis
- Kun colocolpopoiesis
- LANS-RH (liposuction-assisted nerve-sparing radical hysterectomy)
- laparoamnioscopy
- laparohysterectomy
- laparomyomectomy
- laparosalpingectomy
- laparosalpingo-oophorectomy
- laparoscopic-assisted vaginal hysterectomy (LAVH)
- laparoscopic bladder neck suture suspension
- laparoscopic bladder suspension
- laparoscopic fulguration of pelvic endometriosis
- laparoscopic hysterectomy
- laparoscopic laser ablation of pelvic endometriosis
- laparoscopic laser-assisted autoaugmentation

operation *(cont.)*
- laparoscopic lysis of pelvic adhesions
- laparoscopic pelvic lymph node dissection
- laparoscopic pneumodissection
- laparoscopic pyeloplasty
- laparoscopic radical prostatectomy
- laparoscopic resection of uterosacral ligaments
- laparoscopic transcystic lithotripsy (LTCL)
- laparoscopic transcystic papillotomy
- laparoscopic tubal ligation
- laparoscopic urinary diversion
- laparoscopic uterine nerve ablation (LUNA)
- laparoscopy under local anesthesia (LULA)
- laparotomy
- LAP-TAPP (laparoscopic transabdominal preperitoneal) hernioplasty
- large loop excision of the transformation zone (LLETZ)
- Laroyenne pelvic suppuration repair
- laser-assisted tissue welding technique for bladder augmentation
- "Laser Bra" procedure
- laser fulguration of bladder tumor
- laser reduction mammoplasty
- laser uterosacral nerve ablation
- Lash hysterectomy
- Lash internal cervical os repair
- lateral slit of prepuce
- latissimus dorsi flap procedure
- Latzko vesicovaginal fistula repair
- Le Fort colpocleisis
- Leadbetter-Politano ureteral advancement
- Leadbetter-Politano ureteroneocystotomy
- Leadbetter-Politano ureterovesiculoplasty

operation *(cont.)*
- LeDuc anastomosis
- LeDuc-Camey ileocystoplasty
- LEEP (loop electrosurgical excision procedure)
- LeFort uterine prolapse repair
- leiomyomectomy
- Lejour-type breast reduction, modified
- levator muscle sling
- Lich neobladder construction
- Lich ureteral implantation in transplantation surgery
- Lich-Gregoire repair in kidney transplant surgery
- L.I.F.T. (laser-assisted internal fabrication) of breast
- ligation and division of fallopian tubes
- liposuction-assisted nerve-sparing radical hysterectomy (LANS-RH)
- loop electrosurgical excision procedure (LEEP)
- lower pole heminephrectomy
- low flap vertical cesarean section
- low transverse cesarean section
- LULA (laparoscopy under local anesthesia)
- lumbar nephrectomy
- lumpectomy of breast
- LUNA (laparoscopic uterine nerve ablation)
- LUNA (laser uterosacral nerve ablation)
- lymph node dissection
- lysis of intraluminal adhesions
- lysis of perirenal adhesions
- lysis of perivesical adhesions
- Madigan prostatectomy
- Madlener tubal sterilization
- MAGPI (meatal advancement, glanuloplasty, penoscrotal junction meatotomy) hypospadias repair

operation *(cont.)*
mammoplasty
mammotomy
Manchester colpoperineorrhaphy
manual removal of retained placenta
Marshall-Marchetti-Krantz (MMK)
Marshall-Marchetti-Krantz vesicourethral suspension
Marshall-Marchetti procedure
marsupialization of cyst
marsupialization of kidney lesion
marsupialization of ovarian cyst
Martius flap and fascial sling
mastoplasty
mastotomy with abscess drainage
Matsner median episiotomy and repair
Mattox maneuver
Mayo culdoplasty
McCall modified posterior culdoplasty
McCall vaginal vault suspension, high
McDonald cervical cerclage
McGraw gracilis myocutaneous flap vaginal reconstruction
McIndoe vaginal construction
McWhirter simple mastectomy
meatal advancement, glanuloplasty, penoscrotal junction meatotomy (MAGPI)
meatotomy
"mega-pocket" augmentation mammoplasty
metroplasty
metrotomy
microsalpingoplasty
microscopic vasectomy reversal
microsurgical denervation of spermatic cord
microsurgical epididymovasostomy
microsurgical tubal reanastomosis (MTR)
Millen retropubic prostatectomy

operation *(cont.)*
Millin-Read urethrovesical suspension
minilaparotomy pelvic lymph node dissection
minilaparotomy staging pelvic lymphadenectomy
minimally invasive fetal surgery
mirror image breast biopsy
Mitchell epispadias repair
Mitrofanoff appendicovesicostomy
Mitrofanoff appendicovesicotomy
Mitrofanoff continent urinary diversion
Mitrofanoff neourethra procedure
MMK (Marshall-Marchetti-Krantz)
modified Benelli round block mastopexy
modified bulbar urethral sling
modified Kun colocolponeopoiesis
modified Kun colocolpopoiesis
modified Pereyra bladder neck suspension
modified radical hysterectomy
modified radical mastectomy
modified vulvectomy
modified Wertheim procedure for microinvasive carcinoma
morcellated nephrectomy
morcellation vaginal hysterectomy
Moschcowitz culdoplasty
MTR (microsurgical tubal reanastomosis)
Munro and Parker
myomectomy
needle biopsy
needle urethropexy
needling of hydrocephalic head
neobladder construction following total cystectomy
nephrocyst anastomosis
nephropyeloureterostomy
nephroscopy
nephrostomy

operation *(cont.)*
- nephroureterectomy
- nerve-sparing radical cystoprostatectomy
- Nesbit
- Nesbit-Kelami technique for correction of congenital penile curvature
- neurectomy
- Nichol vaginal suspension procedure
- nipple-flap duct resection
- obliteration of caliceal diverticulum
- obstetrical symphysiotomy
- obstetric tamponade
- ochiotomy
- Ombrédanne transseptal orchiopexy
- omentectomy
- omphalotomy
- oophorectomy
- oophorocystectomy
- oophorohysterectomy
- oophoroplasty
- oophorotomy
- open diverticulectomy
- open fetal approach to spina bifida repair
- open resection of bladder diverticulum
- open-womb fetal surgery
- OPERA (outpatient endometrial resection/ablation)
- outpatient endometrial resection/ablation (OPERA)
- orchiectomy
- orchotomy
- oscheoplasty
- outpatient endometrial resection/ablation (OPERA)
- ovarian cystectomy
- ovarian denervation
- ovariohysterectomy
- ovariosalpingectomy
- ovariotomy
- oversewing of ovarian cyst

operation *(cont.)*
- owl incision technique reduction mammoplasty
- Oxford urinary incontinence
- pancreas after kidney (PAK) transplantation operation
- panhysterectomy
- paravaginal hysterectomy
- parovariotomy
- partial cystectomy
- partial hysterectomy
- partial nephrectomy
- partial omentectomy for removal of IUD
- partial penectomy
- partial scrotectomy
- partial vaginectomy
- passage of sound
- Patey modified radical mastectomy
- pelvic evisceration
- pelvic exenteration
- pelvic laparotomy
- pelvic lymphadenectomy
- pelvilithotomy
- pelviolithotomy
- pelvioplasty
- pelviscopy
- penectomy
- penile amputation
- penile reconstruction
- penile vein ligation
- penotomy
- percutaneous aspiration of kidney
- percutaneous bladder neck stabilization (PBNS)
- percutaneous mechanical thrombectomy (PMT)
- percutaneous needle biopsy of kidney
- percutaneous nephrolithotomy
- percutaneous nephrostolithotomy (PCNL)
- percutaneous nephrostomy

operation *(cont.)*
- percutaneous nephrostomy with stent
- percutaneous patent ductus arteriosus closure
- percutaneous resection of transitional cell carcinoma of the renal pelvis
- percutaneous stone dissolution
- percutaneous transluminal angioplasty
- percutaneous transluminal renal angioplasty (PTRA)
- periareolar augmentation mammoplasty
- perineal prostatectomy
- perineal urethroscopy
- perineal urethrostomy
- perineoplasty
- perinotomy
- periprosthetic capsulectomy of breast
- peritoneoscopy
- permanent suprapubic cystostomy
- permanent upper tract diversion
- permanent urinary diversion
- phalloplasty
- phallotomy
- pipelle uterine aspiration
- Piper forceps
- plication of urethrovesical junction
- plication of urinary bladder sphincter
- PMT (percutaneous mechanical thrombectomy)
- Polytef augmentation urethroplasty
- Pomeroy tubal ligation
- Porro hysterectomy
- posterior colporrhaphy
- posterior colpotomy
- posthioplasty
- postpartum tubal ligation
- Prentiss maneuver
- preputiotomy

operation *(cont.)*
- presacral neurectomy
- preventive mastectomy
- primary vaginal hysterectomy
- proctocolpoplasty
- proctocystotomy
- proctoperineoplasty
- promontofixation
- prophylactic mastectomy
- prostatectomy
- prostatolithotomy
- proximal genital reconstruction
- PTFE (polytetrafluoroethylene) suburethral sling procedure
- pubiotomy
- pubococcygeal sling
- pubovaginal repair for urinary incontinence
- pubovaginal sling
- punch suprapubic cystostomy
- pyeloplasty
- pyelostomy
- pyelotomy
- pyeloureterovesical anastomosis
- QUART (quadrantectomy, axillary dissection, and radiotherapy)
- radical cystectomy
- radical cystoprostatectomy
- radical hemivulvectomy
- radical mastectomy
- radical nephrectomy
- radical nephroureterectomy
- radical perineal prostatectomy
- radical prostatectomy
- radical retropubic prostatectomy with nerve-sparing technique
- Raz sling
- reattachment of amputated penis
- Récamier curettage of the uterus
- recanalization
- reconstruction of penis
- rectopexy
- rectosigmoidectomy
- rectovaginopexy

operation *(cont.)*
- rectovesicovaginal fistulectomy
- reduction cystoplasty
- reduction mastopexy
- reimplantation of ovary
- reinsertion of ureteral stent
- removal of dorsal hood
- removal of IUD
- renal angioplasty
- renal autotransplantation
- renal lithotomy
- renipuncture
- resection and fulguration of bladder tumor
- resection and reanastomosis of ureter
- resection of bladder tumor
- retrograde ureteroscopic endopyelotomy
- retrograde urethrography
- retroperitoneoscopy
- retropubic exploration
- retropubic prostatectomy
- retropubic urethral suspension
- revision of episiotomy scar
- revision of stoma
- Ripstein rectal prolapse repair
- rollerball endometrial ablation
- Rutkow sutureless plug-and-patch repair for inguinal hernia
- sacrocolpopexy
- sacrospinous colpopexy
- sacrospinous vaginal vault suspension procedure
- sacrouterine neurectomy
- Saenger cesarean section
- salpingectomy with removal of tubal pregnancy
- salpingo-oophorostomy
- salpingo-ovariotomy
- salpingoplasty
- salpingosalpingostomy
- salpingotomy
- salpingo-uterostomy

operation *(cont.)*
- salvage cystectomy
- Scardino vertical flap pyeloplasty
- "scarless" mastectomy
- Schauta radical vaginal hysterectomy
- Schauta vaginal
- Schroeder excision of diseased endocervical mucosa
- Schuchardt paravaginal rectal displacement incision
- Schwartz-Pregenzer urethropexy
- scrotal exploration
- scrotal fistulectomy
- scrotoplasty
- second-look
- segmental mastectomy
- Semm hysterectomy
- Shirodkar cervical cerclage
- short-scar tumescent reduction mammoplasty
- Simonsen large rectovaginal fistula repair
- Simonsen technique for large rectovaginal fistula repair
- simple mastectomy
- simultaneous areolar mastopexy and breast augmentation (SAMBA)
- skinning vulvectomy
- skin-sparing mastectomy
- sling procedure for stress urinary incontinence
- SMART (surgical myomectomy as reproductive therapy)
- Smith-Boyce
- speculoscopy
- spermatocelectomy
- spermatocystectomy
- sphincterotomy of bladder
- Spinelli reduction of prolapsed uterus
- splenectomy
- split-flap vaginal reconstruction

operation *(cont.)*
- Stamey bladder suspension procedure
- standard vaginal hysterectomy
- stereotaxic core needle biopsy
- Straight-In surgical procedure
- Sturmdorf conical removal of endocervix
- subcutaneous mastectomy
- subtotal hysterectomy
- subtotal thyroidectomy
- suburethral fascial sling
- suburethral sling procedure
- suction curettage
- suction lipectomy
- superficial vulvectomy
- supracervical hysterectomy
- suprapubic catheterization
- suprapubic cystostomy
- suprapubic cystotomy
- suprapubic lithotomy
- suprapubic needle aspiration of bladder
- suprapubic tube insertion
- surgical extirpation of gonads
- surgical repair of atrial septal defect
- sutureless plug and patch repair for inguinal hernia
- symphysiotomy for horseshoe kidney
- syringotomy
- TAH/BSO (total abdominal hysterectomy with bilateral salpingo-oophorectomy)
- Tanagho anterior bladder flap procedure
- TeLinde modified radical hysterectomy
- tension-free vaginal tape (TVT) procedure
- TEP (totally extraperitoneal) hernia repair
- ThermaChoice uterine balloon therapy (UBT)
- Thiersch-Duplay urethroplasty

operation *(cont.)*
- thoracoabdominal radical nephrectomy
- thromboendarterectomy
- Torek two-stage operation for undescended testicle
- total abdominal evisceration (TAE)
- total abdominal hysterectomy (TAH)
- total abdominal hysterectomy with anterior vaginal colporrhaphy
- total cystectomy
- total cystectomy with urethrectomy
- total mastectomy
- trachelotomy
- transabdominal radical nephrectomy
- transabdominal retroperitoneal lymph node dissection
- transaxillary subpectoral mammoplasty
- transcervical balloon tuboplasty (TBT)
- transperineal needle biopsy of prostate
- transperineal prostatic cryoablation
- transplantation of ureter into ileum with external diversion
- transrectal needle biopsy of prostate
- transseptal orchiopexy
- transsexual surgery
- transsphenoidal exploration of pituitary
- transumbilical breast augmentation
- transureteroureteral anastomosis
- transureteroureterostomy (TUU)
- transureteroureterostomy anastomosis
- transurethral balloon Laserthermia prostatectomy
- transurethral biopsy
- transurethral collagen injection
- transurethral cystoscopy
- transurethral enucleation
- transurethral fistulectomy
- transurethral incision of prostate (TUIP)

operation *(cont.)*
- transurethral lysis of adhesions
- transurethral needle ablation (TUNA)
- transurethral prostatectomy
- transurethral resection (TUR)
- transurethral resection of bladder neck
- transurethral resection of bladder tumor (TURBT)
- transurethral resection of prostate (TURP)
- transurethral ultrasound-guided laser-induced prostatectomy (TULIP)
- transurethral ureteroscopic lithotomy
- transurethral ureteroscopic lithotripsy
- transvaginal hysterectomy
- transvaginal sacrospinous colpopexy
- transverse cervical cesarean section
- transvesical prostatectomy
- Triangle gelatin-sealed sling material
- triangular vaginal patch sling
- trigonectomy
- tubal reconstruction
- Tudor "rabbit ear" urethropexy
- TULIP (transurethral ultrasound-guided laser-induced prostatectomy)
- TUMT (transurethral microwave thermotherapy)
- TUNA (transurethral needle ablation)
- TURBT (transurethral resection of bladder tumor)
- Turner-Warwick urethroplasty
- TURP (transurethral resection of prostate)
- two-stage technique of mastectomy
- UAE (uterine artery embolization)
- ultrasound-guided transcervical tuboplasty

operation *(cont.)*
- ultrasound-guided transvaginal aspiration of eggs
- unilateral groin dissection
- unilateral orchiectomy
- UPLIFT (uterine positioning via ligament investment fixation and truncation) procedure
- Urban extended radical mastectomy
- ureteral meatotomy
- ureteral reimplantation
- ureterocaliceal anastomosis
- ureterocystoplasty
- ureteroileocutaneous anastomosis
- ureteroileostomy
- ureterolithotomy
- ureterolysis
- ureteroneocystostomy
- ureteropexy
- ureteroplasty
- ureteroplication
- ureteropyelostomy
- ureteroscopy
- ureterosigmoidostomy
- ureterotomy
- urethral diverticulectomy
- urethral meatoplasty
- urethral meatotomy
- urethral plication
- urethral sling
- urethral sphincter electromyogram
- urethral surgical reconstruction
- urethrectomy
- urethrocystoscopy
- urethrolysis
- urethroperineovesical fistulectomy
- urethroplasty
- urethrotomy
- urinary diversion procedure for intestinal urinary conduit
- urodynamic assessment
- uterine artery embolization (UAE)
- uterine balloon therapy

operation *(cont.)*
- uterine suspension
- uteroplasty
- vaginal celiotomy
- vaginal flap reconstruction and pubovaginal sling procedure
- vaginal flap reconstruction of urethra and vesical
- vaginal hysterectomy
- vaginal hysterectomy and anterior repair
- vaginal hysterotomy
- vaginal interruption of pregnancy with dilation and curettage (VIP-DAC)
- vaginal lengthening
- vaginal lithotomy
- vaginal wall sling procedure
- vaginectomy
- vaginoperineoplasty
- vaginoperineotomy
- vaginoscopy
- vaginotomy
- varicocele ligation
- varicotomy
- vasectomy
- vasoepididymostomy
- vasotomy
- vasovasostomy
- vasovasotomy
- vesical lithotomy
- vesicolithotomy
- vesicopsoas hitch
- vesicosigmoidovaginal fistulectomy
- vesicotomy
- vesicoureterovaginal fistulectomy
- vesicourethropexy
- vesiculotomy
- video-assisted extraperitoneal laparoscopic bladder neck suspension (VELBNS)
- visual laser ablation of the trigone (VLAT)
- voiding cystourethrography

operation *(cont.)*
- vulvar fistulectomy
- vulvectomy
- vulvovaginal
- V-Y plasty of bladder neck
- Walsh radical retropubic prostatectomy
- WAMBA (Wise areola mastopexy breast augmentation)
- Waters extraperitoneal cesarean section with supravesical approach
- Watkins uterine interposition
- wedge resection of bladder
- wedge resection of kidney
- wedge resection of ovary
- Wertheim excision of vagina and wide lymph node excision
- Wertheim radical hysterectomy with pelvic lymph node dissection
- Wertheim-Schauta procedure
- Williams vulvovaginoplasty
- Willy Meyer incision for mastectomy
- Winter procedure
- Wise pattern reduction mammoplasty
- Yachia incisionless bladder suspension
- Y-V-plasty
- Young-Dees-Leadbetter bladder-neck reconstruction
- zipper sphincterotomy
- zygote intrafallopian tube transfer (ZIFT)

operative cystoureteroscope

operative staging

operating staging, laparoscopic pelvic lymph node dissection, and extraperitoneal pelviscopy

operator gene

operon

ophthalmia neonatorum

ophthalmoarthropathy

ophthalmopathy, infiltrative
opisthotonus
Opitz
Opitz C
Opitz FG
Opitz Frias
Opitz G/BBB
Opitz Kaveggia
Opitz trigonocephaly
Opmilas 144 Plus laser system
opodidymus
opportunistic infection
opsoclonus-myoclonus
optical aspirating curette (OAC)
Opticon catheter
Opti-Flow catheter
option, therapeutic
Opti-Plast XT balloon catheter
OptiVu HDVD (high definition video display) system
OPTN (Organ Procurement and Transplantation Network)
OR (operating room)
OR1 electronic endoscopy system
oral antiestrogen
oral contraceptive (OC)
- Alesse (levonorgestrel/ethinyl estradiol)
- Anovlar
- Anovulatorio
- Aviane-28 (levonorgestrel and ethinyl estradiol)
- Brevicon
- Brevinor 21 or 28
- Ciclovulan
- Cyclessa (desogestrel/ethinyl estradiol)
- Demlen
- desogestrel/ethinyl estradiol
- dospirenone/ethinyl estradiol
- Enpresse (levonorgestrel/ethinyl estradiol tablets)
- Estrinor
- Estrophasic

oral contraceptive *(cont.)*
- Estrostep
- ethinyl estradiol/levonorgestrel
- ethynodiol diacetate/ethinyl estradiol
- Gencept
- Genora
- gestodene low dose estrogen/ progestin
- Jenest-28
- Kliovance
- Levlen
- Levlite (levonorgestrel/ethinyl estradiol)
- levonorgestrel/ethinyl estradiol
- Levora (levonorgestrel/ethinyl estradiol)
- Loestrin
- Lo/Ovral
- Low-Ogestrel (norgestrel/ethinyl estradiol)
- Microgestin Fe 1.5/30
- Microgestin Fe 1/20
- Micronor
- Milli
- Minovlar
- Mircette (desogestrel/ethinyl estradiol)
- Modicon
- Modicon-28
- Necon
- Necon 0.5/35 norethindrone/ethinyl estradiol)
- Necon 1/35 norethindrone/ethinyl estradiol)
- Necon 1/50 (norethindrone/ mestranol)
- Necon 10/11 (norethindrone/ethinyl estradiol)
- N.E.E.
- Nelova
- Nelova 10/11
- Nelulen 1/50
- Nodiol
- Norcept-E

oral contraceptive *(cont.)*
- Nordette
- Norethin
- norethindrone/ethinyl estradiol
- norgestrel/ethinyl estradiol
- Norimin
- Norinyl (norethindrone/ethinyl estradiol)
- Norlestrin
- Nor-QD
- Nortrel
- Nortrel 1/35 (norethindrone/ethinyl estradiol)
- Nortrel 7/7/7 (norethindrone/ ethinyl estradiol)
- Nortrel-28 (norethindrone/ethinyl estradiol)
- Orlest
- Ortho-Cept (progesterone desogestrel/ethinyl estradiol)
- Ortho-Cyclen
- Ortho Dialpak
- Ortho-Novum 1/35
- Ortho-Novum 1/50
- Ortho-Novum 7/7/7
- Ortho 1/35
- Ortho 7/7/7
- Ortho Personal Pak
- Ortho Tri-Cyclen (norgestimate/ ethinyl estradiol)
- Ovcon
- Ovral
- Ovrette
- Ovysmen 0.5/35
- Ovysmen 1/35
- Plan B (levonorgestrel, 0.75 mg tablets)
- Preven emergency
- Seasonale
- Synphase
- Synphasic 28
- synthetic estrogen-progestogen combination
- synthetic progestogen

oral contraceptive *(cont.)*
- Triella
- Tri-Levlen
- Tri-Norinyl (norethindrone/ethinyl estradiol)
- Trinovum
- Trinovum 21
- Trivora (levonorgestrel/ethinyl estradiol)
- Trivora-21 (ethinyl estradiol/ levonorgestrel)
- Trivora-28 (ethinyl estradiol/ levonorgestrel)
- Yasmin 28 (dospirenone/ethinyl estradiol)
- Zovia (ethynodiol diacetate/ethinyl estradiol)

oral fertility drugs
oral ganciclovir
oral-genital sexual activity
Oralgen oral aerosol insulin
oral hypoglycemic agent
oral phosphate binders
oral sex
oral stimulation of the penis
oral stimulation of the vulva or clitoris
Orandi flap
orBec (beclomethasone)
orbital cyst with cerebral and focal dermal malformations
orbital reducer seal
orchectomy (see *orchiectomy*)
orchialgia
orchichorea
orchidectomy
orchidic
orchiditis
orchidometer
orchidopexy
orchiectomy
- bilateral
- inguinal

orchiepididymitis
orchiocele

orchiodynia
orchioncus
orchioneuralgia
orchiopathy
orchiopexy
  Fowler-Stephens
  transseptal
orchioplasty
orchiorrhaphy
orchiotherapy
orchis (pl. orchises)
orchitis
  gonococcal
  granulomatous
  metastatic
  mumps
  spermatogenic
  traumatic
  tuberculous
orchitis associated with mumps
orchitis parotidea
orchitis variolosa
orchotomy
Oreopoulos-Zellerman peritoneal dialysis catheter
ORF (open reading frame)
organ
  ancestral
  internal female genital
  internal male genital
  intromittent
  reticuloendothelial
  urinary
organ donor
organ donor card
organelle, cytoplasmic
organic impotence
organic iodides
organism
  flagellated
  motile
  unicellular
  urea-splitting
organogenesis
organomegaly
organ preservation solution, Celsior
Organ Procurement and Transplantation Network (OPTN)
organ-sparing surgery
orgasm
  difficulty in attaining
  failure to experience an
orienting suture
orifice
  bladder
  distal
  external urethral
  filling internal urethral
  golf-hole ureteral
  internal urethral
  ureteral
  ureteric
  ureterovesical
  urethral
  uterine
  vaginal
  vesicourethral
  voiding internal urethral
orificium (pl. orificia)
origin
Origin balloon
Origin Medsystems trocar
Origin Tacker laparoscopic tacking device
Origin trocar
Orlest oral contraceptive
Ormond disease
ornithine carbamoyl transferase deficiency (OTC) (formerly carbamyl)
ornithine transcarbamylase deficiency (OTC)
orocraniodigital syndrome
orofacial clefts
orofaciodigital (OFD) syndrome
orogastric tube
orotic aciduria
orotidinuria

Ortho-Cept (progesterone desogestrel, ethinyl estradiol)
Orthoclone OKT3 monoclonal antibody
Ortho-Cream contraceptive
Ortho-Cyclen oral contraceptive
Ortho Dialpak oral contraceptive pack
Ortho Dienestrol vaginal cream
Ortho-est (estropipate)
Ortho Evra (norelgestromin/ethinyl estradiol) contraceptive patch
orthoglycemic glycosuria
Ortho-Gynol contraceptive cream
orthology
Ortho-Novum 1/35 oral contraceptive
Ortho-Novum 1/50 oral contraceptive
Ortho-Novum 7/7/7 oral contraceptive
Ortho 1/35 oral contraceptive
Ortho Personal Pak
Ortho-Prefest (17-beta-estradiol/ norgestimate) hormone replacement therapy
Ortho-Prefest (estradiol/norgestimate)
orthophosphate
orthopic neobladder
Ortho 7/7/7 oral contraceptive
orthosis, CranioCap for infants
orthostasis
orthostatic blood pressure
orthostatic hypotension
orthostatic proteinuria
orthotoluidine stain
orthotopic neobladder
orthotopic ureter
orthotopic ureterocele
Ortho Tri-Cyclen (norgestimate/ethinyl estradiol) oral contraceptive
Ortolani hip maneuver
os
  cervical
  external
  internal
os uteri, pinpoint
oscheoplasty
osmolality, urine
osmolarity
osmometer
osmometry
osmosis
osmotic dilator
osmotic diuresis
osmotic diuretic
osmotic laxatives
osmotic nephrosis
osmotic shift
osmotic shift of water into intracellular compartment
osmotic ultrafiltration
osseous oculodento dysplasia
ossification, enchondral
osteitis
osteitis deformaris
osteitis fibrosa
osteitis fibrosa cystica, refractory
osteoarthritis
osteoblastic bony metastases
osteochondromatosis
osteochondroplasia
osteoclast-activating cytokine
osteodiastasis, occipital
osteodysplasia of Melnich and Needles
osteogenesis imperfecta (OI)
osteodystrophy
  Albright hereditary
  azotemic
  renal
osteomalacia, aluminum-related
Osteomark monoclonal antibody-based agent
Osteomark test
osteomesopyknosis
osteo-onychodysplasia
Osteopatch transdermal patch
osteopathia hyperostotica multiplex infantalis
osteoporosis, postmenopausal
ostial renal artery stenosis
ostia, tubal

ostiomeatal
ostium (pl. ostia)
O'Sullivan-O'Connor retractor
OTC (ornithine transcarbamylase)
  deficiency
OTC (over-the-counter) pharmaceuticals
Otis urethrotome
otopalatodigital syndrome
OTT intrauterine catheter
OTW (over-the-wire)
OTW Thrombolytic Brush for dialysis
outbreeding
outflow, obstruction of
outflow time
outflow tract
outlet
  pelvic
  relaxation of vaginal
  vaginal
outlet contraction of pelvis
outlet forceps
outlet forceps delivery
outlet resistant
out-of-frame mutation/deletion
outpatient endometrial resection/
  ablation (OPERA) procedure
outpatient endometrial resection/
  ablation (OPERA) specialized tissue
  aspirating resectoscope (STAR)
output, urinary
OV (ovarian)
ovale, patent foramen
ovalis
  anulus
  limbus fossae
oval-shaped glandular gonad
OvaRex MAb immunotherapy
Ovarex vaccine
ovarian follicles
ovarian monitoring
ovarialgia
ovarian (OV)
ovarian ablation
ovarian ablation by radiation
ovarian ablation by surgery
ovarian agenesis
ovarian amenorrhea
ovarian artery
ovarian atrophy
ovarian bisection
ovarian blood supply
ovarian cancer
  advanced
  metastatic
  primary
ovarian carcinoma
ovarian colic
ovarian cortex
ovarian cyst
ovarian cystadenocarcinoma
ovarian cystadenoma
ovarian cystectomy
ovarian cyst
  aspiration of
  drainage of
  hemorrhagic
  ruptured
ovarian denervation
ovarian dermoid cyst
ovarian duct
ovarian dwarfism
ovarian dysgenesis
ovarian dysmenorrhea
ovarian endometrioma
ovarian endometriosis
ovarian epithelium
ovarian estrogen secretion
ovarian failure
  premature
  primary
ovarian fibroma
ovarian fimbria
ovarian follicle
ovarian follicular cyst
ovarian fossa
ovarian function
ovarian granulosa cell tumor
ovarian hernia

ovarian hormone estrogen
ovarian hormone, reduced secretion of
ovarian hyperstimulation
ovarian hyperstimulation syndrome (OHSS)
ovarian infarction
ovarian ligament
ovarian mass
ovarian medulla
ovarian neoplasm
ovarian pain
ovarian pedicle
ovarian pedicle, torsion of
ovarian pregnancy
ovarian preservation
ovarian reimplantation
ovarian remnant syndrome
ovarian steroids, 17-beta-estradiol
ovarian stimulation
ovarian suppression
ovarian teratoma
ovarian tissue implanted in arm
ovarian tumor
ovarian varicocele
ovarian vein phlebitis
ovarian vein syndrome
ovariectomy
ovaries (see *ovary*)
ovaries adherent to ureters
ovaries gland
ovaries left in situ
ovarigenic
ovarii, hydrops
ovarioabdominal pregnancy
ovariocele
ovariocentesis
ovariocyesis
ovariodysneuria
ovariohysterectomy
ovarioleukodystrophy
ovariolytic
ovariopathy
ovariorrhexis
ovariosalpingectomy
ovariosalpingitis
ovariostomy
ovariotomy
ovaritis
ovarium (pl. ovaria)
ovarium bipartitum
ovarium disjunctum
ovarium gyratum
ovarium lobatum
ovarium masculinum
ovary (pl. ovaries)
  abscess of
  adherent
  atrophic
  atrophied
  chocolate cyst of
  complex cystic
  consistency of
  cystic
  developmental cyst of
  displacement of
  dominant follicles in
  embryonic
  endometriosis of
  fetal
  fibroma-thecoma tumor
  fibromyoma of
  follicular cyst of
  free border of
  hematosalpinx of
  hernia of
  infarction of
  ligament of
  mesovarian border of
  mobility of
  mulberry
  neoplastic cyst of
  outline of
  polycystic
  position of
  presumptive
  proper ligament of
  rete cyst of
  retention cyst of

ovary *(cont.)*
  rupture of
  senile involution of
  serous cyst of
  simple cystoma of
  size of
  stroma of
  suspensory ligament of
  torsion of
  tubal extremity of
ovary demarcated by deep furrows into lobes
overlapping clones
overriding head
ovary plastered to sidewall
ovary separated into two distinct parts
ovary stimulation
ovary with curved or irregular grooves or furrows
Ovation falloposcopy system
O-Vax therapeutic vaccine
Ovcon oral contraceptive
over-the-counter (OTC) pharmaceuticals
over-the-needle catheter (ONC)
over-the-wire (OTW) brush
overactive bladder
overdistention
overdistention of hollow viscus
overexcretion of salt
overexpression of HER-2/neu
overflow
overflow incontinence
overflow proteinuria
overhead warmer
overhydration
overinsulinization
overlapping of cranial bones
overload
  circulatory
  fluid
  volume
overlying cortical sclerosis
oversewn
oversew (or oversewing) of ovarian cyst
overt homosexuality
overt urologic disease
Oves conception cap
Oves fertility cap
ovicidal
Ovidrel (choriogonadotropin)
oviducal
oviduct
  fimbriated end of
  rupture of
oviductal pregnancy
oviferous
oviform
ovigenesis
ovigenetic
ovigenic
oviparity
ovoid-shaped calcific density
ovosiston
ovotestis (pl. ovotestes)
Ovral oral contraceptive
Ovrette oral contraceptive
OvuKIT
ovulation
  amenstrual
  anestrous
  infrequent
  oligo-
  paracyclic
  supplementary
ovulation-inducing agent
ovulation induction
ovulation pain
ovulation prediction kit
  Conceive Ovulation Predictor
  Ovuplan
  OvuQuick
  OvuSign
  Persona
ovulation stimulant for women
ovulatory cycle
ovulatory disorder
ovulatory dysfunction
ovulatory pain

ovulatory phase of menstrual cycle
ovum (pl. ova)
  blighted
  fertilized
  holoblastic
  impregnated
  mature
  migration of
ovum retrieval by laparoscope
ovum retrieval by transabdominal approach
ovum retrieval by transvaginal approach
ovum retrieval by transvesicle approach
Ovuplan ovulation prediction kit
OvuQuick ovulation prediction kit
OvuSign midstream ovulation prediction kit
OvuStick
Ovysmen 0.5/35 oral contraceptive
Ovysmen 1/35 oral contraceptive
Ovysmen oral contraceptive
owl incision technique reduction mammoplasty
oxalate-containing food
oxalate absorption, excess
oxalate calculus
oxalate crystals
oxalic acid
oxalosis
oxaluria
Oxford operation for urinary incontinence
oxidation of ethylene glycol to oxalic acid
OxiFirst fetal monitor
OxiFirst fetal oxygen monitoring system
oximeter, ear
oximetry
oxycephaly
oxygen
oxygen analyzer
oxybutynin chloride
oxybutynin chloride syrup
oxybutynin transdermal patch
oxycephaly
Oxydome I-II
oxygenated fetal blood
oxygenated plasma-based perfusate
Oxy-Hood (oxygen hood)
Oxy-Igloo
Oxypod I-II oxygen hood
oxytocic drug
oxytocin
oxytocin augmentation
oxytocin challenge test (OCT)
oxytocin stimulation
Oxytrol (oxybutynin transdermal patch)

P, p

PAC (P1-derived artificial chromosome)
pachygyria
pachysalpingitis
pachytene
Pacis BCG bladder cancer treatment
Pacis BCG immunotherapy
pack, packing
  impregnated vaginal
  Iodoform gauze
  Ortho Personal Pak
  vaginal
packaging RNA
packed cells, transfusion
packed cell volume (PCV)
packed red blood cells
packing off abdominal viscera
paclitaxel
pad
  B-D Sensability Breast Self-Examination Aid
  Depends
  Impress Softpatch foam
  lap
  laparotomy
  maternity
  OB
  perineal ("peri pad")
  Peri-Gel

pad *(cont.)*
  Peri+Pad
  Peri-Warm
  sanitary
  Sontac ultrasound gel
  Soothies glycerin gel
  Telfa
  vaginal
  V-pad
  Weck
PadKit sample collection system
pad test for urinary incontinence
Paget disease, extramammary
Paget disease of breast
Paget syndrome
PAH (para-aminohippuric) acid concentrations
pain
  acyclic pelvic
  bearing-down
  breast
  central pelvic
  chronic pelvic (CPP)
  colicky
  cramplike
  crampy abdominal
  excruciating left flank
  expulsive

pain *(cont.)*
- false
- flank
- incapacitating
- intermenstrual
- intractable
- kidney
- labor
- ovarian
- ovulation
- ovulatory
- pelvic
- periumbilical
- phantom breast
- postoperative
- psychogenic pelvic
- referred pelvic
- sharp stabbing
- testicular
- vaginal
- vulvar (of vestibular origin)

pain at symphysis pubis
pain control, postoperative
pain during intercourse
painful erection of the clitoris
painful hematuria
painful menstruation
painful urination
pain in testicles
painless breast mass
painless cervical effacement
painless dilation
painless mammogram
painless thyroiditis
painless uterine contraction
painless voiding
pain of extragenital origin
pain of gastrointestinal origin
pain of musculoskeletal origin
pain of psychogenic origin
pain of urologic origin
pain on erection
pain on intercourse
pain on urination
pain on voiding
pain radiating down left groin and testicle
painting probe, chromosome-specific
pain with defecation
pain with intercourse
pairing mismatches
PAIS (Psychosocial Adjustment to Illness Scale)
Pajot maneuver
PAK (pancreas after kidney) transplantation
palate, cleft
palato-otodigital syndrome
palladium-103 (^{103}Pd) implantation
palladium (^{103}Pd) prostate implant
palliate
palliation
palliative radiation therapy
palliative therapy
Pallister-Hall syndrome
Pallister-Killian mosaic syndrome
Pallister-Killian syndrome (PKS) or tetrasomy 12p
Pallister mosaic aneuploidy
Pallister mosaic syndrome
Pallister-W syndrome
PALM (premature accelerated lung maturation)
palm leaf arborization of cervical mucus
Palmettx
palpable bladder
palpable mass
palpable thrill
palpable uterine contractions
Palpagraph breast mapping mammography device
Palpagraph breast tissue examination device
palpation
- abdominal
- breast
- intraperitoneal

palpation *(cont.)*
- self-breast
- suprapubic
- uterine
- vaginal

palsy (paralysis)
- brachial
- cerebral (CP)
- Déjérine
- Duchenne
- Erb
- facial
- Klumpke
- maternal obstetric
- obstetric

pamidronate
pampiniform plexus of spermatic cord
Panacryl absorbable suture
P-ANCA or pANCA (perinuclear staining pattern of ANCA)
pancake kidney
pancervical smear
pancreas after kidney (PAK) transplantation operation
pancreas, Christmas tree appearance of
pancreatic exocrine secretions
pancreatic infantilism
pan-cultured
panduriform placenta
panendoscope, McCarthy
panendoscopy
panhypopituitarism
panhysterectomy
panmural fibrosis of bladder
panniculitis
panniculus, hanging
Pap (Papanicolaou)
Papanicolaou smear (Pap smear)
Papanicolaou stain
Pap Plus HPV Screen
Pap Plus Speculoscopy (PPS)
PAP (prostatic acid phosphatase)
paper-doll fetus
paper drape
paper, Nitrazine
papilla (pl. papillae)
- renal
- urethral

papillary cystadenofibroma
papillary damage
papillary necrosis
papillary serous cystadenocarcinoma
papillary tissue necrosis
papillary transitional cell carcinoma
papillary tumor
papillitis, necrotizing renal
papilloma
- benign
- bladder
- intraductal
- serous surface

papillomavirus
Papillon Léfevre syndrome
papillotome, Apollo triple-lumen
papillotonic pseudotabes
PapNet test
PAPP A (pregnancy-associated plasma protein A)
papular dermatitis of pregnancy
papule
- pruritic urticarial
- split

papulosis, bowenoid
papyraceous fetus
para (P)
para-aortic lymph nodes
para-aortic node biopsy
para-aortic/periaortic nodes
paracarcinomatous
paracentric inversion
paracervical block (PCB)
paracervical blood needle
paracervical instillation catheter
paracervical tissue
paracervix
paracolpitis
paracolpium
paracyclic ovulation

paracyesis
paracystic pouch
paracystitis
paracystium
paracytic
paradoxical aciduria
paradoxical incontinence
parafollicular cells
paragenital tubule
paragonorrheal
parallel flow dialyzer
parallel plate dialyzer
parallel to the membrane surface
paralogy
paralysis
  bladder
  Dejerine
  Dejerine-Klumpke
  Duchenne
  Duchenne-Erb
  Erb
  Klumpke
  Klumpke-Dejerine
  phrenic nerve
paralytic ileus
paramammary lymph node
paramedian incision
paramesonephric duct
parameter
parametria
parametrial induration
parametric abscess
parametritis
  acute
  chronic
parametrium (pl. parametria)
paramour
paramyotonia congenita (PC)
paranephric body
paraorchidium
paraorchis
paraovarian cyst
parapelvic cyst
parapelvic region
paraperitoneal nephrectomy
paraphimosis
paraplegia, hereditary spastic
paraquat
pararectal fossa
pararenal abscess
pararenal aortic aneurysm
pararenal aortic atherosclerosis
pararenal fat
parasalpingitis
parasexuality
parasitemia
parasitic disease
parasitic fetus
parasitic infection
parasitic infestation
parasitic urinary tract disease
parasitic uterine leiomyoma
paraspinous muscle attachments
parasympathetic stimulation
parasyphilis
parasyphilitic
parathyroidectomy
parathyroid hormone (PTH)
parathyroid-hormone-related protein (PTHrp)
parathyroid hyperplasia
paratubal cyst
paraumbilical incision
paraurethral duct
paraurethral glands
parauterine lymph node
paravaginal hysterectomy
paravaginal lymph node
paravaginal repair
paravaginitis
paravesical blunt dissection
paravesical fossa
paravesical lymph node
paravesical pouch
parenchyma of lobe of kidney
parenchyma of testis
parenchymal scarring
parenchymal thickness

parenchymatous mastitis
parenchymatous nephritis
parenchymatous neurosyphilis
parenchymatous renal disease
parenchymatous swelling
parenchyma
  breast
  kidney
  prostate
  renal
  testicle
parenchymous goiter
parentage
parentage law
parentage testing
parental balanced chromosomal trans-location
parental cytogenetic abnormality
parental generation
parental obligations
parental responsibilities
parental rights
parenteral antibiotic therapy
parenteral fluids
parenteral nutrition
parent-of-origin studies
paresis
paretic neurosyphilis
parietal peritoneum
parietal pregnancy
parietal presentation
parity
Parkes Weber syndrome
Parkinson disease
parorchidium
parous cervix
parous introitus
parous uterus
parous vagina
parovarian cyst
parovarian region
parovariotomy
parovaritis
parovarium
paroxypropione
paroxysmal nocturnal hemoglobinemia
paroxysmal nocturnal hemoglobinuria
Parrot atrophy of the newborn
Parrot syndrome
Parry disease
Parry-Romberg syndrome
parthenogenesis
partial androgen insensitivity syndrome
partial aneuploidy
partial atelectasis
partial birth abortion
partial cystectomy
partial hysterectomy
partial linkage
partial mastectomy
partial molar pregnancy
partial monosomy
partial nephrectomy
partial obstruction of ureter
partial occlusion of blood outflow line
partial omentectomy for removal of IUD (intrauterine device)
partial penectomy
partial placenta previa
partial salpingectomy
partial scrotectomy
partial tetrasomy
partial tetrasomy 9p
partial upper vaginectomy
partial ureteral obstruction
partial vaginectomy
partial zona dissection (PZD)
particular locus
particulate elements in urine
partner-assisted dialysis
partner, sexual
partners, multiple sexual
partogram
parts, fetal small
parturient
parturifacient
parturition injury of urinary tract
parumbilical

PAS (periodic acid-Schiff) stain
passage
  kidney stone
  renal stone
  sound
  stone
  tissue
  ureteral stone
  urethral false
passes through the membrane as permeate
passing clots and tissue
passing of kidney stone
passing urine
passing water
paste, Monsel
Patau syndrome
patch
  Alora (estradiol) transdermal
  Androderm (testosterone) transdermal
  CombiPatch (estradiol/norethin drone) transdermal
  Dacron
  ERT (estrogen replacement therapy)
  estradiol transdermal
  estradiol/norethindrome
  FemPatch transdermal estrogen replacement
  HRT (hormone replacement therapy)
  Impress Softpatch urinary incontinence
  Kugel Hernia Patch
  Lyrelle
  Ortho Evra (norelgestromin/ethinyl estradiol) contraceptive
  Osteopatch
  oxybutynin transdermal
  Oxytrol (oxybutynin transdermal)
  17-beta-estradiol transdermal
  Testoderm
  Testoderm TTS testosterone
  testosterone transdermal

patch *(cont.)*
  UroMed incontinence
  vascularized gastric tissue
patchy atrophy of renal cortex
patchy endometriosis
patency
patency of fallopian tube
patency of hymenal orifice
patent
patent ductus arteriosus closure, percutaneous
patent fallopian tubes
patent foramen ovale (PFO)
patent hemodialysis access shunt
patent orifice
patent processus vaginalis
patent processus vaginalis peritonei
patent urachus
patent ureter
patent urethra
paternal determination
paternity testing
Patey modified radical mastectomy
Pathfinder DFA (direct fluorescent antigen) test
Pathfinder urologic irrigator
pathogen (see also *bacteria*)
  Acinetobacter lwoffi
  Alcaligenes xylosoxidans
  Döderlein bacillus
  Ducrey bacillus
  E. coli H157:H7
  Gardnerella vaginalis
  group A beta-hemolytic streptococcus
  Herellea vaginicola
  Pseudallescheria boydii
  Salmonella bredeney
  Serratia liquefaciens
  sexually transmitted
  Staphylococcus aureus
  Staphylococcus epidermidis
  Stenotrophomonas
  urinary

pathogenesis of dialysis-related amyloid deposits
pathognomonic
pathologic amenorrhea
pathologic diagnosis
pathologic glycosuria
pathology
pattern
  breast reconstruction
  hypergonadotropic
  hypogonadotropic
  normogonadotropic
  Sertoli-cell-only (SCO)
Patton laparoscopic catheter
pauci-immune crescentic glomerulonephritis
pauci-immune glomerulonephritis
pauci-immune rapidly progressive glomerulonephritis
Paxene (paclitaxel)
PBN hysterosalpingography catheter
PBNS (percutaneous bladder neck stabilization)
PBPI (penile-brachial pressure index) to assess cardiac disease
PC (paramyotonia congenita)
PCB (paracervical block) needle
PCC (propionyl-CoA carboxylase) deficiency
PCL (periventricular leukomalacia)
PCNL (percutaneous nephrolithotomy)
PCNL (percutaneous nephrostolithotomy)
PCO_2
PCO (polycystic ovary) syndrome (PCOS)
PCR (polymerase chain reaction)
PCR-RFLP (polymerase chain reaction restriction fragment length polymorphism)
PC-SPES for advanced prostate cancer
PCT (porphyria cutanea tarda)
PCT (postcoital test)
PCV (packed cell volume)
PD (peritoneal dialysis)
PDA (patent ductus arteriosus)
P.D. Access needle
P.D. Access over-the-needle catheter
P.D. Access peel-away needle introducer
PDC (peritoneal dialysis catheter)
PD (peritoneal dialysis) catheter
PDH (pyruvate dehydrogenase deficiency)
PD plus (peritoneal dialysis combination therapy)
^{103}Pd (palladium) prostatic implant
PDT (photodynamic therapy)
peak and trough levels
peak flow of the urinary bladder
peakometer
peak pairwise score
peak plasma concentration
Pean clamp
Pean hysterectomy forceps
peanut-tip wand
PEARL (physiologic endometrial ablation/resection loop)
Pearl packing forceps
pear-shaped uterus
peau d'orange appearance of breast
PEBB (percutaneous excisional breast biopsy)
Peck disease
pectoral fascia
pectoral muscle
pectoralis fascia
pectoralis major muscle
pectoralis minor muscle
pectoralis muscle
pedal edema, trace
pedal lymphangiography
pederast
pederasty
Pederson vaginal speculum
pediatric cystoscope
pediatrician
pediatric nephrologist

pedicle
  IMA (internal mammary artery)
  muscle
  ovarian
  uterine
  vascular
pedicle compression
pedicle technique reduction mammoplasty
pediculosis pubis
pedigree
PediPort disposable trocar
Pedi vaginal aspirator
pedophilia
pedunculated submucous fibroid
pedunculated subserous fibroid
pedunculated tumor
pedunculated uterine fibroid
pedunculated uterine myoma
pedunculated vesical tumor
Peel-Away access
Peel-Away sheath
peeling skin syndrome
PEEP (positive end-expiratory pressure)
peeping testis
peer education
Pelizaeus-Merzbacher disease
pellagra-cerebellar ataxia-renal aminoaciduria syndrome
pelvic abscess
pelvic adhesions
pelvica, ganglia
pelvicaliceal effacement
pelvicaliectasis
pelvic brim
pelvic cavity
pelvic cellulitis
pelvic congestion syndrome
pelvic deformity
pelvic direction
pelvic endometriosis
pelvic endoscopy
pelvicephalography
pelvic evisceration
pelvic examination
pelvic exenteration
pelvic exploration
Pelvic Flex urinary incontinence program
pelvic floor
pelvic floor electrical stimulation (PFS)
pelvic floor electromyogram (EMG)
pelvic floor exercises
pelvic floor function study
pelvic floor integrity
pelvic floor laceration
pelvic floor muscles
pelvic floor reconstruction
pelvic floor repair
pelvic fundus, incompetence of
pelvic gutters
pelvic hyperemia
pelvic inflammatory disease (PID)
pelvic inlet
pelvic kidney
pelvic laparotomy
pelvic lavage
pelvic lymph node dissection
pelvic lymph nodes
pelvic lymphadenectomy
pelvic lymphatics
pelvic mass
pelvic muscles
pelvic outlet
pelvic pain
  acute
  acyclic
  chronic
  referred
pelvic pain
pelvic pain on intercourse
pelvic peritoneum, endometriosis of
pelvic peritonitis
pelvic plane of outlet
pelvic presentation
pelvic pressure
pelvic pyemia
pelvic relaxation

pelvic rest
pelvic salpingitis
pelvic sepsis
pelvic septicemia
pelvic sidewall
pelvic sonogram
pelvic structures
pelvic support
pelvic surgery
pelvic thrombophlebitis
pelvic ultrasonography
pelvic ultrasound
pelvic vascular thrombosis
pelvic vein congestion
pelvic version
pelvic viscera
pelvic wall
  anterior
  posterior
pelvicaliceal changes
pelvicaliceal collecting system
pelvicaliceal distention
pelvicaliceal echo pattern
pelvicaliceal, pelvicalyceal
pelvicaliceal system
pelvicephalography
pelvicephalometry
pelvic, exenteration
pelvic-floor surgery
pelvifaxation
pelvigraph
pelvilithotomy
pelvimeter
  Collin
  Collyer
  DeLee
  Hanely-McDermitt
  Martin
pelvimetry
  CT
  manual
  radiographic
pelvina, ganglia
pelviolithotomy
pelvioperitonitis
pelvioplasty
pelvioscopy
pelvirectal achalasia
pelvis (pl. pelves)
  android
  anthropoid
  bifid
  borderline
  brachypellic
  contracted
  cordate
  dolichopellic
  dwarf
  elephant
  extrarenal
  false
  flat
  frozen
  funnel-shaped
  gynecoid
  infantile
  inlet contraction of
  kyphotic
  lordotic
  maternal
  mesatipellic
  Otto
  outlet contraction of
  platypellic
  relaxation of
  renal
  round
  simple flat
  true
  ureteral
  ureteric
pelviscope
pelviscopic examination
pelviscopy
pelvis of kidney
pelvis renalis
pelvitherm
pelviureteral junction

pelviureteric junction
pelviureterography
PelvX pelvic support device
pemphigoid gestationis
pemphigus neonatorum
pemtumomab
pencil, electrosurgical
pencil-point suprapubic access catheter
pencil-point suprapubic access needle
Penduloff incision
pendulous abdomen
pendulous breast
pendulous urethra
pendulous urethral stricture
penectomy
 complete
 partial
penetrance, variable
penetrant molecules
penetrant
penetration of egg
penetrating extension of cervical
  carcinoma
penetrating genital injury
Penetrex (enoxacin)
pen, Humalog Pen
penicillin
penile agenesis
penile amputation
penile block
penile-brachial pressure index (PBPI)
penile cellulitis
penile condyloma
penile Doppler study
penile edema
penile ejaculate
penile epispadias
penile fibromatosis
penile foreskin
penile gangrene
penile hypospadias
penile implant, Alpha 1
penile implant cylinders
penile injection therapy
penile length
penile necrosis
penile prosthesis (see also *prosthesis*)
 AMS (American Medical Systems)
 AMS Ambicor
 AMS 200 CX
 AMS 600 malleable
 AMS 600M malleable
 AMS 650 malleable
 AMS 700 CX inflatable
 AMS 700 CXM inflatable
 Dilamezinsert (DMI) penile
  dilator/inserter
 Duraphase inflatable
 Dura-II positional
 Dynaflex
 Finney Flexi-Rod
 GFS Mark II inflatable
 inflatable
 Jonas
 Mentor Alpha 1 inflatable
 Small-Carrion
penile raphe
penile reconstruction
penile rigidity
penile shaft
penile skin inversion
penile stump
penile urethra
penile vein ligation
penile wart
penis (pl. penes)
 abscess of
 atrophy of
 body of
 boil of
 bulb of
 bulbospongiosus muscle of
 buried
 carbuncle of
 carcinoma in situ of
 cavernous body of
 cavernous nerves of
 cellulitis of

penis *(cont.)*
- clubbed
- concealed
- corkscrew
- corpora cavernosa of
- corpus spongiosum of
- crura of
- crus of
- deep artery of
- deep dorsal vein of
- deep fascia of
- deep veins of
- dorsal artery of
- dorsal nerve of
- dorsum of
- double
- edema of
- embolism of
- fibrosis of
- fibrous tissue of
- foreskin of
- glans
- helicine artery of
- hematoma of
- herpetic infection of
- hypertrophy of
- ischiospongiosus muscle of
- kraurosis of
- leukoplakia of
- micropenis
- oral stimulation of
- perforating artery of
- prepuce of
- psoriasis of
- root of
- septum of
- shaft of
- skin of
- spongy body of
- superficial dorsal veins of
- suspensory ligament of
- thrombosis of
- tip of
- webbed

penis lacuna
penischisis
penis palmatus
penis plastica
Penn pouch for continent urinary diversion
penopubic epispadias
penoscrotal hypospadias
penoscrotal junction
penotomy
PenRad mammography clinical reporting system
Penrose drain
pentalogy of Cantrel
pentalogy syndrome
pentamidine
pentasomy (see also *syndrome*)
pentasomy 8 syndrome
pentasomy 8q syndrome
pentasomy sex chromosome syndrome
pentasomy 13q syndrome
pentasomy 21 syndrome
pentasomy X syndrome
penta X syndrome (also pental)
Pentax ECN-1530 choledocho-nephroscope
pentosan polysulfate sodium
pentosuria
- alimentary
- essential

PEP (progestogen-associated endometrial protein)
PEPCK deficiency, mitochondrial and cytosolic
Pepper syndrome
pepsinuria
peptide
peptide hormones
- activin
- inhibin

per primam, healing
perceptual hearing loss
Percocet (oxycodone; acetaminophen)
Percuflex Plus flexible ureteral stent

percutaneous aspiration of kidney
percutaneous biopsy
percutaneous bladder neck stabilization (PBNS)
percutaneous chemolysis
percutaneous epididymal sperm aspiration
percutaneous excisional breast biopsy (PEBB)
percutaneous mechanical thrombectomy (PMT)
percutaneous needle biopsy of kidney
percutaneous nephrolithotomy (PCNL)
percutaneous nephrolithotripsy
percutaneous nephrostolithotomy (PCNL)
percutaneous nephrostomy
percutaneous nephrostomy drainage
percutaneous nephrostomy with stent
percutaneous patent ductus arteriosus closure
percutaneous pyelogram
percutaneous renal biopsy
percutaneous resection
percutaneous resection of transitional cell carcinoma of the renal pelvis
percutaneous sperm aspiration
percutaneous Stoller afferent nerve stimulation system (PerQ SANS)
percutaneous stone dissolution
percutaneous stone manipulation
percutaneous transluminal angioplasty
percutaneous transluminal renal angioplasty (PTRA)
percutaneous transperineal seed implantation
percutaneous umbilical blood sampling (PUBS)
percutaneous umbilical blood transfusion
Pereyra bladder neck suspension, modified
Pereyra ligature carrier
Perez reflex
perfect fungus
perfectly mixed flow
perforated endometrioma
perforating artery of penis
perforating vessels
perforation
  bladder
  blood vessel
  intestinal
  perinatal intestinal
  urethral
  uterine
perforation of vessels, inadvertent
perforator, Baylor amniotic
perfusate, oxygenated plasma-based
perfuse the filtrate side of the membrane
perfuse the membrane
perfusion
  continuous pulsatile hypothermic
  diminished fetal
  ex vivo
  extracorporeal
  fallopian tube
  hypothermic
  placenta
  renal
  uteroplacental
perfusion defect
perfusion kit, Euro-Collins multiorgan
Pergonal (menotropins)
pericarditis
Peri-Colace (casanthranol; docusate sodium)
perianal condyloma
perianal wart
periareolar augmentation mammoplasty
periareolar incision
periareolar mastopexy
pericardial friction rub
pericarditis, uremic
peri (perineal) care
pericentric inversion
pericolpitis

pericystic
pericystitis
pericystium
perididymitis
periductal mastitis
Peri-Gel pad
perihepatic peritoneum
perihepatitis, gonococcal
perihilar glomerulosclerosis
perimenopausal
perimenopause
perimesonephric cyst
perimetric
perimetritic
perimetritis
perimetrium (pl. perimetria)
perimortem delivery
perinatal acidosis
perinatal asphyxia
perinatal center
perinatal death
perinatal evaluation and treatment unit (PETU)
perinatal genetic counseling
perinatal hormone condition
perinatal infection
perinatal injury
perinatal intestinal perforation
perinatal jaundice
perinatal medicine
perinatal morbidity
perinatal mortality
perinatal mortality rate
perinatal pneumomediastinum
perinatal pneumopericardium
perinatal pneumothorax
perinatal outcome
perinatal risk
perinatal torsion
perinate
perinatologist
perinatology
perineal artery
perineal artery fasciocutaneous flap
perineal biopsy
perineal body
perineal care
perineal compression dressing
perineal fluid collection
perineal hematoma
perineal hernia
perineal hypospadias
perineal itching
perineal laceration
perineal lithotomy
perineal muscle laceration
perineal pad ("peri pad")
perineal prostatectomy
perineal raphe
perineal section
perineal space
perineal surgical apron
perineal tear
perineal urethroscopy
perineal urethrostomy
perineal urethrotomy
perineal varicose veins
perineocele
perineometer
perineoplasty
perineorrhaphy
perineoscrotal
perineostomy
perineosynthesis
perineotomy
perineovaginal fistula
perinephrial
perinephric abscess
perinephric fat
perinephric hematoma
perinephric hemorrhage
perinephric space
perinephric tissue
perinephritis
perinephrium (pl. perinephria)
perineum (pl. perinea)
  breakdown of
  fibrosis of

perineum *(cont.)*
  lacerated
  rigid
  urethrostomy through the
  watering-can
perineural lymphatics
perinuclear ANCA
period
  duration of
  heavy
  interval between
  irregular
  last menstrual (LMP)
  last normal menstrual (LNMP)
  menstrual
  regular
  skipped
periodic abstinence
periodic acid-Schiff stain
periodic breathing
periodic fibroadenosis of breast
periodic intermittent catheterization
periodic paralysis, familial
perioophoritis
perioperative obstetrics
periovaritis
periovular
Peri+Pad
"peri pad" (perineal pad)
peripartal corticosteroid prophylaxis
peripartal vaginal hemorrhage
peripartum
peripartum cardiomyopathy
peripartum pubic separation
peripelvic cyst
peripenial
peripheral aromatization of precursor
  steroids
peripheral cyanosis
peripheral dysostosis
peripheral embolism
peripheral estrogen conversion
peripheral neuritis in pregnancy
peripheral neuropathy
"peri prep" (perineal prep)
periprostatic fat
periprostatic tissue
periprosthetic capsulectomy of breast
perirectal lymphatics
perirenal abscess
perirenal fascia
perirenal fat
perirenal hematoma
perirenal hemorrhage
perirenal mass
perirenal septum
perirenal space
perirenal tissue
perisalpingitis
perisalpingo-oophoritis
perisalpinx
perispermatitis
peristalsis
  retrograde
  ureteral
  ureteric
peristaltic activity
Peri-Strips Dry
peritoneal adhesions
peritoneal cavity
peritoneal constriction ring
peritoneal contact time of dialysate
peritoneal cytology
peritoneal dialysate
peritoneal dialysis (PD)
peritoneal dialysis-associated peritonitis
peritoneal dialysis catheter
peritoneal dialysis complications
peritoneal dialysis diffusion across
  semipermeable membrane
peritoneal dialysis solution
peritoneal edge
peritoneal endometriosis
peritoneal equilibration test (PET)
peritoneal fluid
peritoneal fold
peritoneal irritation
peritonealization

peritoneal lavage
peritoneal membrane
peritoneal oocyte and sperm transfer (POST)
peritoneal pregnancy
peritoneal reflection
peritoneal seeding of endometriosis
peritoneal seeding of tumor
peritoneal space
peritoneal washings
peritonei, processus vaginalis
peritoneoscope
peritoneoscopy
peritoneopericardial diaphragmatic hernia
peritoneum (pl. peritonea)
  endometriosis of pelvic
  parietal
  pelvic
  perihepatic
  posterior parietal
  urogenital
  uterine
  vesicouterine
  visceral
peritoneum identified with hemostats
peritoneum urogenitale
peritoneum was reapproximated
peritonitis
  adhesive
  bacterial
  meconium
  pelvic
  peritoneal dialysis-associated
  puerperal
  spontaneous
peritubal adhesions
periumbilical blood sampling (PUBS)
periumbilical incision
periumbilical pain
periumbilical region
periureteral adhesions
periureteral fibrosis
periureteric
periureteritis
periureteritis plastica
periurethral abscess
periurethral cellulitis
periurethral collagen injection
periurethral cystoscopy
periurethral gland
periurethral injection therapy
periurethral phlegmon
periurethral prostate gland
periurethral site
periurethral tear
periurethral tissue laceration
periurethritis
periuterine
perivaginitis
perivascular decidualized stromal cells
periventricular leukomalacia (PVL)
perivesical adhesions
perivesical inflammation
perivesical tissue
perivitelline space
Peri-Warm pad
permanent brachytherapy
permanent infertility
permanent suprapubic cystostomy
permanent upper tract diversion
permanent urinary diversion
Perma-Seal dialysis access graft
PermCath dual-lumen catheter
permeability
  glomerular
  vascular
permeability coefficient, Pi
permeability of asymmetric membrane
permeability to water and solutes
permeance
permeate
permeate flow direction
Permixon (*Serenoa repens* extract)
permutation
pernicious anemia of pregnancy
pernicious vomiting in pregnancy

peroneal muscular atrophy
PerQ SANS (percutaneous Stoller afferent nerve stimulation system) urge incontinence device
Perras breast prosthesis
Perras-Papillon breast implant
Perrault syndrome
PerryMeter anal EMG sensor
Perry sensor for vaginismus
persistent azoospermia
persistent bacteremia
persistent breast abnormality
persistent ductus arteriosus
persistent ectopic pregnancy
persistent fetal circulation
persistent glomerulonephritis
persistent hematuria
persistent hymen
persistent hyperemesis
persistent müllerian duct syndrome
persistent nipple discharge
persistent occipitoposterior position
persistent patency of ductus arteriosus
persistent proteinuria
persistent pulmonary hypertension of the newborn (PPHN)
persistent trophoblastic disease (PTD)
persistent truncus arteriosus
persistent ventral hood
Persist incontinence treatment system
persisting proteinuria
Persona ovulation-prediction monitoring kit
pessary (pl. pessaries)
  Albert-Smith
  Biswas Silastic
  blue ring
  cube
  doughnut
  Dumontpallier
  Dutch
  elastic vaginal
  Emmet-Gelhorn
  Findley folding

pessary *(cont.)*
  Gariel
  Gelhorn
  Guhrung
  Hodge
  Mayer
  Menge
  Prentif
  Prochownik
  ring
  vaginal
  Zwanck
perstraction
pertussis
pervaporation
PET (peritoneal equilibration test)
PET (positron emission tomography)
petechia (pl. petechiae), fetal
PETU (perinatal evaluation and treatment unit)
Peutz-Jeghers syndrome
pexiganan
Peyronie disease
Peyronie plaque
Pfannenstiel incision
Pfeiffer syndrome
p53 adenoviral gene
p53 mutation
p53 protein overexpression
p53 tumor suppressor gene
Pfister-Schwartz stone basket
PFKM (phosphorfrukinase deficiency)
PFO (patent foramen ovale)
PFS (pelvic floor electrical stimulation)
PGAM (phosphorglycerate mutase deficiency)
PGA synthetic absorbable suture
P gene
PGE1 (prostaglandin E1)
PGH (placental growth hormone)
P-glycoprotein
PgR (progesterone receptor)
pH (hydrogen ion concentration)
phage

phagedenic erosion
phagocytic cells
phagocytic system
phallectomy
phallic phase
phallicism
phallism
phallocampsis
phallocrypsis
phallodynia
phalloid
phalloncus
phalloplastic procedure
phalloplasty
phallotomy
phallus
Phaneuf uterine artery forceps
phantom breast pain
phantom breast sensation
phantom pregnancy
phantom, Schultze
pharaonic circumcision
pharaonic female genital circumcision
Pharmaseal cervical dilator
Pharmaseal uterine sound
PharmaSeed iodine-125 (^{125}I) seeds
PharmaSeed palladium-103 (^{103}Pd) seeds
pharyngeal embryonic groove
phase
  alpha
  beta
  embryonic
  excretory
  genital
  growth
  nephrographic (NP)
  ovulatory
  phallic
  postovulatory
  pregenital
  preovulatory
  pseudoglandular
  terminal sac
phase-contrast microscope
phase of acute renal failure
  oliguric
  postoliguric
  prodromal
phases of adjustment to chronic dialysis
phases of labor
  active
  latent
phases of menstrual cycle
  follicular
  luteal
  ovulatory
  postovulatory
  preovulatory
PHD (personal hemodialysis) system
pHEM-ALERT vaginosis screening device
phenazopyridine
Phenergan
phenoluria
phenomenology of the genitalia
phenomenon (pl. phenomena) (see also *syndrome*)
  backflow
  dawn
  escape
  Jod-Basedow
  nutcracker
  Schwartzman
  Somogyi
  vanishing twin
  wind-up
phenotype
phenotypic abnormalities
phenotypic effect
phenotypic variance
phenotyping
phenoxybenzamine
phentermine
phenylalaninemia
phenylketonuria (PKU)
phenylpropanolamine (PPA)
phenylpyruvic oligophrenia

pheochromocytoma, bladder
pheromones
Philadelphia chromosome
Philips catheter with filiform guide
Philips ultrasound with endovaginal transducer
phimosis (pl. phimoses)
  congenital
  penile
  tubal
phimosis clitoridis
phimosis vaginalis
phimosis with adhesions
phimotic
phlebitis, ovarian vein
phlebography, renal
phlebolith, calcified
phlebometritis
phlebothrombosis, deep vein
phlegmasia alba dolens
phlegmon, periurethral
phlorizin glycosuria
phobia
Phocas fibrocystic breast syndrome
Phocas syndrome
phocomelia syndrome
pH of cord blood
PH-1 (primary hyperoxaluria, type 1)
PhosLo (calcium)
phosphate (PO_4)
phosphate absorption
phosphate binder
phosphate-binding compounds
phosphate crystals
phosphate-loading hypocalcemia
phosphaturia
phosphoenolpyruvate carboxykinase deficiency, mitochondrial or cytosolic
phosphoglycerate kinase deficiency (PGK)
phosphoglycerokinase deficiency (PGK)
phosphorfrukinase deficiency (PFKM)
phosphorglycerate mutase deficiency (PGAM)
phosphorylase deficiency (MPD)
phosphorylase 6 kinase deficiency
phosphorus, serum
phosphuresis
photocoagulation, deep
photodynamic therapy (PDT), Levulan
Photofrin (porfimer sodium)
Photon radiosurgery system
photoradiation
photosensitivity, cutaneous
phototherapy
  ultraviolet
  Wallaby
phrenic nerve paralysis
phthiriasis
pH, urinary
phylogenesis
phylon
physical chemical structural alterations
physical intersex conditions
physical map
physiological measures of sexual arousal
physiologic amenorrhea
physiologic cycle
physiologic delay of menarche
physiologic derangement
physiologic endometrial ablation/ resection loop (PEARL)
physiologic erection
physiologic hydremia of pregnancy
physiologic icterus
physiologic jaundice of neonate
physiotherapy, chest
phytanic acid storage disease
phytotherapy
pica
PICC (peripherally inserted central catheter)
Pick disease
pickups
  DeBakey
  rat-tooth

PID (pelvic inflammatory disease)
PIE (pulmonary interstitial emphysema)
Pierre-Marie disease
Pierre Robin anomalad, complex, or sequence
Pierre Robin syndrome
piezoelectric
piezoelectric transducer
Piezolith-EPL (extracorporeal piezoelectric lithotriptor)
pigmentary retinal degradation
pigmented casts
pigmented epulis
PIGN (postinfectious glomerulonephritis)
pigtail ureteral catheter
PIH (pregnancy-induced hypertension)
pile, sentinel
pill (pl. pills)
  abortion
  birth control (BCP)
  morning after
pilosebaceous unit
Pilot suture guide
PiM (protein inhibitor type M)
pimagedine
PIN (prostatic intraepithelial neoplasia)
Pinard maneuver
Pinard sign of breech presentation
ping-ponging
pinhole meatus
pinhole urethral opening
pinpoint cervical os
pinpoint os uteri
Pinpoint stereotactic arm for delivery of radioactive seed implants
pin vise handle
pinworm vaginitis
pioglitazone
Pipelle endometrial sampling device
Pipelle endometrial suction catheter
Piper forceps
Piper forceps operation
Piper obstetrical forceps
piperacillin
pipette, Wallace
PIPP (Premature Infant Pain Profile)
piritrexim
Pitocin (oxytocin)
Pitocin augmentation of labor
Pitocin induction of labor
Pitocin stimulation
Pitocin therapy
Pitressin (vasopressin)
pitting edema
Pitt-Rogers-Danks syndrome
pituitary amenorrhea
pituitary down-regulation
pituitary dwarfism
pituitary dysfunction
pituitary failure
pituitary gigantism
pituitary gland
pituitary-gonadal axis
pituitary gonadotropins
pituitary hypothyroidism
pituitary infantilism
pituitary testing
pituitary tumor
pityriasis rubra pilaris
Pivet-Cook double lumen needle
Pixie fiberoptic scope
PiZ (protein inhibitor type Z)
PKD (polycystic kidney disease)
PKS (Pallister-Killian syndrome)
PKU (phenylketouria) test
placement, ureter
placenta
  abnormal adherence of
  accessory
  adherent
  annular
  anular
  battledore
  bidiscoidal
  bilobate
  bilobed
  bipartite

placenta *(cont.)*
- central placenta previa
- chorioallantoic
- chorioamnionic
- chorioamniotic
- choriovitelline
- circumvallate
- cirsoid
- cotyledonary
- cup-shaped
- deciduate
- deciduous
- detachment of
- dimidiate
- discoid
- discoplacenta
- disperse
- Duncan
- duplex
- endotheliochorial
- epitheliochorial
- fetal
- first trimester
- fundal
- furcate
- hemochorial
- hemoendothelial
- horseshoe
- incarcerated
- intact
- kidney-shaped
- labyrinthine
- lobed
- low implantation of
- low-lying
- marginal
- maternal
- monochorionic diamnionic
- monochorionic diamniotic
- monochorionic monoamnionic
- monochorionic monoamniotic
- multilobate
- multilobed
- nondeciduate

placenta *(cont.)*
- nondeciduous
- panduriform
- premature detachment of
- premature separation of
- retained
- ring-shaped
- Schultze
- second trimester
- succenturiate
- supernumerary
- syndesmochorial
- third trimester
- trapped
- trilobate
- tripartite
- twin
- uterine
- velamentous
- villous
- yolk-sac
- zonary
- zonular

placenta accreta
placenta accreta vera
placenta biloba
placenta bipartita
placenta circumvallata
placenta cirsoides
placenta diffusa
placenta dimidiata
placenta discoidea
placenta duplex
placenta extrachorales
placenta fenestra
placenta fenestrata
placenta fetalis
placenta gonadotropin
placenta increta
placental abruption
placental alkaline phosphatase test (PLAP)
placental barrier
placental circulation

placental dysfunction
placental dysfunction syndrome
placental dysmature
placental dystocia
placental edema
placental forceps
placental formation
placental fragments
  infected
  retained
placental grade
placental growth hormone (PGH)
placental infarct
placental infarction
placental infection
placental insufficiency
placental lobes
placental localization
placental location
placental membrane
placental perfusion
placental polyp
placental position
placental presentation
placental septa
placental sign of endometrial bleeding
placental site trophoblastic tumor
placental souffle
placental stage labor
placental sulfatase deficiency
placental thrombosis
placental transfusion syndrome
placenta manually separated and extracted
placenta marginata
placenta membranes
placenta multiloba
placenta multipartita
placenta nappiformis
placenta of fetus
placenta panduriformis
placenta percreta
placenta previa
  central
  complete

placenta previa *(cont.)*
  incomplete
  lateral
  low implantation
  marginal
  partial
  total
placenta previa centralis
placenta previa marginalis
placenta previa partialis
placenta protein
placenta reflexa
placenta reniformis
placenta separated spontaneously
placenta spuria
placenta succenturiata
placentation
placenta triloba
placenta tripartita
placenta triplex
placenta uterina
placenta velamentosa
placenta was delivered spontaneously and intact
placentitis
placentogenesis
placentogram
placentography
placentoid
placentologist
placentology
placentoma
placentopathy
placentotherapy
plagiocephaly
plain sutures
Plan B (levonorgestrel) postcoital contraceptive
plane
  anterior-posterior
  coronal
  fascial
  fat
  pelvic canal
  sagittal

plane *(cont.)*
  subfascial
  transverse
Planned Parenthood
plantar crease
PLAP (placental alkaline phosphatase) test
Plaquase (lyophilized collagenase)
plaques of pregnancy
plasma
plasma ACTH concentration
plasma cell balanitis
plasma cell dyscrasia
plasma cell mastitis
plasma phosphate
plasma renin
plasma urate
plasmacrit screening test for syphilis
plasmapheresis
plasmid
plastid
Plasmodium falciparum
Plasmodium malariae
Plastibell
plastica, induratio penis
plate
  axial
  chorionic
  prechordal
  urethral
platelet membrane phospholipid
platelet storage pool disorder
platelet thromboxane synthesis
Platinol (cisplatin)
platybasia
plastypellic pelvis
PLD (polycystic liver disease)
pleiotropy
plesiotherapy
plethora of newborn
plethysmography
pleural space
plexus
  aortic
  celiac
  pampiniform
  prostatic venous
  renal
  superior mesenteric
  uterovaginal
  vaginal
  vesical
  vesical venous
plexus of Santorini
plicamycin
plicate
plicated vaginal wall
plication
  albuginea
  fascial
  Kelly-Kennedy urethral
  Kelly-Stoeckel urethral
  sphincteric
  ureterovesical junction
  urethral
  urethrovesical junction
  vaginal wall
ploidy
plug
  Avina female urethral
  "butt"
  catheter
  Herniamesh
  Marlex PerFix
  meconium
  R-Med
plume
  laser
  smoke
Plummer disease
plunging goiter
plural pregnancy
PMDD (premenstrual dysphoric disorder)
PML (progressive multifocal leuko-encephalopathy)

PMN (polymorphonuclear leukocyte)
PMS (premenstrual syndrome)
PMS-Conjugated Estrogens
PM 60/40 infant formula
PMT (percutaneous mechanical thrombectomy)
pneumaturia
pneumococcal pneumonia vaccine
pneumococcosuria
pneumococcus
pncumococcus nephritis
pneumocystography
pneumogram
pneumomediastinum, perinatal
pneumonia
  congenital, in the newborn
  double
  infective
pneumonitis
  congenital rubella
  fetal aspiration
  meconium
pneumopericardium, perinatal
pneumoperitoneum
pneumoperitoneum needle (see *needle*)
pneumopyelograph
pneumopyelography
pneumoscrotum, ipsilateral
Pneumo Sleeve laparoscopic airlock
Pneumo Sleeve laparoscopic assist device
pneumothorax, perinatal
Pneu-Stick needle
PO_4 (phosphate)
PO_4 binding agent
PO_4 binding effect
PO_4 infusion
pocket
  breast reconstruction
  fluid
  pus
  subcutaneous
PocketDop handheld Doppler monitor
podalic version
podocyte
  effacement of
  epithelial
  foot process of
podofilox
podofilox gel
podophyllin
podophyllum
poikilocytosis
point deletion
point mutation
poisoning
Poland anomaly
Poland syndactyly
Poland syndrome
polar body
polar presentation
polarized light microscopy
pole
  cephalic
  epididymal
  fetal
  inferior (of kidney)
  kidney
  lower (of testis)
  middle
  superior (of kidney)
  temporal
  upper (of testis)
polio (poliomyelitis)
poliodystrophic cerebri progressiva
polio vaccine
Pollack bead chain cystourethrogram
polio vaccine
pollakiuria
pollination
polyacrylonitrile
polyacrylonitrile hemofiltration membrane
polyamine
polyantibiotic ointment (neomycin-polymyxin-bacitracin)
poly A RNA
polyarteritis, microscopic

polyarteritis nodosa
polyarthritis enterica
polybutester suture
polychondritis, relapsing
Polycitra-K (potassium citrate; sodium citrate; citric acid)
polyclonal antibody
polycyesis
polycystic kidney
polycystic kidney disease (PKD)
  autosomal dominant
  autosomal recessive
polycystic liver disease
polycystic ovary
polycystic ovary disease
polycystic ovary (PCO) syndrome (PCOS)
polycythema neonatorum
polycythemia
polycythemia neonatorum
polycythemia, post-transplant
polydactyly, postaxial
polydipsia
polydrug therapy
polydystrophic dwarfism
PolyFlo peripherally inserted central catheter (PICC)
polygenic disorders
polygenic/multifactorial disorder
polygenic/multifactorial inheritance
polyglactin 910 suture material
polyglandular deficiency syndrome
polyglandular disorder
polyhydramnios
polyhypermenorrhea
polyhypomenorrhea
polymenorrhea
polymerase chain reaction
polymerase technique
polymerase chain reaction (PCR)
polymeric IgA
polymeric IgA antigen complex
polymeric molecules
polymicrobial bacteremia
polymicrogyria
polymorphic genetic marker
polymorphic region of DNA
polymorphic variation
polymorphism
polymorphonuclear leukocyte cells
polymorphonuclear leukocytes (PMN, polys)
polymyositis
polyneuritis
polyostotic sclerosing histiocytosis
polyovular ovarian follicle
polyp
  adenomatous
  broad ligament
  cervical
  corpus uteri
  endocervical
  endometrial
  fibrinous
  inflammatory fibroid
  mucous
  nasal
  placental
  ureteral
  ureteric
  uterine
  urethral
polypectomy
polypeptides
polyp forceps
polyphrenic gene
polyploid
polyploidy
polyp of corpus uteri
polypoid calcified irregular mass
polypoid filling defect
polypoid lymphoid hyperplasia
polypoid tissue
polyposis, familial
polyp removal by hysteroscope
polyprophylene button
polyp snare, hysteroscopic
polys (polymorphonuclear leukocytes)

polysiloxone capsules
polysomy
polysulfone
polysulfone hemofiltration membrane
Polytef augmentation urethroplasty
Polytef Teflon paste
polytene chromosome
polytetrafluoroethylene (PTFE) graft
polyurethane pail-handle coiled-tip
  peritoneal dialysis catheter
polyuria
  diabetic
  massive
  vasopressin-resistant
  vasopressin-sensitive
Poly-Vi-Sol infant vitamin supplement
polyzygotic twins
Pomeroy tubal li
gation
Pompe disease
P1-derived artificial chromosome
  (PAC)
P-170 glycoprotein
Ponsky Endo Sock retrieval bag
Ponstel (mefenamic acid)
Ponticelli protocol
Poole suction tip
pool, vaginal
poor clearances of small solutes
poor venous drainage
poor contractions
poor fetal growth
poor tissue turgor
poor urinary flow rate
poor visualization
popliteal pterygium syndrome
popliteal pulse
pop-off suture
population
population genetics
population risk
porencephaly
Porges-Meier flocculation test for
  syphilis
porous kidney
porous membrane
porous polyethylene dialysis catheter
porphyria
  acute intermittent (AIP)
  congenital
  congenital erythropoietic (CEP)
  congenital hematoporphyria
  copro-
  erythropoietic (EPP)
  hardero-
  hematoerythropoietic (HEP)
  idiosyncratic
  pyrroloporphyria
  Swedish
  symptomatic
porphyria cutanea symptomatica
porphyria cutanea tarda (PCT)
porphyrinuria
Porro cesarean section
Porro hysterectomy
port
  access
  flushing
  Port-A-Cath
  venous
portable blood irradiator
Port-A-Cath
Portagen infant formula
Portagen medium-chain triglyceride diet
portio vaginalis
port site, 12 mm
port-wine birthmark
port-wine mark
port-wine stain
position
  dorsal lithotomy
  dorsal recumbent
  dorsal supine
  English
  fetal
  flank
  frog-leg
  frontoanterior

position *(cont.)*
- frontoposterior
- frontotransverse
- knee-chest
- lateral decubitus
- lateral recumbent
- leapfrog
- left flank
- left frontoanterior (LFA)
- left frontoposterior (LFP)
- left frontotransverse (LFT)
- left mentotransverse (LMT)
- left occipitoposterior (LOP)
- left occipitotransverse (LOT)
- left sacroposterior (LSP)
- lithotomy
- mentoanterior (MA)
- mentoposterior (MP)
- mentotransverse
- modified dorsal lithotomy
- Noble
- occipitoanterior (OA)
- occipitoposterior
- occiput-anterior (OA)
- occiput left anterior (OLA)
- occiput-posterior (OP)
- persistent occipitoposterior
- prone
- right frontoanterior (RFA)
- right frontoposterior (RFP)
- right frontotransverse (RFT)
- right mentoanterior (RMA)
- right mentotransverse (RMT)
- right occipitoanterior (ROA)
- right occipitoposterior (ROP)
- right occipitotransverse (ROT)
- right sacroanterior (RSA)
- right sacroposterior (RSP)
- right sacrotransverse (RST)
- sacroposterior (SP) breech
- sacrotransverse (ST)
- sacrum right posterior (SRP)
- Scultetus
- semiprone

position *(cont.)*
- Simon
- Sims
- supine
- Trendelenburg
- Valentine

positional cloning
positional stasis
positive acetowhite test
positive antibody screen
positive beta hCG
positive end-expiratory pressure (PEEP)
positive family history
positive interference
positive Marshall test
positive predictive value
positive pregnancy test
positive pressure ventilation (PPV)
positive, Rh
positive surgical margins
positron emission tomography (PET)
POST (peritoneal oocyte and sperm transfer)
post-Amadori intermediate
postanesthesia recovery room
postartificial menopausal syndrome
postaugmentation mammoplasty bra
postaxial acrofacial dysostosis
postaxial polydactyly
postcatheterization stricture of urethra
postcaval ureter
postcoital bleeding
postcoital spotting
postcoital test (PCT)
postcoital test on cervical mucus at ovulation
postcoitus
postcystectomy
postdate intrauterine pregnancy
post dates
postdatism
postdrainage cystogram
postdrainage cystography
postejaculatory urinalysis

posterior choanal atresia
posterior bladder wall
posterior border of testis
posterior colpoperineorrhaphy
posterior colporrhaphy
posterior colpotomy
posterior commissure
posterior cul-de-sac
posterior exenteration
posterior fontanelle
posterior fornix
posterior labial artery
posterior labial veins
posterior leaf of broad ligament
posterior, left mentoanterior (LMA)
posterior lie
posterior lip of cervix
posterior lip of external os of uterus
posterior nephrectomy
posterior nuchal echolucency
posterior part of vaginal fornix
posterior pelvic exenteration
posterior pelvic wall
posterior retractor
posterior scapular vessels
posterior scrotal veins
posterior surface of prostate
posterior tributaries
posterior urethra
posterior urethral valve
posterior urethritis
posterior urethrovesical angle
posterior vaginal fornix
posterior vaginismus
posterior vulvar commissure
posterior wall defect
posterior wall of urinary bladder
posterior wall of vagina
postevacuation duration
postevacuation films
postfertilization occurrence
postglomerular arteriolar constriction
posthemorrhagic anemia
posthemorrhagic hydrocephalus
posthetomy
posthioplasty
posthitis
postholith
posthysterectomy vaginal vault prolapse and enterocele formation
postinfectious glomerulonephritis (PIGN)
postinfectious glomerulopathy
postinfective glomerulonephritis
postirradiation vaginitis
postmastectomy lymphedema syndrome
postmastectomy radiation therapy
postmature infant
postmaturity
postmeiotic segregation
postmenopausal atrophic vaginitis
postmenopausal bleeding
postmenopausal osteoporosis
postmenopausal vaginitis
postmenopausal woman
postmicturition residual urine volume
postmortem delivery
postnatal care
postnatal life
postobstetric urethral stricture
postobstructive diuresis
postoliguric phase of acute renal failure
postoperative angulation of ureter
postoperative complications
postoperative constriction of ureter
postoperative cystography
postoperative dialysis
postoperative neophallus
postoperative pain
postoperative pain control
postoperative pelvic hematoma
postoperative settling of breast
postoperative shock
postoperative transsexual
postoperative urethral stricture
postovulatory phase of menstrual cycle
postparathyroidectomy hypocalcemia
postpartum alopecia

postpartum amenorrhea
postpartum atony
postpartum cardiomyopathy
postpartum care
postpartum complication
postpartum course
postpartum day
postpartum deep-vein phlebothrombosis
postpartum depression
postpartum events
postpartum hemoglobin
postpartum hemorrhage
postpartum hepatorenal syndrome
postpartum hypertension
postpartum maternal thyroid dysfunction
postpartum mood disorder
postpartum pelvic thrombophlebitis
postpartum pituitary necrosis syndrome
postpartum psychosis
postpartum recovery
postpartum spinal headache
postpartum sterilization
postpartum subinvolution of uterus
postpartum tetanus
postpartum transient hyperthyroidism
postpartum tubal ligation
postpartum uterine atony
postprandial blood glucose level
postprandial hypoglycemia
postprandial rise in peripheral glucose
postprocedural tubal spillage
postprocedure nephrostogram
postprostatectomy incontinence
postpuberty
postpubescent
postpyelonephritis cortical scarring
postradiation adhesions
postrenal anuria
postrenal azotemia
postrenal factors
postrenal obstructive azotemia
poststreptococcal glomerulonephritis (PSGN)
post-term birth
post-term infant
post-term pregnancy
post-transfusion hepatitis
post-transplant acute renal failure (ARF)
post-transplant diabetes mellitus
post-transplant graft thrombosis
post-transplant polycythemia
post-traumatic renal failure
post-traumatic stress disorder
postural proteinuria
postural version
posture, frog-leg
postuterine
postviral fatigue syndrome
postvoid film
postvoiding film
postvoid residual (PVR)
postvoid residual urine
postvoid residual urine volume
postvoiding cystogram
postvoiding cystography
postvoiding residual
postvoiding urethral catheterization
postzygotic event
Potaba (aminobenzoate)
potassium (K)
potassium bitartrate
potassium deficiency
potassium depletion nephropathy
potassium depletion syndrome
potassium excretion
potassium hydroxide (KOH)
potassium ion (K+)
potassium losing nephritis
potassium replacement
potassium retaining diuretic
potassium sparing diuretic
potency, sexual
potential for fluid accumulation and overhydration
potential to void while standing
potential teratogens

Potter facies
Potter version
Potts-Smith forceps
pouch (also see *reservoir*)
  anterior uterovesical
  blind vaginal
  Broca
  Camey urinary
  deep perineal
  Denis Browne
  Douglas rectouterine
  Florida
  GraBag retrieval
  hepatorenal
  Indiana
  Indiana urinary
  intestinal
  inverted U-shaped
  Kock continent ileostomy
  Kock U-shaped urinary
  laparoscopic instrument
  Mainz urinary
  marsupial
  marsupial drain
  paracystic
  paravesical
  Penn
  Ponsky Endo Sock retrieval
  Reality vaginal
  rectal
  rectouterine
  rectovaginal
  rectovaginouterine
  rectovesical
  renal
  Rowland
  superficial inguinal
  superficial perineal
  UCLA
  uterovesical
  vesicoureteral
  vesicouterine
  Wallaby
pouchitis
pouch of Douglas
  abscess of
  blood in
  free fluid in
  pus in
pouchogram
pouchography, evacuation
Poupart ligament
povidone-iodine
povidine-iodine douche
powder burn spots
Powell forceps
power magnification, loupe
power mode color Doppler imaging
power of attorney for healthcare
power setting
Pozzi uterine tenaculum forceps
PPHN (persistent pulmonary hypertension of the newborn)
PPROM (preterm premature rupture of membranes)
PPV (positive-pressure ventilation)
Prader-Labhart-Willi syndrome
Prader-Willi syndrome
praecox, ejaculatio
Prague maneuver
Pramet FA prenatal vitamins
Pramilet prenatal vitamins
pramlintide
Prandase (acarbose)
Prandin (repaglinide)
Pratt uterine dilator
prazosin
pre-betalipoproteinemia
prebiopsy mammogram
prebirth waiver
PreCare Conceive nutritional supplement
Preceptin contraceptive cream
precervical sinus
precipitate delivery
precipitate labor
precipitated amorphous phosphate salts
precipitated urates

precipitated by immersion
precipitated dissolved polymer
precipitated phosphates
precipitating cause
precipitation of dissolved polymer
precipitous labor
Precision Office TUNA system
Precision Tack transvaginal anchor system
Precision Twist transvaginal anchor system
preclimacteric menorrhagia
precocious pseudopuberty
precocious puberty
precordium, hyperdynamic
Precose (acarbose)
precosity, sexual
precursor
predecidual changes in endometrium
prediabetes
predialysis
predialysis phase
predictive testing
predictor (see *ovulation prediction*)
predisposing cause
predisposing mutation
predispositional testing
prednisolone
preeclampsia
  mild
  severe
  superimposed
preeclamptic edema
preeclamptic precautions
Preemie SMA 20 infant formula
Preemie SMA 24 infant formula
preequilibration
preference, sexual
preformed nuclei
pregenital phase
Pregestimil infant formula
pregnancy
  abdominal
  aborted

pregnancy *(cont.)*
  aborted ectopic
  acute yellow atrophy of liver in
  ampullar
  bigeminal
  broad ligament
  cervical
  chemical
  chloasma occurring in
  clinical
  combined
  compound
  cornual
  ectopic
  edema of
  extra-amniotic
  extrachorial
  extramembranous
  extrauterine
  fallopian
  fallopian tube
  false
  gemellary
  hemorrhage in ectopic
  heterotopic
  higher order
  high risk
  hydatid
  hydatidiform mole
  hysterical
  interstitial
  intrahepatic cholestasis of
  intraligamentary
  intraligamentous
  intramural
  intraperitoneal
  intrauterine (IUP)
  isthmic tubal
  late vomiting of
  luteoma
  macrocytic anemia of
  mask of
  membranous
  mesenteric

pregnancy *(cont.)*
- mesometric
- molar
- multiple
- mural
- nephropathy in
- nervous
- octuplet
- ovarian
- ovarioabdominal
- oviductal
- parietal
- peripheral neuritis in
- peritoneal
- pernicious anemia of
- persistent ectopic
- phantom
- plaques of
- plural
- postdate intrauterine
- post-term
- prolonged
- pseudointraligamentary
- quadruplet
- quintuplet
- rape-induced
- recurrent jaundice of
- ruptured ectopic
- sarcofetal
- sarcohysteric
- secondary abdominal
- septulet
- sextuplet
- spurious
- stump
- term
- termination of
- toxemia of
- toxemic retinopathy of
- transient hypertension of
- triplet
- tubal
- tuboabdominal
- tuboligamentary

pregnancy *(cont.)*
- tubo-ovarian
- tubouterine
- twin
- ureteral calculi in
- uterine
- uterine muscular wall
- uteroabdominal
- uterotubal
- viable
- vomiting of

pregnancy at term
pregnancy estimated at term
pregnancy history
pregnancy hormone
pregnancy-induced hypertension (PIH)
pregnancy interruption, vaginal, with dilation and curettage (VIP-DAC)
pregnancy loss
pregnancy phobia
pregnancy-related venous thromboembolism (VTE)
pregnancy sign
- Chadwick
- Jacquemier

pregnancy test
- AccuPoint hCG Pregnancy Test Disc
- Affirm one-step
- Answer
- Be Sure One Step
- Biocept-5
- Biocept-G
- Brite-Life One Step
- CARDS Q.S. hCG serum/urine
- ClearBlue Easy
- Clearblue Easy One-Step
- Concise Performance Plus
- Concise Performance Plus hCG-Combo
- Confirm 1-Step
- CVS
- DBest
- e.p.t.
- Fact Plus

pregnancy test *(cont.)*
  Fact Plus Pro
  HealthCheck One-Step One Minute
  LifeSign1 midstream
  PrePaQ
  QuickVue one-step hCG-Combo
  SelfCare
  serum
pregnancy-induced hypertension (PIH)
pregnancy-related nausea
pregnancy tumor
pregnanediol glucuronide
pregnanetriol
pregnant uterus
pregnant woman
Pregnyl (chorionic gonadotropin)
preimplantation diagnosis
preimplantation genetic diagnosis
preinvasive lesion
preinvasive lesion of cervix
preinvasive lesion of vulva
preinvasive urothelial neoplasia
preliminary diagnosis
preliminary drainage
Prelone (prednisone)
premalignant lesion of cervix
premalignant state
premammary abscess
Premarin (conjugated estrogens)
premature accelerated lung maturation (PALM)
premature alopecia
premature birth
premature delivery
premature detachment of placenta
premature ejaculation
premature infant
Premature Infant Pain Profile (PIPP)
premature labor
premature menopause
premature ovarian failure
premature rupture of membranes (PROM)
premature senility syndrome
premature separation of placenta
premature sloughing
prematurity
  anemia of
  hyperbilirubinemia of
  interstitial pulmonary fibrosis of
premenopausal amenorrhea
premenstrual dysphoric disorder (PMDD)
premenstrual edema
premenstrual salivary syndrome
premenstrual syndrome (PMS)
premenstrual tension
premenstrual tension syndrome
premenstruum
PremesisRX prenatal vitamin
Premier Type-Specific HSV-1 IgG ELISA test
Premier Type-Specific HSV-2 IgG ELISA test
Premier vaginal retractor
Premilene suture
premonitory symptoms
Premphase (conjugated estrogens and medroxyprogesterone)
Premphase (medroxyprogesterone)
Prempro (conjugated estrogens; medroxyprogesterone)
prenatal care
prenatal course
prenatal diagnosis
prenatal diagnostic services
prenatal exposure to the anticonvulsant drugs
prenatal genetic diagnosis
prenatal history
prenatal hormone condition
prenatal life
prenatal tests
prenatal vitamins (see *vitamins*)
Prenavite prenatal vitamins
Prentif pessary
Prentiss maneuver
preoperative renal angiography

preovulatory mucus
preovulatory phase of menstrual cycle
preovulatory surge of luteinizing hormone
PrePaQ pregnancy test
prepared and draped in sterile fashion
prepared and draped in the usual sterile manner
preparturient
Prepidil (dinoprostone)
Prepidil Gel (dinoprostone cervical gel)
prep, KOH
prepped and draped in sterile fashion
prepped and draped in the usual sterile manner
preprostate urethral sphincter
preprostatic part of male urethra
PREP System for Pap smear
prepuberal (prepubertal)
prepubertal
prepubescent
prepuce (see also *foreskin*)
  adherent
  clitoral
  frenulum of
  hooded
  nonretractable
  penile
  redundant
  tight
  ventral apron
prepuce of clitoris
prepuce of penis
preputial calculus
preputial sac
preputial washings
preputiotomy
preputium (pl. preputia)
prerectal lithotomy
prerenal azotemia
prerenal factors
prerenal uremia
presacral edema
presacral neurectomy
Prescott-Brodie stain
presenile dementia
presenile tremor syndrome
presentation of fetus
  acromion
  breech
  brow
  cephalic
  complete breech
  compound
  double-footling breech
  Duncan
  face
  foot
  footling
  footling breech
  frank breech
  full breech
  head
  incomplete foot
  incomplete knee
  knee
  mentum
  oblique
  occiput-anterior
  occiput-posterior
  parietal
  pelvic
  placental
  polar
  shoulder
  sincipital
  single-footling breech
  transverse
  twin
  vertex
presentation of cord
presentation of fertility
presenting part
preservation of solid material
preservation, ovarian
presomite embryo

pressure
  bimanual
  carbon dioxide
  CDP (continuous descending)
  CPAP (continuous positive airway)
  detrusor
  fundal
  intra-abdominal
  intravesical
  intravesicular
  leak-point
  low urethral (LUP)
  maternal abdominal
  maximum urethral closure (MUCP)
  pelvic
  suprapubic
  tubal perfusion
pressure atrophy of renal parenchyma
pressure collapse of lung
pressure difference across membrane thickness
pressure dressing
pressure flow nomogram
pressure transducer
presumption of legitimacy
presumptive diagnosis
presumptive ovaries
presumptive preovulatory follicle
presymptomatic testing
preterm birth
preterm delivery
preterm infant
preterm infant formula
preterm labor
preterm premature rupture of membranes (PPROM)
pretibial area
pretibial edema
Preven emergency contraception kit
preventive mastectomy
prevesical
prevesicle space
previa
  incomplete placenta
  marginal placenta

previa *(cont.)*
  partial placenta
  placenta
  total placenta
  vasa
previable fetus
previllous embryo
priapism
priapus
Pribnow box
primary adhesion
primary agammaglobulinemia
primary amenorrhea
primary atelectasis
primary cachexia
primary cesarean section
primary chemotherapy
primary ciliary dyskinesia
primary closure
primary closure of myelomeningocele in utero
primary complaint
primary craniosynostosis
primary dysfunctional labor
primary dysmenorrhea
primary follicle
primary hematuria
primary herpetic infection
primary hydrocephalus
primary hyperhidrosis
primary hyperoxaluria and oxalosis
primary hyperoxaluria, type 1 (PH-1)
primary hypogonadism
primary immunodeficiency
primary infertility
primary juxtaglomerular cell hyperplasia
primary megaloureter
primary megaureter
primary neoplasm
primary neutrophil granules
primary oocyte
primary ovarian cancer
primary ovarian failure
primary ovarian follicle

primary reanastomosis of vas
primary renal calculus
primary renal candidiasis
primary renal disease
primary renal tubular acidosis
primary renal vein thrombosis
primary sex character
primary sex characteristics
primary syphilis
primary teeth
primary uterine inertia
primary vaginal hysterectomy
primary vascular causes of ARF
primary vesical calculus (pl. calculi)
primer
primigravida (gravida 1)
primigravida, elderly
primipara ("primip")
primiparity
primiparous
primordial duct
primordial follicle
primordial germ cells
primordial gigantism
primordial uteroplacental circulation
Primus hemodialyzer model 1350
Primus hemodialyzer model 2000
principle
  constant infusion
  Mitrofanoff
Pringle syndrome
Priscilla White classification of diabetes
Prisma CRRT system
private mutation
private placement adoption
Privet coaxial catheter
PRL (prolactin level)
pRNA
probability
proband
Pro-Banthine (propantheline)
probe
  AccuProbe 600 system cryotherapy
  athVysion HER-2 DNA

probe *(cont.)*
  BiLAP bipolar cutting and coagulating
  biplane sector
  Bruel-Kjaer transvaginal ultrasound
  Check-Flo suprapubic wanding
  Circon-ACMI electrohydraulic lithotriptor
  Corson
  Eder
  electrosurgical
  Fine-Lap
  intrauterine
  latex balloon
  LCx
  Mammotome
  Modulap coagulation
  PROSURG
  Savannah
  Surgiflex
  ultrasonic lithotripsy
  Versadopp 10
  YSI neonatal temperature
probenecid
probond
Procar introducer
procedure (see *operation*)
Proceed hemostatic surgical sealant
process (pl. processes)
  cuprammonia
  excretory
  metabolic
processus vaginalis
processus vaginalis peritonei
Prochownik pessary
procidentia
Proclim (medroxyprogesterone)
procreate
procreation
procreative freedom
Procrit (epoetin alfa)
proctitis
  acute
  chronic
  factitial

proctocele
proctocolitis, venereal
proctocolpoplasty
proctocystocele
proctocystotomy
proctoperineoplasty
prodromal labor
prodromal phase of ARF
production of urine
production, renin
productive nephritis
products of conception, retained
proemial breast
Profasi (chorionic gonadotropin)
profile
  biophysical (BBP)
  Dianon prostate
  fetal biophysical
  lung maturity
  PIPP (Premature Infant Pain)
  urethral pressure
Profile Mammography system
profluens, hydrops tubae
profuse uterine hemorrhage
progenitalis
progenitor
progeny
progeria
progeria of adulthood
progeroid nanism
progestational challenge
progestational hormone
Progestasert (progesterone) intrauterine device
progestens
progesterone
progesterone challenge test
progesterone gel, Crinone
progesterone receptor (PgR)
progesterone-receptor analysis
progesterone-receptor-positive tumor
progesterone-receptor status
progesterone replacement therapy
progesterone secretion
progestin
progestogen
progestogen-associated endometrial protein (PEP)
prognostic indicator
prognostic marker
prognostic value
Prograf (tacrolimus)
program
  gene therapy
  START SMART (for assisted reproduction)
programmed cell death
progression of uremic neuropathy
progressive autonomic failure
progressive bladder outlet obstruction
progressive bulbar paralysis
progressive carboxylate dehydrogenase deficiency
progressive choroidal atrophy
progressive decompensation of urinary system
progressive diaphyseal dysplasia
progressive facial hemiatrophy
progressive hemifacial atrophy
progressive hepatolenticular degeneration
progressive hypertrophic interstitial neuropathy
progressive infantile poliodystrophy
progressively worsening respiratory function
progressive multifocal leukoencephalopathy (PML)
progressive muscular atrophy
progressive osseous heteroplasia
progressive pallid degeneration syndrome
progressive poliodystrophy
progressive tapetochoroidal dystrophy
progressive systemic sclerosis
progressive uterine dilation
prohormone, synthetic vitamin D
Project, Human Genome

prokaryote
prolactin
prolactin level (PRL)
prolactinoma, estrogen-induced
prolactin-producing adenoma
prolactin, serum
prolapse
  anal
  bladder
  cord
  first degree
  genital
  gravid uterus
  massive genital
  neovaginal
  rectal
  second degree
  third degree
  umbilical cord, occult
  umbilical cord, overt
  urethral
  urethral meatus
  uterine
  uterovaginal
  vaginal
  vaginal vault
  vaginal wall
prolapsed cord
prolapsed fetal arm
prolapsed fetal foot
prolapsed hemorrhoid
prolapsed umbilical cord
prolapsed urethral mucosa
prolapsed uterus repair
prolapsed vaginal vault
ProLease encapsulated sustained-release growth hormone
Prolene mesh tape
Prolene suture
Proleukin (aldesleukin; interleukin-2, recombinant)
proliferation
  cellular
  ductal

proliferation *(cont.)*
  mesangial
  renal cellular
  stromal
  vascular
proliferative endarteritis
proliferative glomerulonephritis
proliferative phase
proliferative poststreptococcal
proliferative retinopathy
proline dehydrogenase deficiency
proline oxidase deficiency
prolonged depression of fetus
prolonged erection of the clitoris
prolonged fetal depression
prolonged labor
prolonged pregnancy
prolonged rupture of membranes (PROM)
prolonged second stage of labor
prolonged uterine contractions
PROM (premature rupture of membranes)
PROM (prolonged rupture of membranes)
Promensil nutritional supplement
pro-metaphase stage of mitosis
Prometrium (micronized progesterone)
prominent nose
promontofixation
promoter
promoter region
prone position
pronephric duct
prongs
Pronova nonabsorbable suture
pronuclear-stage embryo transfer (PROST)
pronucleus
propantheline
Propaq Encore neonatal vital signs monitor
proper ligament of ovary
properdin

prophase
prophylactic antibiotic irrigating solution
prophylactic anticoagulation in pregnancy
prophylactic coverage
prophylactic dialysis
prophylactic digitalization
prophylactic intravenous antibiotics
prophylactic mastectomy
prophylactic preoperative anticoagulation with subcutaneous heparin
prophylactic subcutaneous mastectomy
prophylactic vasectomy
prophylaxis
  antibiotic
  antimicrobial
  long-term
  peripartal corticosteroid
propionic acidemia
propionyl CoA carboxylase (PCC) deficiency
proportionate infantilism
propositus
propranolol
propylthiouracil (PTU)
Proscar (finasteride)
ProSobee infant formula
PROST (pronuclear-stage embryo transfer)
ProstaCoil self-expanding urethral stent
prostacyclin
prostaglandin (pl. prostaglandins)
prostaglandin E_1 (alprostadil; PGE_1)
prostaglandin E_2 (dinoprostone; PGE_1)
prostaglandin gel or cream
prostaglandin synthesis
prostaglandin synthetase inhibitor
ProstaJect ethanol injection system
Prostalase laser system
ProstaScint (CYT-356 radiolabeled with ^{111}In) monoclonal antibody imaging agent
ProstaSeed ^{125}I prostate brachytherapy seeds
ProstaSeed ^{125}I radiation treatment
ProstAsure Index
ProstAsure test
prostate
  abscess of
  adenocarcinoma of
  adenofibromatous hypertrophy of
  apex of
  atrophy of
  benign
  benign adenoma of
  benign enlargement of
  boggy
  boggy and tender
  calculus of
  carcinoma of
  congestion of
  diffusely swollen
  ductal carcinoma of
  enlarged
  exquisitely tender
  female
  fibroadenoma of
  fibroma of
  fibromuscular
  firm
  fistula of
  Gleason score for carcinoma of
  hemorrhage of
  high-riding
  high-riding ballotable
  holmium laser resection of the (HoLRP)
  hyperplasia of
  hyperplastic
  indurated
  infarction of
  inferolateral surface of
  laser resection of
  lateral lobe of
  lymph vessels of

prostate *(cont.)*
    median lobe of
    microwave thermotherapy of
    myoma of
    nodular
    non-nodular
    obstructive
    posterior surface of
    rock-hard
    rubber consistency
    smooth
    stony-hard
    stricture of
    swollen
    tender
    transurethral incision of (TUIP)
    transurethral resection of (TURP)
prostate adenocarcinoma
prostate apex
prostate cancer
    hormone-refractory
    localized
    metastatic
prostate chips
prostatectomy
    Campbell radical retropubic
    cryoprostatectomy
    cystoprostatectomy
    laparoscopic radical
    Madigan
    McDougal
    Millen retropubic
    nerve-sparing radical
    perineal
    radical
    radical perineal
    radical retropubic
    retropubic
    transurethral balloon Laserthermia
    transurethral ultrasound-guided laser-induced prostatectomy (TULIP)
    transvesical
    Walsh radical retropubic
prostate enlargement
prostate gland
prostate implant
prostate infarction
prostate seeding
prostate-specific antigen bound to alpha$_1$-antichymotrypsin (PSA-ACT)
prostate-specific antigen (PSA) free/total index
prostate-specific membrane antigen (PSMA)
prostate stroma
prostate tumorigenesis
prostatic acid phosphatase (PAP)
prostatic adenoma
prostatic androgen metabolism
prostatic apex
prostatic atrophy
prostatic bed
prostatic calculus
prostatic capsule, surgical
prostatic catheter
prostatic chips
prostatic concretion
prostatic cyst
prostatic duct
prostatic ductule
prostatic enlargement
prostatic enlargement with bladder elevation
prostatic fistula
prostatic fluid
prostatic fossa
prostatic hemorrhage
prostatic hyperplasia
prostatic induration
prostatic intraepithelial neoplasia (PIN)
prostatic lobules
prostatic malignancy
prostatic massage
prostatic nodule
prostatic obstruction
prostatic plexus

prostatic resection
prostatic sarcoma
prostatic secretions
prostatic shaving
prostatic sheath
prostatic sinus
prostatic stone
prostatic stricture
prostatic urethra
prostatic uterus
prostatic utricle
prostatic varices
prostatic venous plexus
prostaticovesical
prostatism
  obstructive
  silent
prostatitis
  acute
  acute bacterial
  allergic
  bacterial
  cavitary
  chronic
  chronic bacterial (CBP)
  chronic nonbacterial
  congestive
  diverticular
  eosinophilic
  gonococcal
  granulomatous
  monilial
  nonbacterial
  nonspecific granulomatous
  trichomonal
prostatocystitis
prostatodynia
prostatolith
prostatolithotomy
prostatomegaly
prostatomembranous urethra
prostatorrhea
prostatoseminal vesiculectomy
prostatovesiculectomy
prostatovesiculitis
Prostatron mobile microwave thermotherapy device
prosthesis (see also *implant*)
  Amoena breast prosthesis
  AMS Ambicor penile
  AMS Securo-T urinary
  AMS 600 malleable penile
  AMS 600M malleable penile
  AMS 650 malleable penile
  AMS 700 CXM penile
  AMS 700 CX inflatable penile
  AMS 700 CXM inflatable penile
  AMS 800 sphincter urinary
  Becker breast
  Becker tissue expander/breast
  Belle-Amie breast
  bladder neck support
  breast
  CUI gel breast
  Dilamezinsert (DMI) penile dilator/inserter
  Dow-Corning silastic
  Duraphase inflatable penile
  Dura-II positional penile
  Dynaflex penile
  fallopian tube
  Finney Flexi-Rod penile
  GFS Mark II inflatable penile
  inflatable penile (IPP)
  Introl bladder neck support
  Jonas penile
  Mentor Alpha 1 inflatable penile
  multichannel implantable urinary
  NOA implanted urinary
  penile
  Perras breast
  Scott-Bradley penile
  700 Ultrex Plus penile
  Small-Carrion semirigid penile
  testicular
  ureterovesical
  UroLume endoprosthesis
prosthesis exchange

prosthesis sizer
prosthetic breast
prosthetic device
prosthetic woven Dacron graft
Prostin (alprostadil)
prostitution
PROSURG probe
protamine/heparin infusion
protanomaly
protanopia
protease
protease-mediated tissue destruction
protein analysis
protein functional assay
protein product
protein truncation test (PTT)
Protectaid contraceptive sponge with
  F-5 Gel
Protect-a-Pass suture passer
protector, BabyShades eye
ProteGen vaginal sling procedure
protein, proteins
  AFP (alpha-fetoprotein)
  alpha-fetoprotein (AFP)
  angiogenic
  anti-Tamm-Horsfall
  aquaporin 1
  Bence Jones
  carrier
  complement
  estrogen receptor (ER)
  filtered
  human complement factor H-related
    (hCFHrp)
  mammastatin
  Novel erythropoiesis-stimulating
  nuclear matrix
  placenta
  progestogen-associated endometrial
    (PEP)
  purified placental
  thyroxine-binding
proteinaceous ground substance
protein C
protein-caking
protein/creatinine ratio
protein excretion
protein inhibitor type M (PiM)
protein inhibitor type Z (PiZ)
protein in urine
protein kinase C
protein matrix
protein overexpression, p53
protein receptor, HER2
protein-restricted diet
protein S
protein solder for tissue welding
proteinuria
  asymptomatic
  Bence Jones
  benign postural
  constant
  exercise
  gestational
  heavy
  intermittent
  isolated
  nephrotic-range
  nonisolated
  orthostatic
  overflow
  persistent
  persisting
  postural
  Tamm-Horsfall
proteolytic enzymes
proteome
proteomics
proteus syndrome
Proteus mirabilis
protocol
  chemotherapy (see *chemotherapy
    protocol)*
  Costello
  Pitocin augmentation
  Yuzpe
proton density images (MRI)
proton magnetic resonance
  spectroscopy

proto-oncogene
protoporphyria, erythrohepatic
protoporphyrin
protozoa
protracted active phase of labor
protraction disorder
protrusion
  anal
  bladder
  uterine
  vaginal
protuberance, intrauterine
Provenge vaccine
Provera (medroxyprogesterone)
proximal convoluted tubule
proximal genital reconstruction
proximal hydronephrosis
proximal part of prostatic urethra
proximal renal tubular acidosis
proximal RTA type 2
proximal splenorenal shunt
proximal tubal occlusion
proximal tube
proximal tubules
proximal urethral resistance
proximal urethral sphincter
proximal urethritis
proximate cause
Proximate skin staples
Prozac
prune-belly syndrome
pruritic urticarial papule
pruritic urticarial papules and plaques of pregnancy (PUPPP)
pruritus
pruritus gravidarum
pruritus vulvae
PSA (prostate-specific antigen)
  complex
  free
PSA-ACT (prostate-specific antigen bound to alpha$_1$-antichymotrypsin)
PSA4 home blood test for prostate cancer
PSA velocity
psammoma bodies
psammomatous calcification, stippled
PSC Fertility Monitor
PSD Gel
Pseudallescheria boydii
pseudobulbar palsy
pseudocholinesterase deficiency
pseudocyesis
pseudofollicular salpingitis
pseudogene
pseudogestational sac
pseudogout
pseudohemaphroditism, male
pseudohematuria
pseudohermaphrodite
pseudohermaphroditism
  familial incomplete male
  female
  male
pseudohernia
pseudo-Hurler polydystrophy
pseudohydronephrosis
pseudohyphae, filamentous
pseudohypoparathyroidism
pseudointraligamentary pregnancy
pseudomasturbation
pseudomembranous enterocolitis in newborn
pseudomenstruation
Pseudomonas aeruginosa
pseudonephritis, athlete's
pseudo-obstruction
pseudopolydystrophy
pseudopolyp
pseudopregnancy
pseudopuberty, precocious
pseudothalidomide syndrome
pseudoxanthoma elasticum (PXE)
pseudovagina creation
pseudovaginal hypospadias
PSGN (poststreptococcal glomerulonephritis)

PSMA (prostate-specific membrane antigen)
PSN (polysynthane) hemodialyzer
psoas hitch
psoas muscle
psoriasis of the penis
psychogenic dysmenorrhea
psychogenic dyspareunia
psychogenic incontinence
psychogenic pain
psychogenic pelvic pain
psychogenic vaginismus
psychologic status
psychomotor development
psychosexual development
psychosexual dysfunction
psychosexual outcome
psychosexual status
psychosis, postpartum
Psychosocial Adjustment to Illness Scale (PAIS)
psychosocial sequelae
psyllium hydrocolloid
PTD (persistent trophoblastic disease)
PTEN cancer gene
pterygium Colli syndrome
pterygium syndrome, multiple
pterygium universale
PTFE (polytetrafluoroethylene) graft
PTFE suburethral sling procedure
PTH (parathyroid hormone)
pthiriasis pubis
P-32 (^{32}P) chromic phosphate suspension for ovarian cancer
PTHrp (parathyroid-hormone-related protein)
PTK gene
ptosis
    Aries-Pitanguy correction of mammary
    breast
    kidney
    mammary
    testicular
ptotic breasts
ptotic kidney
PTRA (percutaneous transluminal renal angioplasty)
PTT (protein truncation test)
PTU (propylthiouracil)
p21 (Kip1) protein prostate cancer tumor marker
ptyalism
pubarche
pubertal menorrhagia
pubertal process
pubertal psychosexual milestones
puberty
    delayed
    precocious
    true precocious
pubes
pubescence
pubescent uterus
pubic bone
pubic bone anchor
pubic hair
pubic hairline
pubic lice
pubic symphysis
pubic tubercle
pubiotomy
pubis
    mons
    separation of symphysis
pubis symphysis
pubocervical fascia
pubocervical ligament
pubococcygeal muscle exercises
pubococcygeal sling operation
puboprostatic ligament
pubovaginal operation for urinary incontinence
pubovaginal sling procedure
pubovesical ligament
PUBS (percutaneous umbilical blood sampling)
PUBS (periumbilical blood sampling)

pudendal anesthesia
pudendal apron
pudendal artery
pudendal block
pudendal canal
pudendal cleft
pudendal hernia
pudendal lips, frenulum of
pudendal neurogram
pudendal sac
pudendum (pl. pudenda)
pudendum femininum
puerpera (pl. puerperae)
puerperal abscess of breast
puerperal complication
puerperal endometritis
puerperal fever
puerperal hemoglobinemia
puerperal infection
  breast
  femoral thrombophlebitic
  parametrial
  renal
  uterine
  vaginal
puerperal mastitis
puerperal morbidity
puerperal pulmonary embolism
puerperal pyrexia
puerperal sepsis
puerperal septicemia
puerperal tetanus
puerperant
puerperium (pl. puerperia)
pulmonary alveolar basement membrane
pulmonary atresia
pulmonary capillary hypertension
pulmonary capillary pressure
pulmonary collapse
pulmonary edema
pulmonary embolism
pulmonary hemosiderosis
pulmonary hypertension
pulmonary hypoperfusion syndrome
pulmonary immaturity
pulmonary infarction secondary to bony spicule embolization
pulmonary interstitial emphysema (PIE)
pulmonary maturity
pulmonary necrotizing granulomas
pulmonary-renal complex
pulmonary renal syndromes, diseases associated with
  congestive cardiac failure with uremia
  drug reactions
  Goodpasture syndrome
  Henoch-Schönlein purpura
  hypersensitivity angiitis
  idiopathic immune complex glomerulonephritis
  legionnaires disease
  mixed connective tissue disease
  mixed cryoblobinemia
  pauci-immune rapidly progressive
  polyarteritis nodosa
  renal vein thrombosis with pulmonary emboli
  right-sided bacterial endocarditis
  sarcoidosis
  silicon nephropathy
  systemic lupus erythematosus
  Wegener granulomatosis disequilibrium
pulmonary stenosis
pulmonary toilet
pulpal dysplasia
pulp stones
Pulsalith lithotripter
pulsatile GnRH secretion
pulse
  brachial
  carotid
  dorsalis pedis
  femoral
  popliteal
  posterior tibial

pulse *(cont.)*
    radial
    thready
pulsed-dye laser therapy for ureteral
    stone lithotripsy
pulsed laser
pulse mode
pulse steroid therapy
pulse therapy
Pulsolith laser lithotriptor
pump
    breast
    CMS vacuum
    computerized peristaltic
    D-Modem and insulin
    Dahedi 25 insulin
    Egnell breast
    H-TRON plus V100 insulin infusion
    insulin
    MultApump disposable
    Niagara high flow
    vacuum
    vacuum-type breast
    Zimmer automatic
pump system
punch
    Eppendorfer biopsy
    Gaylor biopsy
    Gelhorn biopsy
    mini Tischler delicate biopsy
    Schubert-Van Doren biopsy
    Sklar Kevorkian biopsy
    Thoms-Gaylor biopsy
    Tischler biopsy
    Wittner uterine biopsy
punch biopsy
punch suprapubic cystostomy
punctate areas
punctuation
puncture
    renipuncture
    venipuncture
    viscus
puncture aspiration of breast cyst
puncture incision
puncture sites
PUPPP (pruritic urticarial papules
    and plaques of pregnancy)
pure-breeding
Puregon (follitropin beta)
pure hereditary
pure red cell aplasia
purified placental protein
purine
purine autism
purine metabolic disorders
purpura
    Henoch-Schönlein
    thrombocytopenic
    thrombotic thrombocytopenic
purpuric rash
pursestring mastopexy
pursestring mouth of neonates with
    congenital syphilis
pursestring suture
purulent-appearing leukorrhea
purulent mastitis
purulent salpingitis
purulenta, lochia
pus from pelvic abscess
push-back and ESWL (extracorporeal
    sound wave lithotripsy)
pusher, MetraTie knot
pushing in labor
pus in abdominal cavity, dissemination
    of
pus in cul-de-sac
pus in pouch of Douglas
putative father
putative parents
putty kidney
PVR (postvoid residual)
PXE (pseudoxanthoma elasticum)
pyelectasia
pyelectasis
pyelitic

pyelitis
  acute
  calculous
  chronic
  defloration
  encrusted
  hematogenous
  hemorrhagic
  suppurative
  urogenous
pyelitis cystica
pyelitis glandularis
pyelitis granulosa
pyelitis gravidarum
pyelocaliceal
pyelocaliectasis
pyelocalyceal
pyelocystitis
pyelofluoroscopy
pyelogenic cyst of kidney
pyelogram, pyelography (see also *urogram, urography*)
  antegrade
  excretory intravenous
  intravenous (IVP)
  percutaneous
  rapid-sequence intravenous
  retrograde
pyelographic appearance time
pyelography (see *pyelogram; urogram*)
pyelolithotomy, coagulum
pyelolymphatic
pyelonephritic kidney
pyelonephritis
  acute
  acute bacterial
  ascending
  atrophic
  bacterial
  calculous
  chronic
  chronic bacterial
  emphysematous
pyelonephritis *(cont.)*
  medullary
  red-hot ascending
  xanthogranulomatous
pyelonephritis of pregnancy
pyelonephrosis
pyeloplasty
  capsular flap
  Culp
  disjoined
  dismembered
  Foley Y-plasty
  open
  Scardino vertical flap
pyeloscopy
pyelostogram
pyelostomy
pyelotomy, extended
pyelotubular backflow
pyelotubular reflux
pyeloureterectasis
pyeloureteritis cystica
pyeloureterography
pyeloureterovesical anastomosis
pyelovenous backflow
pyemia, pelvic
pyemic embolism
pygodidymus
pygomelus
pygomorphus
pygopagus
pyknochysostosis
pyloric stenosis
pyocele
pyocolpocele
pyocolpos
pyocystitis
pyoderma
pyogenic salpingitis
pyometra
pyometritis
pyonephritis
pyonephrolithiasis

pyonephrosis
  acute
  chronic
pyonephrotic
pyo-ovarium
pyophysometra
pyopyelectasis
pyosalpingitis
pyosalpingo-oophoritis
pyosalpingo-oothecitis
pyosalpinx
pyosemia
pyospermia
pyoureter
pyramidal calcium deposits
pyramidal cavity
pyramids, renal
pyrexia
  maternal
  puerperal
pyrexia of unknown origin
Pyridium (phenazopyridine)
Pyridorin
Pyridorin XR
Pyrilinks-D screening urine test
pyrimidine
pyroglutamicaciduria
pyropoikilocytosis
pyruvate carboxylase deficiency
pyruvate dehydrogenase deficiency (PDH)
pyruvate dehydrogenase phosphatase
pyruvate kinase deficiency
pyuria
PZD (partial zona dissection)

Q, q

Qb-blood flow
QDR-1500 or QDR-2000 bone densitometer
QOL (quality of life)
Q-tip test for determining urethral mobility
QTL (quantitative trait loci)
Q-TWiST (time without symptoms or toxicity)
quadrangular fontanelle
quadrant
  left lower (LLQ)
  left upper (LUQ)
  right lower (RLQ)
  right upper (RUQ)
quadrant of breast
  lower inner
  lower lateral
  lower medial
  lower outer
  upper inner
  upper lateral
  upper medial
  upper outer
quadrantectomy, axillary dissection, and radiotherapy (QUART) for breast cancer
quadrantectomy mastectomy
Quadripolar electrosurgical cutting forceps
Quadripolarity
quadruplet
quadruplet pregnancy
qualitative evaluation
quality of contractions
quality of life (QOL)
quantitative analysis
quantitative culture
quantitative evaluation
quantitative genetics
quantitative measurement of protein excretion
quantitative molecular technique
quantitative trait
quantitative trait loci (QTL)
quantitative urine culture
Quantum PD night exchange system
QUART (quadrantectomy, axillary dissection, and radiotherapy)
quartan malaria
quarter-strength formula
quartz rod and laser scalpel
questionable calcifications
Queyrat, erythroplasia of
Quick-Core II biopsy needle
quickening

QuickVue one-step hCG-Combo pregnancy test
QuickVue UrinChek 10+ urine test strips
quinacrine (Q) chromosome staining method
quinestrol
Quintero amniocentesis needle
Quinton catheter
Quinton Mahurkar dual-lumen hemodialysis catheter
Quinton PermCath (*not* PermaCath) vascular access catheter
Quinton-Scribner double-lumen shunt
quintuplet
quintuplet pregnancy

R, r

RA (rheumatoid arthritis)
RAB (remote afterloading brachytherapy)
rachischisis
rachischisis posterior
racial differences
radial aplasia-amegakaryocytic thrombocytopenia syndrome
radial artery anastomosis
radial artery to cephalic vein anastomosis
radiant warmer
radiation
  heavy particle
  supervoltage
  whole pelvis
radiation changes
radiation cystitis
radiation exposure
radiation infertility
radiation necrosis
radiation oncology
radiation proctitis
Radiation Therapy Oncology Group (RTOG) trials
radiation therapy, palliative
radiation therapy system (RTS)
radiation therapy to pelvis
radiation vaginitis
radical abdominal hysterectomy and vaginectomy with extraperitoneal lymphadenectomy
radical cystectomy
radical cystoprostatectomy
radical hemivulvectomy
radical hysterectomy
radical mastectomy
radical nephrectomy
radical nephroureterectomy
radical perineal prostatectomy
radical prostatectomy (RP)
radical retropubic prostatectomy
radical vaginal hysterectomy and vaginectomy with extraperitoneal lymphadenectomy
radical vulvectomy with bilateral inguinal-femoral lymphadenectomy
radioactive agent (see *imaging agent*)
radioactive gallium
radioactive seed implants
radioactive seeds for cervical cancer therapy
radiocontrast agents
  iodinated benzoic acid derivative
  organic iodides
  protein iodides

radiofrequency catheter ablation system, AngeCool RF
radiofrequency interstitial tissue ablation (RITA) system
radiogram
radiograph
radiographic pelvimetry
radiographic urodynamic assessment
radioimmunoassay (RIA)
  CA15-3 RIA
  Truquant BR RIA
radioimmunoluminography
radioisotope
radioisotope bone scan
radioisotope renal excretion test
radioisotope, technetium
radiolabeled peptide alpha-M2
radiolucency
radiolucent filling defect
radiolucent stone
radionuclide bladder scan
radionuclide cystography (RNC)
radionuclide-labeled leukocytes
radionuclide-labeled platelets
radionuclide mammography
radionuclide renography
radionuclide scan
radionuclide testicular scintigraphy
radionuclide uptake
radiopacity
radiopaque calculus
radiopaque fluid extravasation
radiopaque medium
radiopaque stone
radiopaque urine
radiopaque vesical calculus
radiopharmaceutical study
radioresistant tumor
radiosensitivity testing
radiotherapeutic castration
radiotherapy
  adjuvant
  extended-field
  external beam

radiotherapy *(cont.)*
  hyperfractionated
  interstitial
  intracavitary
  neoadjuvant
  preoperative
radium
radium applicators
radium insertion, vaginal candle
radium needle implants
radius, absent
raffinate (retentate)
RAINBO (Resource and Information Network for Bodily Integrity of Women)
Raji cell assay
raloxifene
Ramathibodi tubal hook
Ramathibodi uterine elevator
Ramirez vascular access shunt
Randall endometrial suction biopsy curette
Randall kidney stone forceps
Randall stone forceps
randomized controlled trials (RCT)
randomized trial
randomly amplified polymorphic DNA (RAPD)
random mating
ranitidine
Rapamune (sirolimus, formerly rapamycin)
rapamycin (now sirolimus)
RAPD (randomly amplified polymorphic DNA)
rape
  forcible
  marital
rape crisis center
rape crisis intervention
rape crisis team
rape-induced pregnancy
rape treatment center

raphe
- amniotic
- anogenital
- median
- penile
- perineal
- scrotal

raphe penis
raphe scroti
Rapicide
Rapide suture
rapidly progressive glomerulonephritis (RPGN)
rapid plasma reagin circle-card test (RPR-CT)
rapid plasma reagin (RPR) test
rapid premature sexual development
rapid refilling of bladder
rapid second stage of labor
rapid sequence intravenous pyelogram (IVP)
rapid ultrafiltration
Raplon adjunct to general anesthesia
Rapoport differential ureteral catheterization test
Rapp-Hodgkin syndrome
rare benign X-linked disorder
rare-cutter enzyme
rasburicase
rash
- butterfly
- hydatid
- macular
- maculopapular
- maculovesicular
- papular
- purpuric
- vesicular

rate
- abortion
- baseline fetal heart
- birth
- conception
- fetal death

rate *(cont.)*
- fetal heart (FHR)
- GFR (glomerular filtration)
- glomerular filtration (GFR)
- maternal death
- neonatal mortality
- perinatal mortality
- stillbirth
- voiding flow

rating, Dubowitz-Ballard
ratio
- antigen-antibody
- BUN/creatinine
- Hybritech Tandem PSA
- KtV
- LH:FSH
- protein/creatinine
- scarf
- thyroid hormone binding (THBR)
- urea reduction (URR)
- urine creatinine/serum creatinine

ratio of abortions to live births
ratio of permeate concentration
rat-tooth pickups
Raz double-prong ligature carrier used in bladder neck suspension
Raz repair for stress urinary incontinence
Raz sling operation
Rb tumor suppressor gene
RBC casts
RBC (red blood cell)
RBF (renal blood flow)
RCC (renal cell carcinoma)
RCF infant formula
RCT (randomized controlled trials)
RDS (respiratory distress syndrome)
reaction
- acquired immunodeficiency immune
- antibody-mediated immune
- Bittorf
- cell-mediated immune
- congenital complement component deficiency immune

reaction *(cont.)*
  cytotoxic immune reaction
  decidual
  deciduoid
  direct-complement-activated immune
  Herxheimer
  IgE-mediated immune
  immune complex (IC)
  Jarish-Herxheimer
  startle
  transfusion
  type 1-4
reactive hypoglycemia
reactive oxygen species (in sperm)
reactive, reparative atypia
reading frame
reagent, Millon
reagent strip, Tes-Tape
Reality vaginal pouch
real-time ultrasonography
reanastomose
reanastomosis
reanastomosis of oviduct
reanastomosis of vas
reanastomosis, tubal
rear tip extenders for penile implant
reasonable diet
reattachment of amputated penis
rebound tenderness
Récamier curettage of the uterus
recanalization
recanalization of vasectomy
recanalization reducible mass
receptor status
receptor
  estrogen
  nuclear steroid
recess
  hepatorenal
  splenorenal
recession, clitoral
recessive X-linked ichthyosis
recipient
recipient immune modulation
reciprocal cross
reciprocal translocation
recirculation, access (AR)
Recklinghausen disease (NF1)
Reclus disease
recoil, arm and leg
recombinant clone
recombinant DNA
recombinant DNA molecule
recombinant DNA techniques
recombinant human erythropoietin (rhEPO or r-HuEPO)
recombinant human relaxin
recombinant interleukin-2
recombinase
recombination
recombination frequency
Recombivax
reconstruction
  bladder
  breast
  pelvic floor
  penile
  renovascular
  vaginal
  vaginal wall
  vulvar deformity
reconstructive mammoplasty
recovery of ultrafiltrate
recovery phase
rectal ampulla
rectal endometriosis
rectal examination
rectal examination confirmatory
rectal gonorrhea
rectal mucosa tear
rectal multiplane transducer
rectal neovagina
rectal pouch
rectal pressure catheter
rectal prolapse
rectal stricture
rectal vascular system

rectocele, second degree
rectolabial fistula
rectopexy
Rector-Gordon-Healey-Mendoza-Spitzer type 4 renal tubular acidosis
rectosigmoid colon
rectosigmoidectomy
rectourethral fistula
rectourethralis
rectouterine fold
rectouterine muscle
rectouterine pouch
rectovaginal endometriotic nodules
rectovaginal examination
rectovaginal examination is confirmatory
rectovaginal fascia
rectovaginal fistula
rectovaginal fistula repair
rectovaginal pouch
rectovaginal septum
rectovaginal septum tear
rectovaginopexy
rectovaginouterine pouch
rectovesical fascia
rectovesical fistula
rectovesical fold
rectovesical lithotomy
rectovesicalis muscle
rectovesical muscle
rectovesical pouch
rectovesical septum
rectovesicovaginal fistula
rectovestibular fistula
rectovulvar fistula
rectum
  endometriosis of
  prolapse of
rectus fascia
rectus muscle
rectus muscle fascia
rectus muscle was divided
rectus muscle was separated
rectus sheath
  anterior
  posterior
rectus urethralis muscle
recurrence risk
recurrent abortion
recurrent bladder infections
recurrent bladder neck obstruction
recurrent cervicitis
recurrent infections
recurrent jaundice of pregnancy
recurrent pregnancy loss
recurrent spontaneous abortion (RSA)
recurrent UTI (urinary tract infection)
red blood cell cast
red blood cells (RBCs), packed
red blood cells in urine
red cell aplasia, pure
red cell casts
red cell mass, increased
Reddick-Saye suture grasper
red-free filter
red-hot ascending pyelonephritis
red reflex
red Robinson catheter
red rubber catheter
reduced acid excretion
reduced enzymatic activity
reduced gene transcription
reduced GFR (glomerular filtration rate)
reduced hindbrain herniation
reduced secretion of ovarian hormones
reduced urine excretion
reduced urine flow
reduction
  clitoral
  embryonic
  selective
reduction cystoplasty
reduction glansplasty with preservation of neurovascular bundle
reduction in glomerular permeability
reduction in urinary stream

reduction mammoplasty
reduction mastopexy
reduction of chromosomes
reduction of fetuses
reduction of urinary volume
redundant copies
redundant prepuce
redundant renal pelvis
redundant tissue
refeeding gynecomastia
referred pelvic pain
reflection
  bladder
  peritoneal
  vaginal
  vesicouterine
  vesicouterine peritoneal
reflection of peritoneum from rectum to upper vagina and uterus
reflection of vagina
reflex (pl. reflexes)
  Babinski
  bladder
  blink
  cremasteric
  deep tendon (DTRs)
  embrace
  gag
  Galant
  grasp
  latching on
  letdown
  micturition
  milk let-down
  Moro
  Perez
  red
  renal
  rooting
  tonic neck
reflex detrusor contraction
reflexic neurogenic bladder
reflex testing
reflux (pl. refluxes)
  intrarenal
  pyelotubular
  ureteral
  ureteral-vesical
  ureterorenal
  ureterovesical
  urine
  vesicoureteral
  vesicoureteric (VUR)
refluxing spastic neurogenic bladder
reflux nephropathy
reflux of urine
reflux treatment, Chondrogel vesicoureteral
refractive index
refractometer
refractory pulmonary edema
refrigeration palsy
Refsum disease
regenerated cellulose
regimen
  chemotherapy
  cyclic estrogen-progestin
  medical
  treatment
region
  paracervical
  parapelvic
  parovarian
  periumbilical
  suprapubic
regional anesthesia
regional anticoagulation with sodium citrate
regional heparinization
regional ileitis
regional ileitis
Regional Organ Procurement Agency (ROPA)
regional paracervical block
Regnault type B mastopexy
Regranex gel (becaplermin) recombinant platelet-derived growth factor B

Regressin tumor growth inhibitor
regressor, fetal
regularity of menstruation
regulator gene
regulatory region
regulatory sequence
regurgitation of food in newborn
regurgitation, syphilitic aortic (AR)
Reifenstein syndrome
Reiger anomaly-growth retardation (SHORT syndrome)
Reiger syndrome
reimplantation
  extravesical
  ovary
  tapered
  ureteral
  ureteral stent
Reiter complement-fixation test for syphilis
Reiter syndrome
rejection
  antibody mediated
  chronic renal allograft
  hyperacute
  renal transplant
rejection factor, R
rejection of transplanted kidney
relapse
  clinical
  mucocutaneous
  serologic
relapsing infection
relapsing polychondritis
relapsing urinary tract infection
relative
  first degree
  second degree
relative amenorrhea
relative contraindications
relative recovery
relaxation of anterior vaginal wall
relaxation of pelvis
relaxation of posterior vaginal wall
relaxation of vaginal outlet
relaxation, pelvic
relaxed vaginal outlet
Release-NF (nitrofurazone Foley) catheter
releasing hormone
Reliance urinary control insert catheter
Reliance urinary control stent
ReLibra (testosterone gel)
relinquishing parental rights to contracting couple
Relpax (eletriptan) for migraines
REMEEX urethral sling
Remifemin over-the-counter menopause relief
remittent disease
remote afterloading brachytherapy (RAB)
removal of dorsal hood
removal of fallopian tube
removal of intact mammary implant
removal of kidney through laparoscope
removal of retained placenta
removal of retained products of conception
removal of urinary bladder
Renacidin bladder and catheter irrigant
RenaClear dialyzer cleaning system
Renagel (sevelamer)
renal ablation glomerulopathy
renal adenocarcinoma
renal agenesis, bilateral
renal allograft
renal allograft recipient
renal allotransplant
renal amyloidosis
renal angiogram
renal angiography
renal angiomyolipoma
renal angioplasty, percutaneous transluminal (PTRA)
renal anomaly
renal antigen
renal anuria

renal arteriogram
renal arteriography
renal artery
renal artery aneurysm
renal artery embolism
renal artery hemorrhage
renal artery necrosis
renal artery, obstruction of
renal artery occlusion
renal artery stenosis
renal artery thrombosis
renal atrophy
renal autotransplantation
renal axis
renal azotemia
renal biopsy
renal blood flow (RBF)
renal bone disease
renal calculi, multiple
renal calculus
renal capillary endothelium
renal capsule
  fatty
  fibrous
renal carbuncle
renal carcinoma
renal cast
renal cell carcinoma (RCC)
renal cells with fat inclusions
renal cellular proliferation
renal circulation imaging
renal cirrhosis
renal cocktail
renal colic
renal collecting system
renal column
renal column of Bertin
renal compromise
renal concentrating capacity
renal concentrating defect
renal contusion
renal corpuscle
renal cortex, patchy atrophy of
renal cortical adenoma
renal cortical isotope scanning agent
renal cortical necrosis
renal cortical stenosis
renal cross-fused ectopia
renal cyst
  complex
  simple
renal cyst study
renal deterioration
renal dialysis
renal diluting capacity, limited
renal disease with edema
renal drawfism
renal duct
renal duplex scan
renal dysfunction
renal dysplasia
renal dysplasia-blindness, hereditary
renal edema
renal epithelial transport
renal excretion, impaired
renal failure
  acute
  chronic
  chronic end-stage
  end-stage
  end-stage chronic
  fulminant
  nonoliguric
  post-traumatic
  terminal
renal failure index
renal failure with acute tubular necrosis
renal fascia
renal fat
renal fibrosis
renal flares
renal flow curve
renal fossa
renal function
  compromised
  impaired
renal functional adaptation
renal functional impairment

renal function impairment
renal function test
renal glomerulus
renal glucose transport
renal glucosuria
renal glycosuria
renal hamartoma
renal helical CT (RHCT)
renal hemangiopericytoma
renal hematuria
renal hemorrhage
renal hilum
renal hypertension
renal hypoperfusion
renal hypoplasia
renal imaging
renal imaging technique
renal impression on liver
renal infantilism
renal infarct
renal infarction
renal injury
renal insufficiency, chronic progressive
renal interstitium
renalis, fascia
renal ischemia
renal isthmus
renal labyrinth
renal-limited ANCA-associated
  crescentic glomerulonephritis
renal-limited disease
renal-limited glomerulonephritis
renal lithiasis (also renolithiasis)
renal lithotomy
renal lobe
renal loss of protein
renal mass
renal mass lesion
renal medulla
renal medullary necrosis
renal mesangium
renal obstruction
renal osteodystrophy
renal outline
renal papilla
renal papillary damage
renal papillary necrosis
renal parenchyma
renal parenchymal disease
renal pedicle
renal pelvic urothelial carcinoma
renal pelvis
  mucosa of
  muscular layer of
  redundant
  subepithelial hematoma of
renal perfusion, decreased
renal perfusion scan
renal phlebography
renal plasma flow
renal plexus
renal PO_4 reabsorption
renal pouch
renal preservation during reconstruction
renal pyramids
renal reflex
renal reserve, diminished
renal resistive index
renal-retinal dysplasia
renal-retinal dystrophy
renal-retinal syndrome
renal revascularization
renal rickets
renal scan, diuretic
renal scarring
renal scintigraphy
renal sclerosis
renal segment
renal shadow
renal shutdown
renal sinus
renal sinus echo
renal sinus fat
renal size
renal sodium excretion
renal sonogram
renal-splenic venous shunt
renal stone

renal substitution therapy
renal surface of spleen
renal tomography
renal transplant
renal transplant center
renal transplant donor
renal transplant rejection, hyperacute
renal transplant team
renal transplantation
renal trauma
renal tuberculosis
renal tubular acidosis (RTA)
  distal
  gradient-limited
  proximal
  types 1-4
renal tubular defect
  acquired
  intrinsic
renal tubular defect for reabsorption of phosphate
renal tubular defect for reabsorption of potassium
renal tubular dysfunction
renal tubular ectasia
renal tubular function
renal tubular lumen
renal tubular necrosis
renal tubular plug
renal tubule
renal ultrasound
renal underperfusion
renal unit
renal vascular damage
renal vascular hypertension (RVH)
renal vascular resistance (RVR)
renal vasculitis
renal vein
renal vein renin assay
renal vein thrombosis (RVT)
renal venous occlusion
Re/Neph dietary supplement
Re-New forceps
Re-New laparoscopic scissors
reniculus (pl. reniculi)
renin, plasma
renin production
renin secretion, increased
renin study
renipuncture
RenoCal-76
Reno-Dip
renogastric
renogenic
Renografin contrast medium
Renografin-60 contrast medium
renogram curve
renogram, scintirenography
renography
  captopril
  DTPA
renointestinal
renolithiasis (also renal lithiasis)
Reno-M contrast medium
Reno-M-Dip (now Reno-Dip)
renomegaly
Reno-M-30 (now Reno-30)
Reno-M-60 (now Reno-60)
renoprival
renopulmonary
Reno-30
Reno-60
renotrophic
renotrophin
renotropic
renovascular disease
renovascular hypertension
renovascular procedure
renovascular reconstruction
renovascular stent
Renovist II contrast medium
Renovue-Dip contrast medium
Renpenning syndrome
rent (tear or rupture)
Rentrop infusion catheter
repaglinide

repair
  anterior
  bottle
  enterocele
  episiotomy
  hernia
  paravaginal
  pelvic floor
  posterior
  rectocele
  rectovaginal fistula
  vesicovaginal fistula
repair of prolapsed uterus
repair of vaginal eversion
repeated segments
repeat mammogram
Repel bioresorbable barrier film
reperitonealization
reperitonealize
reperitonealized
repetitive DNA
replacement, hormone
Replens vaginal gel
replication analysis
replication banding
replication, viral
replicon
Repliderm collagen-based wound dressing
Repliform tissue graft
repressor
repressor gene
reproduction
  asexual
  assisted
  cytogenic
  gross
  sexual
  third-party
reproductive endocrinologist
reproductive endocrinology
reproductive sterilization by tubal ligation
reproductive surgeon
reproductive technology
  ART (assisted reproductive technology)
  SMART (surgical myomectomy as reproductive therapy)
  sperm aspiration
  STARRT (selective tubal assessment to refine reproductive therapy) falloposcopy
  START SMART Program for assisted
Repronal
Repronex (menotropins for injection)
repulsion
rerupture of aneurysm
resectable lesion
resected malignant breast tumor
resected, surgically
resection
  en bloc
  endometrial
  loop
  OPERA (outpatient endometrial resection/ablation)
  percutaneous
  segmental
  transurethral
  wedge
resection and fulguration of bladder tumor
resection and reanastomosis of ureter
resection electrode
resection of bladder tumor
resector, StarBAR resection electrode
resectoscope (see also *endoscope*)
  ACMI rotating continuous flow
  Baumrucker
  Iglesias
  Iglesias fiberoptic
  Nesbit
  OPERA STAR
  STAR (specialized tissue aspirating)
  Stern-McCarthy
  Storz

resectoscope electrode
reserve, diminished renal
reservoir
  Camey
  Camey continent
  conduit
  continent supravesical bowel urinary diversion
  continent urinary diversion
  Duke pouch
  ileal conduit
  ileal neobladder
  intra-abdominal
  inverted U-pouch ileal reservoir
  Kock pouch
  LeBag ileocolic urinary
  Mainz pouch urinary
  Rowland pouch
  sigmoid colon
  W-stapled urinary
reservoir ileostomy
residual
  fibrocystic
  large postvoid
  moderate postvoid
  postvoid (PVR)
  postvoiding
residual calculous material
residual dysplasia
residual glomeruli
residual ovary syndrome
residual renal function
residual tumor
residual urine
residual urine accumulation
residual urine volume
residual volume (RV)
residue
  filter
  sediment
resin compound
resins, cation exchange
Resipump
resiquimod
resistance
  proximal urethral
  urinary sphincter
resistant ovary syndrome
resolution
Resolve (support group for infertile couples)
resorption, water
Resource and Information Network for Bodily Integrity of Women (RAINBO)
RespiGam
respiration, Kussmaul
respirator (see *ventilator*)
respiratory acidosis
respiratory alkalosis
respiratory decompensation
respiratory distress
respiratory distress syndrome (RDS)
respiratory failure
respiratory syncytial virus (RSV)
response to exogenous vasopressin
response
  immune
  lactation letdown
  vasovagal
rest
  kidney
  pelvic
restless legs syndrome
Restore orthobiologic soft-tissue implant
restriction
  fetal growth
  symmetric fetal growth
restriction enzyme cutting site
restriction enzymes
restriction fragment
restriction fragment length polymorphism (RFLP)
restriction landmark genomic scanning (RLGS)
restriction map
restriction site

resulting offspring
retained bladder syndrome
retained dead fetus
retained decidua
retained menstrual blood
retained menstruation
retained placenta
retained placental fragments
retained portions of placenta
retained products of conception
retained secundines
retained testis
retained tissue within uterine cavity
retained urine
retardata, ejaculatio
retardation
  fetal growth
  intrauterine growth
retarded ejaculation
rete cyst of ovary
retentate
retentate stream
retention
  nitrogen
  urinary
retention cyst of ovary
retention factor (rF)
retention of dead fetus
retention suture
rete testis
reticulocyte count
reticulum, sarcoplasmic
retinal dysplasia-retinal aphasia, Loken-Senior-type
retinal sheen in nephrotic syndrome
retinitis, hemorrhagic
retinitis pigmentosa (RP)
retinitis pigmentosa and congenital deafness
retinoids
retinoblastoma
retinocerebral angiomatosis
retinopathy of prematurity (ROP)
retinopathy, proliferative
retinoschisis
RET proto-oncogene
retractable foreskin
retracted nipple
retractile testis
retraction
  intercostal
  nipple
  skin of breast
  subcostal
retraction of skin
retraction ring
retractor
  Airlift balloon
  Army-Navy
  Balfour
  Bookwalter
  bowel
  Breisky-Navratil
  circular self-retaining
  curved ribbon
  Deaver
  Eccentric "Y"
  Finochietto
  Gazayerli endoscopic
  Guttmann
  Heaney hysterectomy
  Kitner (also Kittner)
  laser Jackson
  lateral vaginal
  Lone Star
  Magrina-Bookwalter vaginal
  malleable
  narrow lateral Heaney
  Navratil
  Newport lateral vaginal
  O'Connor-O'Sullivan
  O'Sullivan-O'Connor
  Olivier
  Omni-Lift
  Omni-Tract
  posterior
  Premier vaginal
  R-Med mini

retractor *(cont.)*
- Rosenkranz pediatric
- Rosenkranz wire-basket
- self-retaining
- SJM Rosenkranz pediatric
- Space-OR
- Thompson
- Turner-Warwick self-retaining
- vaginal-cervical Ahluwalia retractor-elevator (VCARE)
- weighted posterior

retraining
- bladder
- toilet

retrieval, transvaginal oocyte
retroareolar dysplasia, sheetlike
retroareolar mass
retrocaval ureter
retrocecal appendix
retroflexed uterus
retroflexion
retroflexion of uterus
retrograde cystography
retrograde cystourethrogram
retrograde ejaculation
retrograde filling
retrograde introduction of contrast agent
retrograde menstruation
retrograde pyelogram
retrograde pyelography
retrograde sclerotherapy
retrograde studies
retrograde ureteral catheterization
retrograde ureterogram
retrograde ureteropyelogram
retrograde ureteropyelography
retrograde ureteroscopic endopyelotomy
retrograde urethrocystography
retrograde urethrogram
retrograde urethrogram catheter
retrograde urethrography
retrograde uretography
retrograde urography
retroiliac ureter
retrolental fibroplasia (RLF)
retromammary mastitis
retromammary space
retromembranous hematoma
retropectoral mammary implant
retroperineal lymphadenopathy
retroperitoneal fibrosis
retroperitoneal fixation
retroperitoneal lymph nodes
retroperitoneal mass lesion
retroperitoneal space
retroperitoneoscopy
retroperitoneum
retroperitonitis, idiopathic fibrous
retroplacental bleeding
retropubically
retropubic exploration
retropubic prostatectomy
retropubic space
retropubic urethral suspension operation
retropubic urethropexy, Burch
retrotransposon
retrovirus
retrourethrocystography
retrouterine cul-de-sac
retrouterine pouch of Douglas
retroversion of uterus
retroverted gravid uterus
retroverted uterus
retrovirus, human mammary tumor
Rett syndrome
returned to the patient through the venous access
Retzius, space of
Reuter suprapubic trocar and cannula system
revascularization, renal
ReVele
reverse conversion
reversed ductus arteriosus
reverse genetics
reverse Giemsa (R) chromosome staining method
reverse osmosis separations

reverse osmosis water purification
system
reverse transcriptase
reverse transcription
reverse surgical sterilization in women
reverse T3 or rT3
reversible postrenal factors
reversible prerenal factors
revision of episiotomy scar
revision of stoma
Rezulin (troglitazone)
rF (retention factor)
RF (rheumatic fever)
RF (rheumatoid factor)
RFA (right frontoanterior) position
RFLP (restriction fragment length polymorphism)
RFP (right frontoposterior) position
R.F. tissue ablation device
RFT (right frontotransverse) position
Rh (Rhesus)
rhabdomyolysis
rhabdomyosarcoma of testicle
rhagades seen in congenital syphilis
RHCT (renal helical CT)
Rheomacrodex (dextran 40)
rhEPO (recombinant human
erythropoietin)
Rhesus isoimmunization
rheumatic fever (RF)
rheumatism, gonorrheal
rheumatoid arthritis (RA)
rheumatoid factor (RF)
Rheumatrex (methotrexate)
Rh factor
Rh immune globulin
Rh incompatibility
Rh isoimmunization
Rh negative
Rh-negative blood
Rh negative, unsensitized
Rh sensitization
RhoC gene
RhoC GTPase gene
Rho(D) immune globulin
Rho(D)-positive
RhoGAM (Rh0(D) immune globulin)
Rh positive
r-HuEPO or rHuEPO (recombinant
human erythropoietin)
rhythmic uterine contractions
RIA (radioimmunoassay)
ribbon uterus
rib gap defects with micrognathia
ribonucleic acid (RNA)
ribonucleotides
ribosomal RNA
ribosome
rice water stools
Richardson technique, modified
Richards-Rundle syndrome
rickets
hypophosphatemic
renal
rickettsial infection
ridge
cervicovaginal
genital
interureteric
intratrigonal
mammary
mesonephric
urethral
urogenital
wolffian
Rieger syndrome
rifampin
right-angle clamp
right-angle lens
right-angle scissors
right atrial extension of uterine
leiomyosarcoma
right flank incision
right flank pain
right frontoanterior (RFA) position
right frontoposterior (RFP) position
right frontotransverse (RFT) position
right internal mammary anastomosis

right lower quadrant (RLQ)
right lower quadrant tenderness
right mentoanterior (RMA) position
right mentotransverse (RMT) position
right midback
right occipitoanterior (ROA) position
right occipitotransverse (ROT) position
right of procreation
right ovarian veins
right pelvic sidewall
right sacroanterior (RSA) position
right sacroposterior (RSP) position
right sacrotransverse (RST) position
right-sided bacterial endocarditis
right testicular vein
right upper quadrant (RUQ)
right ureter
rigid biopsy forceps
rigid cervix
rigid cystoscope
rigid endoscopic access
rigid fiberoptic hysteroscope
rigid hymen
rigid hysteroscope
rigidity in erèctile dysfunction
rigid pelvic floor
rigid perineum
rigid suction curet
rigid ureter
rigid ureterorenoscopy
rigid ureteroscope
rigid ureteroscopy
RigiScan for evaluation of penile
  tumescence
rigors
Riley-Day syndrome
ring
  amnion
  anorectal
  Bandl
  contraction
  estradiol-loaded silicone
  external
  Falope

ring *(cont.)*
  gestational
  hymenal
  internal
  intravaginal (IVR)
  NuvaRing (etonogestrel/ethinyl
    estradiol) contraceptive vaginal
  peritoneal constriction
  retraction
  stiff
  tubal
  umbilical
  urethral marking
  vaginal constriction
  Yoon fallopian tube ligation
ring chromosome 20
Ringer lactate solution
ring forceps
Ring-McLean sump drain
ring pessary
ring-shaped placenta
ripe cervix
ripening of cervix
Ripstein operation for rectal prolapse
risk assessment
risk communication
risk factors
risk for prematurity and low birth
  weight
risk modification
risk, NMR (neonatal mortality)
RITA (radiofrequency interstitial tissue
  ablation) system
Ritgen maneuver
ritodrine
Riza-Ribe grasper needle
RLF (retrolental fibroplasias)
RLGS (restriction landmark genomic
  scanning)
RLS (restless leg syndrome)
RLQ (right lower quadrant)
RMA (right mentoanterior) position
R-Med mini-retractor
R-Med plug

RNA (ribonucleic acid)
RNA polymerase
RNA splicing
RNC (radionuclide cystography)
RNP (registered nurse practitioner)
ROA (right occipitoanterior position)
robertsonian translocation
Roberts syndrome
Robin anomalad, sequence, or syndrome
Robinow syndrome
Robinson straight urethral catheter
robotic surgery device, AESOP (automated endoscopic system for optimal positioning)
robotics, SurgiScope
Rocaltrol (calcitriol)
ROC and ROC XS suture fasteners
Rocephin (ceftriaxone)
Rochester-Pean forceps
rocker-bottom feet
Rockey-Davis incision
rock-hard prostate gland
ROC suture fastener
ROC XS suture fastener
rodent ulcer
Roeder loop
Roe v. Wade
rogletimide
rollerbar or roller bar
rollerbar electrode endometrial ablation
rollerbar endometrial ablation
RollerLOOP surgical electrode
Romano-Ward Syndrom
Romberg hemifacial atrophy
room
  birthing
  delivery
  labor and delivery
  LDR (labor, delivery, and recovery)
  recovery
room air
rooming in
rooting reflex
rootless teeth
root of penis
ROP (retinopathy of prematurity)
ROP (right occipitoposterior position)
ROPA (Regional Organ Procurement Agency)
ropivacaine
roquinimex
Rosch-Thurmond fallopian tube catheter
Rose-Bradford kidney
Rosenberg-Chutorian syndrome
Rosenkranz pediatric retractor
Rosenkranz wire-basket retractor
roseola infantum
Rosewater syndrome
rosiglitazone
Rossavik fetal growth equation
Rossavik fetal growth model
ROT (right occipitotransverse position)
rotation
  Benenenti
  DeLee
  fetal head
  key-in-lock
  Kielland
  manual
  Scanzoni
rotavirus
Rothmund-Thomson (RTS) syndrome
Rotor syndrome
round block technique of mastopexy
round catheter tip
round ligament of uterus
round pelvis
Roussy-Lévy syndrome
Rowasa enema
Rowland pouch
Royal Women's coaxial catheter
RP (radical prostatectomy)
RP (retinitis pigmentosa)
RPGN (rapidly progressive glomerulonephritis)

RPR (rapid plasma reagin) test
RPR-CT (rapid plasma reagin circle-card test) for syphilis
rRNA
RSA (recurrent spontaneous abortion)
RSA (right sacroanterior) position
RSP (right sacroposterior) position
RST (right sacrotransverse) position
RSV (respiratory syncytial virus)
RTA (renal tubular acidosis)
RTOG (Radiation Therapy Oncology Group) trials
RTS (radiation therapy system)
RU 486 (mifepristone) early abortion pill
rubber dam
rubbery consistency prostate
rubella
  congenital
  maternal
rubella titer
rubella titer immune
Rubens flap for breast reconstruction
Rubenstein syndrome
Rubenstein-Taybi syndrome
Rubin cannula
Rubin maneuver
Rubin test
rubitecan
rubra, lochia
rudimentary gonads
rudimentary uterine horn
ruga (pl. rugae)
  scrotal
  tubal
rugal folds
rugated vaginal mucosa
rugation
rugous, vagina
Ruhr syndrome
rule, Nägele's
rule out sepsis
ruler, laser depth
RUMI uterine manipulator
run-in time
running locking sutures
running sutures
rupture
  amnion
  amniotic membrane
  aneurysm
  appendiceal
  bladder
  liver
  large bladder
  marginal sinus
  matured graafian follicle
  ovarian
  plaque
  splenic
  urethral
  uterine
ruptured abdominal aortic aneurysm
ruptured aortic atheromatous plaque
ruptured appendix
ruptured bladder
ruptured dermoid cyst
ruptured ectopic pregnancy
ruptured membranes
ruptured ovarian cyst
ruptured renal cyst
ruptured tubal pregnancy
ruptured tubo-ovarian abscess
ruptured urethra
rupture from endometrioma
rupture of membranes
  artificial
  premature (PROM)
  preterm premature (PPROM)
  prolonged
  spontaneous
RUQ (right upper quadrant)
Russell-Silver syndrome
Russell syndrome
Russian tissue forceps
Rutkow sutureless plug-and-patch repair for inguinal hernia
Rutner biopsy needle

Rutner percutaneous suprapubic balloon catheter
Ruvalcaba syndrome
Ruysch glomerulus
RV (residual volume)
RVH (renal vascular hypertension)
RVR (renal vascular resistance)
RVT (renal vein thrombosis)

S, s

Saber BT blunt-tip surgical trocar
saber cut incision
sac
  abnormal gestational
  allantoic
  amnionic
  amniotic
  chorionic
  cystic
  embryonic
  fetal
  gestational
  hernia
  intrauterine
  monoamniotic
  preputial
  pseudogestational sac
  pudendal
sacciform kidney
saccular mass
saccus vaginalis
saclike outpouching of the urethral wall
sacral agenesis, congenital
sacral backache
sacral colpopexy
sacral edema
sacral nerve stimulation (SNS) therapy
sacral plexus
sacral promontory
sacral sensory nerve ganglia
sacral teratoma
sacrocolpopexy, abdominal
sacrogenital fold
sacroposterior (SP) position
sacrospinous colpopexy
sacrospinous ligament
sacrospinous scarring
sacrospinous vaginal vault suspension procedure
sacrotransverse (ST) position
sacrouterine fold
sacrouterine ligament
sacrouterine neurectomy
sacrovaginal fold
sacrovesical fold
saddle bags flap
saddle block anesthesia
saddle sensation
saddle-shaped uterus
Sadowsky breast marking system
Sadowsky hook wire
Saenger cesarean section
Saethre-Chotzen syndrome
safe sex
Safetex cervical spatula
Safety AV fistula needle

Safil synthetic absorbable surgical
  suture
sagging of breasts
sagittal fontanelle
sagittal plane
sagittal septum of rectus sheath
sagittal suture
sagittal synostosis
sago spleen
Sahara Clinical Bone Sonometer
Sahara portable bone densitometer
Sakati syndrome
Saldino-Noonan syndrome
SalEst salivary estriol measurement
  system
SalEst system for preterm labor
salicylate
salicylate poisoning
saline abortion
saline breast implant
saline diuretic
saline induction
saline, normal
saline-resistant alkalosis
saline slush
saline solution
saline wash
Salmonella
Salmonella bredeney
salpingectomy, abdominal
salpingectomy with removal of tubal
  pregnancy
salpinges (pl. of salpinx)
salpingioma
salpingitic
salpingitis
  bacterial
  chlamydial
  chronic interstitial
  follicular
  foreign body
  gonococcal
  gonorrheal
  hemorrhagic
salpingitis *(cont.)*
  interstitial
  mural
  nodular
  parenchymatous
  pelvic
  pseudofollicular
  purulent
  tuberculous
salpingitis and oophoritis
  acute
  chronic
salpingitis follicularis
salpingitis gonorrhoica
salpingitis in previously occluded tubes
  (SPOT)
salpingitis isthmica nodosa (SIN)
salpingitis profluens
salpingocele
salpingocentesis
salpingocyesis
salpingogram
salpingography
  selective
  selective ostial
salpingolithiasis
salpingolysis
salpingoneostomy
salpingo-oophorectomy
  bilateral
  unilateral
salpingo-oophoritis
salpingo-oophorocele
salpingo-oophorostomy
salpingo-oothecitis
salpingo-oothecocele
salpingo-ovariectomy
salpingo-ovariotomy
salpingoperitonitis
salpingopexy
salpingoplasty
salpingorrhagia
salpingorrhaphy
salpingosalpingostomy

salpingoscopy
salpingostomatomy
salpingostomatoplasty
salpingostomy, linear
salpingotomy, abdominal
salpingo-uterostomy
salpinx (pl. salpinges)
salpinx uterina
Salpix contrast medium
salt-losing nephritis
salt-losing syndrome
salt restriction
saluresis
saluretic
Salute tissue fixation system
salvage cystectomy
SAM (subcutaneous augmentation material)
SAMBA (simultaneous areolar mastopexy and breast augmentation)
sampler
  Multispatula cervical
  PadKit collection system
sample, dilute urine
sampling
  axillary node
  chorionic villus
  cord blood
  endocervical
  fetal blood
  feetal scalp blood
  fetal skin
  percutaneous umbilical blood
Sandimmune (cyclosporine)
Sandhoff disease
Sanfilippo syndrome
SangCya (cyclosporine)
sanguinolenta, lochia
sanitary pad
San Luis Valley syndrome
SANS (Stoller afferent nerve stimulation) urinary incontinence device
Santavouri disease
Santorini plexus
saphenous vein fistula
saphenous vein shunt
Sarafem (fluoxetine)
sarcofetal pregnancy
sarcohysteric pregnancy
sarcoidosis
sarcoma
  embryonal
  endometrial stromal
  Kaposi
  prostatic
sarcoplasmic reticulum
Sarrett suture carrier
SART (Society for Assisted Reproductive Technology)
Sassone score of transvaginal ultrasound
satellite DNA
satellite hemodialysis unit
satellite nodules
satisfaction with sexual activity
sats (O_2 saturations)
satumomab pendetide monoclonal antibody
saturated potassium iodide solution
satyriasis
Savannah steerable probe
SAVVY contraceptive vaginal gel
SAVVY vaginal microbicide
Saxtorph maneuver
Saxtorph-Pajot maneuver
SBGM (self blood glucose monitoring)
SBP (spontaneous bacterial peritonitis)
SC (separation coefficient)
SCAD (short chain acyl-CoA-dehydrogenase) deficiency
scale
  Bethesda rating
  Brazelton Neonatal Behavioral Assessment
  Cranley Maternal-Fetal Attachment Scale
  Dubowitz infant maturity
  ECOG (Eastern Cooperative Oncology Group) performance status

scale *(cont.)*
- Karnofsky rating
- masculinity-femininity
- NIPS (Neonatal Infant Pain Scale)
- Tanner Developmental

scalpel
- Cobalt Scalpel
- Harmonic
- LaserSonics Nd:YAG LaserBlade
- Shaw electrical
- Shaw I and Shaw II hemostatic

scalp electrode
scalpel wound
scalp pH
scalp-skull and limbs, absence defect of
scan (also see *imaging*)
- abdominopelvic CT
- BladderScan
- bone
- computerized tomographic (CT)
- contrast-enhanced
- CT (computerized tomographic)
- DEXA (dual-energy x-ray absorptiometry)
- diuretic renal
- kidney
- magnetic resonance imaging (MRI)
- non-contrast-enhanced
- radioisotope bone
- radionuclide bladder
- radionuclide renal
- renal
- renal duplex
- renal perfusion
- TechneScan MAG3
- technetium-labeled sulfur colloid
- thyroid
- unenhanced

scanner
- Bruel-Kjaer ultrasound
- T-Scan 2000 transpectral impedance
- TransScan TS2000 electrical impedance breast

scanning electron microscopy
scant amount of tissue
scant mucoid material
scanty menstruation
scanty vaginal bleeding
Scanzoni maneuver
scaphocephaly
scaphoid abdomen
scapula elevata
scar
- inframammary
- surgical
- traumatic
- uterine

SCAR (sequence characterized amplified region)
Scardino vertical flap pyeloplasty
scarf ratio
scarf sign in neonate
scarlatinal nephritis
"scarless" mastectomy
Scarpa fascia
scarred kidney
scar revision
scarring
- cortical
- endometrial
- postpyelonephritis cortical scarring
- renal
- uterine lining

scar tissue in ureter
SCD (seminal collection device)
SCF 24 infant formula
Schatz maneuver
Schauta radical vaginal hysterectomy
Schiller solution
Schiller staining of cervix
Schiller test for cervical carcinoma
Schimmelbusch bladder syringe
Schimmelbusch disease
Schimmelbusch syndrome
Schindler disease
Schinzel acrocallosal syndrome
Schinzel-Giedion syndrome
Schinzel syndrome

Schistosoma mansoni
Schistosoma haematobium
schistosomal bladder carcinoma
schistosomiasis
schizencephaly
Schmidt syndrome
Schmidt-type metaphyseal chondrodysplasia
Schmidt-type metaphyseal dysostosis
Schönlein-Henoch purpura
Schroeder-Braun uterine tenaculum forceps
Schroeder excision of diseased endocervical mucosa
Schroeder tenaculum
Schubert uterine biopsy forceps
Schubert-Van Doren biopsy punch
Schuchardt paravaginal rectal displacement incision
Schüller duct
Schultze phantom
Schultze placenta
Schwachman-Diamond syndrome
Schwachman syndrome
schwannoma
Schwartz formula/equation
Schwartz-Jampel syndrome
Schwartzman phenomenon
Schwartz-Pregenzer urethropexy
Schweizer uterine forceps
sciatic endometriosis
SCID (severe combined immunodeficiency)
scintigraphy
  cortical
  radionuclide testicular scintigraphy
  renal
  stress perfusion
  vesicoureteral
scintimammography (SMM)
scintirenography
scintiscan
scirrhous carcinoma of breast
scissor dissection
scissors
  bandage
  bladder
  Braun episiotomy
  curved unipolar
  dissecting
  Electroscope
  endoscopic
  enterotomy
  Evershears II bipolar curved
  Ferguson
  Heaney-Mayo
  Jameson
  Jorgenson
  Mayo
  Metzenbaum
  Re-New laparoscopic
  right-angle
  Sims uterine
  Sovereign bipolar
  Take-apart
  umbilical
  Waldman episiotomy
  Yankauer
  Z-Scissors hysterectomy
sclerema neonatorum
scleroderma
sclerosing adenosis of breast
sclerosing disease
sclerosing membranous glomerulonephritis
sclerosis
  diffuse mesangial
  overlying cortical
  renal
  systemic
sclerotherapy
  antegrade scrotal
  retrograde
sclerotic area
sclerotic kidney
SCNB (stereotaxic core needle biopsy)
scope (see *endoscope*)

Scopette device to reduce genital prolapse
score
 American Urological Association (AUA) Symptom Score
 Apgar
 AUA (American Urological Association) Symptom
 Bishop cervical ripening
 "bother" prostatic symptoms
 extreme drug resistance (EDR)
 Gleason carcinoma of the prostate
 International Prostate Symptom Score (IPSS)
 IPSS (International Prostate Symptom Score)
 NACS (Neurologic and Adaptive Capacity Score)
 NASS (Neonatal Abstinence Scoring System)
 Sassone
scotoma (pl. scotomata)
Scott-Bradley penile prosthesis
Scott craniodigital syndrome with mental retardation
scraping the uterine cavity
scrapings
 cervical
 ulcer
 uterine
 vaginal wall
screen
 Pap Plus Speculoscopy (PPS)
 PAPNET cervical smear
 STD (sexually transmitted disease)
 Virgo ANCA (antineutrophil cytoplasmic antibodies)
screen-film mammogram
screen-film mammography
screening
 cancer
 carrier
 endometrial
 genetic
screening *(cont.)*
 mammography
 newborn
 STD
screw
 hysteroscopic myoma
 laparoscopic myoma
Scribner shunt
scrotal abscess
scrotal contents
scrotal defect
scrotal dermatitis
scrotal elevation
scrotal exploration
scrotal fistulectomy
scrotal fold
scrotal hematoma
scrotal hernia
scrotal hydrocele
scrotal hypospadias
scrotal ice packs
scrotal ligament
scrotal mass
scrotal neck
scrotal part of ductus deferens
scrotal raphe
scrotal rugae
scrotal sac
scrotal septum
scrotal suspensory
scrotal swelling
scrotal-testicular trauma
scrotal testis
scrotal veins
scrotectomy, partial
scrotiform
scrotoplasty
scrotum (pl. scrota, scrotums)
 bifid
 chimney sweep's cancer of
 skin of
 transillumination of
 watering-can
SCUF (slow continuous ultrafiltration)

Scultetus position
SDNS (steroid-dependent nephrotic syndrome)
SDP (shared decision-making program)
SDS-PAGE (sodium dodecyl sulfate-polyacrylamide gel electrophoresis)
Sea-Band acupressure wristband
seal, orbital reducer
search for affirmation
Seasonale oral contraceptive
sebaceous cyst of breast
sebaceous gland
sebaceous miliaria
seborrheic dermatitis
Seckel syndrome
secondary abdominal pregnancy
secondary adhesion
secondary amenorrhea
secondary arrest of dilation
secondary atelectasis
secondary blepharospasm
secondary dysmenorrhea
secondary dyspareunia
secondary follicle
secondary gout
secondary hyperparathyroidism
secondary hypertension
secondary hypogonadism
secondary infection
secondary infertility
secondary megaureter
secondary membranous disease
secondary oocyte
secondary perineal tear
secondary renal calculus
secondary renal tubular acidosis
secondary sex character
secondary sex characteristics
secondary stricture formation
secondary syphilis
secondary testicular damage
secondary to trauma
secondary uterine inertia
second degree cystourethrocele
second degree prolapse of uterus
second degree perineal laceration
second degree rectocele
second degree relative
second degree uterine prolapse
second-look laparoscopy
second-look laparotomy
second-look procedure
second stage of labor
second trimester
second trimester abortion
second trimester bleeding
second trimester placenta
secrecy
secretory phase
secreted molecules
secretion
  altered hormone
  Bartholin gland
  cleansing acid
  endogenous gonadotropin
  excessive
  inappropriate gonadotropin
  increased androgen
  mucus
  ovarian estrogen
secretory duct of Bartholin gland, obstruction of
secretory endometrium
section (also see *cesarean section*)
  cesarean (C-section)
  classical cesarean
  extraperitoneal cesarean
  frozen
  Latzko cesarean
  low cervical cesarean
  low transverse cesarean
  lower uterine segment cesarean
  lower uterine segment transverse cesarean
  perineal
  primary cesarean
  supravesical cesarean
  transperitoneal cesarean

section *(cont.)*
  transperitoneal classical cesarean
  vaginal cesarean
Secu ("C-Q") clip
secundigravida (gravida 2)
secundines, retained
sedation
  Demerol
  intravenous
  Versed
sediment residue
sediment, spun urine
seeding
  metastatic
  prostate
  tumor
seed points
seeds
  BrachySeed iodine-125
  BrachySeed palladium-103
  EchoSeed (iodine-125) brachytherapy
  gold marker
  IoGold radioactive
  I-Plant radioactive iodine-125
  PharmaSeed iodine-125
  PharmaSeed palladium-103
  ProstaSeed I-125
  radium
  Symmetra ^{125}I brachytherapy
seepage of urine
segment
  aperistaltic distal ureteral
  lower uterine
  renal
  upper uterine
segmental artery
segmental fibroadenosis of breast
segmental glomerulonephritis
segmental hyalinosis
segmental ischemia
segmental mastectomy
segmental necrotizing glomerulonephritis
segmental renal artery waveform
segmental resection
segmental resection of bladder
segmental resection of diseased renal artery
segregation
segregation distortion
Segura stone basket
Seiler colposcope
Seip syndrome
Seitelberger disease
Seitzinger tripolar cutting forceps
seizure prophylaxis
seizures in newborn
Seldinger approach
Seldinger technique
SelectCells endometrial sampling device
Select GT blood glucose system
selection
selective adrenal vein angiography
selective estrogen receptor modulator (SERM)
selective fetal reduction
selective membrane skin
selective mutism, or elective mutism
selective ostial salpingography
selective ovarian vein angiography
selective reduction
selective renal artery angiography
selective renal artery embolization
selective salpingography
selective termination
selective tubal assessment to refine reproductive therapy (STARRT) falloposcopy system
selective tubal occlusion procedure (STOP) contraceptive device
selenium yeast
selenomethionine
self blood glucose monitoring (SBGM)
self-care dialysis
SelfCare pregnancy test
self-catheterization, intermittent

self-incompatibility
self-induced abortion
self-pollination
self-retaining catheter
self-retaining retractor
self-sterility
self-stimulation of the genitals
Selikowitz endoscopic knife
sella turcica
Sellick maneuver for aspiration prevention
semen (pl. semina, semens)
semen analysis
semen donor
semen fructose test
semenuria
semiconservative
semilunar incision
seminal collection device (SCD)
seminal colliculus
seminal duct
seminal fluid
seminal gland
  mucosa of
  muscular layer of
seminal granule
seminal lake
seminal vesicle, cellulitis of
seminal vesiculitis
seminal vesiculography (SVG)
seminal vesiculopathy
seminiferous tubule dysgenesis
seminiferous tubules
seminoma
seminomatous
seminoma, spermacytic
seminuria
semipermeable membrane
semiprone position
semirigid uteroscope
Semkin forceps
Semm hysterectomy
senile atrophy of vulva
senile involution of ovary
senile melanoderma
senile nephrosclerosis
senile vaginitis
senility
Senographe 2000D digital mammography imaging system
SenoScan mammography system
sensate flap
sensation
  bladder
  incomplete bladder emptying
  saddle
sensitivity
sensor, anal EMG PerryMetor
sensorineural deafness in hereditary nephritis
sensory paralytic bladder
sentinel lymph node (SLN)
sentinel node biopsy
sentinel pile
SEPA (soft enhancer of percutaneous absorption)/testosterone gel
separation anxiety
separation coefficient, SC
separation factor, SF
separation of streams of feed, permeate, and retentate
separation of symphysis pubis
separation process
separation, symphyseal
Sephardic Jew
Sepracoat coating solution
Seprafilm (sodium hyaluronate and carboxymethylcellulose) bioresorbable membrane
Sepragel bioresorbable gel
Sepramesh biosurgical composite
sepsis (pl. sepses)
  instrumentation
  neonatal
  pelvic
  puerperal
septate hymen
septate uterus

septate vagina
septectomy, uterine
septic abortion
septic embolism
septicemia
  pelvic
  puerperal
  transient
septic shock
septic syndrome
septo-optic dysplasia
Septra, Septra DS (trimethoprim; sulfamethoxazole)
septula of testis
septulet pregnancy
septum (pl. septa)
  glans penis
  penile
  perirenal
  rectovaginal
  rectovesical
  scrotal
  transverse
  urethral
  urogenital
  uterine
  vaginal
septum penis
sequelae
  serious fetal
  serious maternal
sequelae of rape
  emotional
  psychologic
  social
sequence characterized amplified region (SCAR)
sequence of nucleotides
sequence tagged microsatellite (STMS)
sequence tagged site (STS)
sequence, twin reversed arterial perfusion (TRAP)
sequencing
sequential clamp and suture technique
sequential clamp, cut, and tie technique
sequential compression device
sequential intravesical air
sequential intravesical air and contrast agent
sera, immune
Serenoa repens extract
serial dilation
serial dilators
serial estriol determinations
serial fetal magnetic resonance imaging
serial sonograms
serial ultrasound examinations
serial x-ray films
serious fetal sequelae
serious maternal sequelae
SERM (selective estrogen receptor modulator)
serologic relapse
serologic test for syphilis (STS) (see also *syphilis*)
  fluorescent treponal antibody absorption (FTA-ABS)
  hemagglutination test for syphilis (HATTS)
  microhemagglutination assay for antibodies to *T. pallidum* (MHA-TP)
  rapid plasma reagin (RPR)
  Venereal Disease Research Laboratory (VDRL)
serology nonreactive
Seroma-Cath wound drainage system
seromuscular graft
seromuscular intestinal patch graft
seronegative
Serophene (clomiphene citrate)
seropositive
serosa of urinary bladder
serosa of uterine tube
serosa of uterus
serosal surface of uterus
serosanguineous fluid
serosa, lochia

serotype
serous adenocarcinoma
serous covering
serous cyst of ovary
serous cystadenocarcinoma
serous cystadenoma
serous surface papilloma
serrated curet
Serratia liquefaciens
Serratia marcescens
serrations, Kapp-Beck
serratus anterior muscle
Sertoli cells of testis
Sertoli-cell-only (SCO) pattern
Sertoli-cell-only syndrome
Sertoli-Leydig cell ovarian tumor
Sertoli-stromal cell ovarian tumor
serum 1,25-dihydroxyvitamin D3 (calcitriol)
serum accumulation in pelvis
serum accumulation in wound
serum albumin
serum alpha-fetoprotein
serum amylase
serum bicarbonate
serum chemistry
serum complement levels
  C3
  C4
  CH50
serum creatinine
serum creatinine concentration
serum hCG (human chorionic gonadotropin)
serum hepatitis
serum iron
serum iron and ferritin
serum nephritis
serum phosphorus
serum pregnancy test
serum prolactin
serum prolactin level
serum protein changes
serum protein electrophoresis (SPE)
serum proteins, properdin
serum-sensitive strains
serum testosterone
serum urea and creatinine levels
serum urea nitrogen
sessile hydatid
S.E.T. hemodialysis catheter
Setleis syndrome
setting sun sign in newborn
sevelamer
7p deletion syndrome
7q21.3 deletion syndrome
7q21-q22 deletion syndrome
7q36 deletion syndrome
7 duplication syndrome
7p11.2-p13 duplication syndrome
7p15.1-p21.3 duplication syndrome
7p21.1-p14.2 duplication syndrome
17-alpha-hydroxylase deficiency
17-beta-estradiol hormone replacement therapy
17-beta-estradiol/norethindrone
17-beta-estradiol transdermal patch
17 duplication syndrome
17-epitestosterone
17-hydroxycorticosteroid (17-OHCS)
17-hydroxyprogesterone (17-OHP)
17-ketosteroids (17-KS)
17p11.2 duplication syndrome
700 Ultrex Plus penile prosthesis
severe acidemia
severe combined immunodeficiency (SCID)
severe dysnatremia
severe preeclampsia
severe toxemia
sex (pl. sexes)
  anal
  gay
  homosexual
  oral
  safe
  straight
  vaginal

sex assignment
sex chromatin
sex chromatin mass
sex chromosome
sex chromosome imbalance
sex-determining chromosomes
sex hormone-binding globulin (SHBG)
sex hormones
sex-influenced
sex-influenced inheritance
sex-limited inheritance
sex-linked
sex-linked inheritance
sex-linked locus
sex of rearing
sex reassignment surgery
sex steroid
sex steroid-binding globulin
sex surrogate
sextuplet pregnancy
sexual abstinence
sexual abuse
sexual activity
  frequency of
  oral-genital
  satisfaction with
sexual assault
sexual characteristics, secondary
sexual contact
sexual desire
sexual development, rapid premature
sexual differentiation
sexual dimorphism
sexual disorder
sexual dwarfism
sexual dysfunction agents
sexual encounters with prostitutes
sexual endurance
sexual excitation
sexual experimentation
sexual generation
sexual gratification
sexual history
sexual identity conflict
sexual infantilism
sexual intercourse
sexual intercourse phobia
sexuality
sexualization
sexual love phobia
sexually active patient
sexually active with multiple partners
sexually differentiated cognitive abilities
sexually stimulated hair
sexually transmitted disease (STD)
  AIDS (acquired immunodeficiency syndrome)
  chancroid
  chlamydia
  Chlamydia trachomatis
  cytomegalovirus (CMV)
  genital condyloma (or condylomata)
  giant anal wart
  giant anorectal condyloma acuminatum
  gonorrhea
  granuloma inguinale
  herpes simplex
  herpes simplex virus (HSV)
  herpesvirus
  human immunodeficiency virus (HIV)
  lymphogranuloma venereum
  syphilis
  trichomonas
  Trichomonas vaginalis
  venereal warts
sexually transmitted infection
sexually transmitted pathogens
sexual maturation, early
sexual maturity
sexual partners, number of different
sexual potency
sexual precosity
sexual preference
sexual procreative conduct
sexual reproduction
sexual transmission

SF (separation factor)
SGA (small for gestational age)
shadow
  breast
  butterfly breast
  kidney
  renal
shadowing, acoustical
shadowing stone
shaft of penis
shaggy grayish exudate
shake test
shake test for maturity of fetal lungs
shaken baby syndrome
shaking chill
shallow discrete ulcers
shame and isolation
Shapiro intrauterine insemination catheter
shared decision-making program (SDP)
sharp curettage
sharp dissection
sharp stabbing pain
sharp trocar
shaving, prostatic
Shaw electrical scalpel
Shaw I and Shaw II Teflon-coated hemostatic scalpel
SHBG (sex hormone-binding globulin)
shears
  Evershears II bipolar curved
  LaparoSonic coagulating
sheath
  endometrial resection and ablation (ERA) resectoscope
  fibrin
  Futura resectoscope
  hysteroscopy
  laparoscopic access
  Microgyn resectoscope safety
  MicroSpan
  O'Connor
  prostatic
  rectus
shedding
  cyclic endometrial
  viral
shedding of bloody fluid
Sheehan syndrome
sheen, retinal
sheetlike retroareolar dysplasia
shelf, Blumer rectal
shelled out
shell out a cyst
Shepard intrauterine insemination catheter
Shereshevskii-Turner syndrome
Sherwood intrascopic suction/irrigation system for laparoscopic procedures
shield, CapSure continence
shift of intravascular fluid volume into peritoneal space
Shigella
Shilder disease
Shilder encephalitis disease
Shirodkar cervical cerclage procedure
Shirodkar clamp
Shirodkar suture
shock
  bacterial
  endotoxic
  obstetric
  postoperative
  septic
  toxic
"shock" bladder
shocklike state
shocks, lithotripsy
shock wave generator
shock wave lithotripsy (SWL)
shoemaker's breast
Shohl solution (sodium citrate; citric acid)
Sholkoff balloon hysterosalpingography catheter
short arm of chromosome (p)
short arm syndrome

short chain acyl-CoA-dehydrogenase
deficiency (SCAD)
short cord
shortening of urethra
shortening of vagina
short-scar procedure in breast reduction
technique
short-scar technique of mastopexy
short-scar tumescent reduction
mammoplasty
short stature homeobox (SHOX)-
containing gene
short stature-onychodysplasia
short stature, telangiectatic erythema
of the face syndrome
SHORT syndrome
short tandem repeats
short-term incontinence
short-term lymphocyte culture
short-time dialysis
short umbilical cord
shotgun method
shotgun sequencing
shotgun vitamin therapy
shotty breast
shoulder dystocia
shoulder impaction
shoulder presentation
shoulders, impacted
SHOX (short stature homeobox)-
containing gene)
Shprintzen syndrome
shriveled kidney
shunt
Allen-Brown
Allen-Brown vascular access
arteriovenous (AV)
arteriovenous bovine
Blalock-Taussig
Brescia-Cimino
Buselmeier vascular access
Cimino
corpora cavernosa-corpus
spongiosum

shunt *(cont.)*
dialysis
distal splenorenal (DSRS)
glans to cavernosum
hemodialysis access
LeVeen
proximal splenorenal
Quinton-Scribner double-lumen
Ramirez vascular access
renal-splenic venous
saphenous vein
Scribner
splenorenal
Thomas vascular access
VPS (ventriculoperitoneal)
Warren
Warren splenorenal
Winter
shunt-dependent hydrocephalus
shunted blood
shutdown, renal
Shwachman Diamond syndrome
Shwachman syndrome
Shy-Drager syndrome
SI (International System of Units)
sialidosis
Siamese twins
sibutramine
sickle cell crisis
sickle cell disease
sickle cell nephropathy
sickle cell thalassemia
sickle cell trait
sickle gene
side effects of chemotherapy
Side-Fire reflecting dish
side-to-side anastomosis
sidewall, pelvic
SIDS (sudden infant death syndrome)
Siemens Servo 300 ventilator
Siemens Servo 900C ventilator
Siewerling-Creutzfeldt disease
sigmaS serum tumor marker for breast
cancer

sigmoid colon
sigmoid colon reservoir
sigmoid colon segments
sigmoid colon vaginoplasty using
  modified technique
sigmoid kidney
sigmoid neovaginal construction
sigmoidocolpoplasty
sigmoidovaginal fistula
sigmoidovesical fistula
sigmoid pedicle
sigmoid segment
sigmoid vaginoplasty
sign
  abnormal cerebral
  banana
  blue dot
  Branham
  brim
  Chadwick
  chandelier
  Chaussier
  Cullen
  Dalrymple
  Danforth
  drooping lily
  Gauss
  Goodell
  Grey-Turner
  Guyon
  halo (of hydrops)
  Hegar
  Hoehne
  Homans
  Jacquemier
  Jello
  lemon
  linguine
  natural fertility
  Nicoladoni-Branham
  Pinard
  placental
  scarf
  setting sun

sign *(cont.)*
  Sister Mary Joseph
  Spalding
signs of life
SIHC (surgically implanted hemodialysis catheter)
SIL (squamous intraepithelial lesion)
Silastic band
Silastic catheter
Silastic condom
Silastic tube
Silber aspiration catheter
sildenafil citrate
silent cervical dilation
silent prostatism
silent thyroiditis
silicone breast implant
silicone catheter
silicone Foley catheter
silicone gel breast implant
silicone Penrose drain
silicone Pezzer drain
silicone retention disk
silicone rubber
silicone stent
silicone vaginal ring
silicon nephropathy
Silitek stent
Silken Secret vaginal moisturizer
silk sutures
Siltex silicone gel breast implant
Silver impregnation stain
silver nitrate
silver nitrate drops
Silver-Russell dwarfism
Silver-Russell syndrome
Silver stain
Silver syndrome
simian crease
Similac Improved infant formula
Similac infant formula
Similac Lactose Free infant formula
Similac Natural Care human milk
  fortifier

Similac PM 60/40 infant formula
Similac Special Care
Similac Special Care 20 infant formula
Similac Special Care 24 infant formula
Similac Special Care with Iron 24
Similac 13 infant formula
Similac 20 infant formula
Similac 24 infant formula
Similac 27 infant formula
Similac with Iron 20
Similac with Iron 24 infant formula
similarity
Simmonds disease
Simon position for vaginal examination
Simonsen large rectovaginal fistula repair
Simonsen technique for large rectovaginal fistula repair
Simons syndrome
simple cystoma of ovary
simple endometrial hyperplasia
simple flat pelvis
simple goiter
simple kidney cysts
simple mastectomy
simple mastopexy
simple renal cyst
simple sequence repeat (SSR)
simple urethritis
simplex
  congenital herpes
  herpes
Simpson dysmorphia syndrome
Simpson forceps
Simpson-Golabi-Behmel syndrome
Simpson uterine sound
Sim SC-20 formula
Sim SC-40 formula
Sims-Huhner sperm-mucus interaction test
Sims position for vaginal examination
Sims speculum
Sims uterine curette
Sims uterine scissors
Sims uterine sound
Sims vaginal speculum
simulation radiography
Simulect (basiliximab) monoclonal antibody
simultaneous areolar mastopexy and breast augmentation (SAMBA)
SIMV (synchronized intermittent mandatory ventilation)
SIN (salpingitis isthmica nodosa)
Sinding-Larsen-Johansson disease
SIN (squamous intraepithelial neoplasia)
sincipital presentation
SingleBAR electrode cautery
single base
single base pair substitution
single copy
single-cuff dialysis catheter
single-gene disorder
single-lumen catheter
single-lumen breast implant
single-lumen silicone breast implant
single nucleotide polymorphism (SNP)
single nucleotide substitutions
single photo emission tomography (SPECT)
single primer amplification reaction (SPAR)
single sequence polymorphism (SSP)
single-stranded conformational polymorphism (SSCP)
Singleton Marten syndrome
single-tooth tenaculum
single-toothed tenaculum
single umbilical artery
single-walled incubator
Singley forceps
sinovaginal
sinus
  marginal
  precervical
  prostatic
  renal

sinus *(cont.)*
  urachal
  urogenital
  venous
Sipple syndrome
sireniform fetus
sirenomelia
sirolimus
SIS (small intestine submucosal) technology urethral sling
Sister Mary Joseph sign
site
  incision
  port
  puncture
  stoma
  tenaculum
SiteSelect percutaneous breast biopsy system
situs inversus, bronchiectasis, and sinusitis syndrome
sitz bath, hot
6-mercaptopurine
6p deletion syndrome
6p24 deletion syndrome
6p duplication syndrome
6q23 duplication syndrome
sixth and seventh nerve palsy
size
  estimated fetal
  gestational
size-selective barrier
SJM Rosenkranz pediatric retractor system
Sjögren-Larsson syndrome
Sjögren syndrome
skeletal dysplasia
skeletal metastases
skeletonized
Skene duct
Skene gland adenitis
Skene glands
skenitis
skin, anogenital
skin approximation
skin crease incision
skin defect
skin induration
skin markings of lymphedema
skinning vulvectomy
skin of breast, superficial thrombophlebitis
skin of penis
skin of scrotum
skin-sparing mastectomy
skin staples
skin striae
skin thickening
skin turgor
skin ulcers
skipped generation
Sklar Cervex brush (*not* Cervix)
Sklar Kevorkian biopsy punch
SLE (systemic lupus erythematosus)
SLE-like syndrome
sleep apnea
sleeve
  built-in reduction
  laparoscopic
sliding lock
sliding scale for insulin dosage
slight costovertebral angle tenderness
slight cystocele
slightly retroflexed uterus
sling (see also *urethral sling*)
  Aldridge-Studdiford urethral
  AlloSling
  autologous urethral
  bioabsorbable urethral
  BioSling urethral
  Bio-Vascular remodelable tissue urethral
  bulbar urethral
  bulbourethral
  Cook Stratasis urethral
  fascia lata suburethral
  fascial
  FortaPerm surgical

sling *(cont.)*
  implantable urethral
  in situ urethral
  in vivo urethral
  laparoscopic urethral
  levator muscle
  modified bulbar urethral
  musculofascial
  ProteGen vaginal
  PTFE (polytetrafluoroethylene)
    suburethral
  pubococcygeal
  pubovaginal
  Raz
  REMEEX urethral
  SPARC urethral
  Straight-In male
  Stratasis urethral
  suburethral fascial
  SurgiSis pubourethral
  SurgiSis sling/mesh
  Suspend
  takedown of urethral
  TVT (tension-free vaginal tape)
    modified urethral
  transpelvic urethral
  TriAngle
  triangular vaginal patch
  UltraSling
  urethral
  Veritas urethral
  Vesica urethral
  woven
sling procedure for stress urinary
  incontinence
slipped umbilical ligature
slit
  dorsal
  lateral
slit pore
slope, slow
SLO (Smith-Lemli-Opitz) syndrome
sloughed urethra syndrome
sloughing, premature
slough of endometrium
slough of nipple
slough of skin
slow continuous ultrafiltration (SCUF)
slow fetal growth
Slow-K (potassium chloride)
slowly progressive glomerular disease
slow-slope active phase of labor
Slow/Stop Flow Recirculation method
slow urinary stream
sludging, capillary
slushing procedure
slush, cooling
Sly syndrome
small atrophic kidney
small bladder capacity
small bowel mesentery
small-capacity bladder
Small-Carrion penile prosthesis
Small-Carrion semirigid penile
  prosthesis
small for dates
small for gestational age (SGA) infant
small kidney
small parts of fetus
small penis
small single copy
small solutes
small-vessel vasculitis
SMA Lo-Iron 13 infant formula
SMA Lo-Iron 20 infant formula
SMA Lo-Iron 24 infant formula
SMA 13 infant formula
SMA 20 infant formula
SMA 24 infant formula
SMA 27 infant formula
SmartBeam IMRT
SMART (sperm microaspiration
  retrieval technique)
SMART (surgical myomectomy as
  reproductive therapy)
smear
  auramine-stained buffy coat
  buffy coat

smear (*cont.*)
- cervical
- cul-de-sac
- cytologic
- ectocervical
- endocervical
- endometrial
- lateral vaginal wall
- pancervical
- Pap (Papanicolaou)
- Tzanck
- urinary
- vaginal
- vaginal cuff
- VCE (vagina, cervix, endocervix)

smegma clitoridis
smegma, entrapment of
smegmalith
smegma preputii
Smellie method of delivery
Smellie-Veit maneuver
smile incision
Smith-Boyce operation
Smith-Lemli-Opitz (SLO) syndrome
Smith-Magenis syndrome
SMM (scintimammography)
smoke evacuation pencil, ExtendEVAC
smoke evacuation unit, Crystal Vision
smoke plume
SmokEvac electrosurgical probe
SmokEvac trumpet-valve smoke evacuator
smoky urine
smooth prostate
smooth-muscle gene expression
SMS coaxial catheter
SMX/TMP (sulfamethoxazole/trimethoprim)
snap-cap septa
snap gauge band for impotence testing
snare
- hysteroscopic polyp
- polyp
- stone

SnET2 (tin ethyl etiopurpurin)
SnMP (tin mesoporphyrin)
SNP (single nucleotide polymorphism)
SnPP (tin protoporphyrin)
SNS (sacral nerve stimulation) therapy
Snugs mastectomy bandage wrap
Soaker Catheter
social worker
Society for Assisted Reproductive Technology (SART)
Society for Urodynamics and Female Urology (SUFU)
sodium (Na)
sodium bicarbonate
sodium cellulose phosphate
sodium chloride (NaCl)
sodium chloride solution
sodium citrate
sodium dodecyl sulfate (SDS)-polyacrylamide gel electrophoresis (PAGE)
sodium ion (Na 2+)
sodium estrone sulfate
sodium iothalamate I-125
sodium polystyrene sulfonate
sodium propionate
sodium retention
sodomy
SofDraw amniocentesis syringe
Sof-Flex laparoscopic basket
Sof-Flex loop suprapubic catheter
Sofsilk nonabsorbable silk suture
Sof-Tact glucose monitor
Soft-Cell catheter
soft coaxial catheter
soft enhancer of percutaneous absorption (SEPA)
softening of cervix
softening of uterus
Soft-Pass laparoscopic catheter
SoftScan laser mammography system
Soft Seal cervical catheter
Soft Seal transcervical balloon catheter
soft silicone rubber dialysis catheter

soft tissue mass
soft tissue necrosis
Soft Torque uterine catheter
soft uterus
software
  BrachyVision
  VariSeed software for prostate brachytherapy
  XPlan radiation treatment
Sohval-Soffer syndrome
Solera thrombectomy catheter
sole therapy for CRF (chronic renal failure)
sol-gel membrane formation
solid mass
solid organ transplant
solid renal lesion
solids
solitary cyst of breast
solitary functioning kidney
solitary kidney
solitary mass
Solos cystoscope
Solu-Medrol (methylprednisolone)
soluble, solubility
solute (pl. solutes)
  nitrogenous
  uremic
solute clearance
solute concentration of urine
solution
  antibiotic
  balanced electrolyte
  Belzer
  Betadine
  betastarch
  Bicarbolyte bacteriostatic
  Celsior organ preservation
  Euro-Collins
  Extraneal peritoneal dialysis
  FRED (fog reduction elimination device) anti-fog
  gentamicin
  isotonic

solution *(cont.)*
  isotonic saline
  Lugol
  mannitol
  Monsel hemostatic
  peritoneal dialysis
  Ringer lactate
  saturated potassium iodide
  Schiller
  Sepracoat coating
  Shohl
  sodium chloride
  Suby G
  ViaSpan organ preservation
solution-diffusion
solvent nephrotoxicity
somaclonal variation
somatic cell genetics
somatic cells
somatic hybrid
somatic mosaicism
somatomedin-C
somatostatin
somatropin
Somer uterine elevator
Somite embryo
Somogyi phenomenon
Sonablate 200 ultrasound system
SonoCT real-time compound imaging
sonogram, pelvic
sonographer
sonographic guidance
sonographic planning of oncology treatment (SPOT)
sonographic techniques
  transabdominal full-bladder
  transvaginal empty-bladder
sonography (see *imaging*)
  Acuson computed
  Acuson transvaginal
  endovaginal
  fetal
  transvaginal
sonohysterography

sonohysterography catheter (see *catheter*)
Sonolith 3000 lithotriptor
Sonolith 4000 lithotriptor
Sonolith 4000+ lithotriptor
Sonolith Praktis portable lithotriptor
sonolucent cystic lesion or mass
sonolucent rim around the fetal skull
sonometer, Sahara Clinical Bone
Sonopsy 3-D ultrasound breast biopsy system
SonoSite 180 hand-carried ultrasound system
Sontac ultrasound gel pad
Soothies glycerin gel pads for nursing mothers
Sopher ovum forceps
Soprano cryoablation system
sorbapheresis
sorbitol
sore, venereal
sorption-diffusion
SOS gene
Sotos syndrome
souffle
  fetal
  mammary
  placental
  systolic mammary
  umbilical
  uterine
Soules intrauterine insemination catheter
sound
  adventitious
  bladder
  Blutton bladder
  coaxial uterine
  Greenwald
  LeFort urethral
  Linder-Golomb SP introducer
  passage of
  Pharmaseal uterine
  Simpson uterine

sound *(cont.)*
  Sims uterine
  TFE uterine
  urethral
  uterine
  Van Buren
sounding of uterus
sounding, urethral
Souques-Charcot syndrome
Southern blot
Southern blotting
Sovereign bipolar forceps
Sovereign bipolar scissors
SOX9 gene
Soyalac infant formula
soy infant formula
SP (sacroposterior) breech presentation of the fetus
SP (sacroposterior) position
SPA (sperm penetration assay)
space
  adnexal
  Bowman
  dead
  extraperitoneal
  intervillous
  perineal
  perinephric
  perirenal
  peritoneal
  perivitelline
  pleural
  prevesicle
  retromammary
  retroperitoneal
  retropubic
  vesicovaginal
Spacemaker balloon dissector
space-occupying mass
space of Retzius
Space-OR retractor
spacing, third
Spalding sign
span, fertilizable life

SPAR (single primer amplification reaction)
SPARC urethral sling
spasm
  bladder
  cervical
  tubal
spasmodic croup
spasmodic dysphonia
spasmodic torticollis
spastic bladder
spastic dysmenorrhea
spasticity, detrusor
spastic paraparesis
spastic paraplegia
spastic pseudosclerosis
spatula
  Ayre cervical
  bladder
  Kocher bladder
  Safetex cervical
spatulate, spatulated
SPE (serum protein electrophoresis)
specialized gender team
specialized tissue aspirating resectoscope (STAR)
speciation
species
specific gravity
specificity
specimen
  breast core biopsy
  catheterized urine
  clean-catch urine
  double-voided
  double-voided a.m. urine
  first a.m. urine
  first morning
  24-hour urine
specimen retrieval bag (see *bag*)
SPECT (single photon emission computed tomography)
spectral karyotype (SKY)
SpectraScience biopsy forceps
SpectraScience reusable biopsy forceps
spectrophotometric determination
Spectrum breast implant
Spectrum silicone Foley catheter
Speculite
speculoscopy, Pap Plus
speculum
  Amko vaginal
  Berlind-Auvard weighted vaginal
  Collin vaginal
  Cusco "Swiss pattern" vaginal
  endocervical
  Freeway Graves
  Garrigue weighted vaginal
  Graves
  Graves vaginal
  GRAVESPEC vaginal
  Graves Wide View
  Guttmann vaginal
  Gynex
  Henrotin weighted vaginal
  Jonas Graves vaginal
  Kleenspec disposable vaginal
  Kogan endocervical
  laser Auvard weighted
  laser Graves
  Miltex-Kogan endocervical
  Moore Graves vaginal
  Pederson vaginal
  Sims
  Sims vaginal
  SRT (smoke removal or retrieval tube) vaginal
  Steiner
  Steiner-Auvard
  vaginal
  Vantage Graves vaginal
  Vusco vaginal
  weighted
  weighted Sims
  Weisman Graves vaginal
  Welch Allyn vaginal
speculum examination
Spee embryo

spells, apneic
Spence, tail of
Spenco breast implant
sperm
  anonymous donor (ADS)
  frozen
  microsurgical extraction of ductal (MEDS)
  poor motility of
  viable
  washed
sperm activity
sperm agglutination
sperm antibodies
sperm aspiration
  epididymal (ESA)
  microsurgical epididymal (MESA)
  percutaneous epididymal
spermacytic seminoma
Sperma-Tex preshaped mesh
spermatic cord
  hydrocele of the
  torsion of
spermatic cyst
spermatic duct
spermatic fistula
spermatic vein
spermatic vessels
spermatid
spermatocele
spermatocelectomy
spermatocidal
spermatocide
spermatocyst
spermatocystectomy
spermatocyte
spermatocytic granuloma
spermatogenesis
spermatogenesis stimulant
spermatogenic
spermatogenic arrest
spermatogonia
spermatoid
spermatophobia
spermatorrhea
spermatozoa
spermatozoon
spermaturia
sperm bank
sperm buffer
SpermCheck test
sperm collection for artificial insemination
sperm count
sperm density
sperm-egg interaction in vivo
sperm-egg transport
sperm extraction from epididymis
sperm filter
sperm granuloma
spermicidal contraceptive
spermicide
sperm injection, intracytoplasmic (ICSI)
sperm microaspiration retrieval technique (SMART)
sperm morphology
sperm motility, decreased
sperm-mucus interaction
spermolytic
sperm pellet
sperm penetration assay (SPA)
sperm plasma membrane
sperm-oocyte interaction test
sperm recovery
sperm retrieval
  nonsurgical
  surgial
sperm washing
S-phase fraction of cells
sphenoidal fontanelle
spherical mass
spherical neoplasm
spherocytosis
spherophakia-brachymorphic syndrome
sphincter
  anal
  artificial
  AS-800 artificial urinary

sphincter *(cont.)*
  esophageal
  external
  external anal
  external urethral
  gastroesophageal
  Hyrtl
  inguinal
  internal
  internal os
  internal urethral
  Nelaton
  plication of
  preprostate urethral
  proximal urethral
  rectal
  urethral
  urethrovaginal
  vaginal
sphincteral achalasia
sphincter atony
sphincter competency
sphincter dysfunction
sphincter dyssynergia
sphincter electromyogram
sphincter EMG
sphincteric megaureter
sphincter muscles
sphincterotomy of bladder
sphincter tone normal
sphincter urethrae
sphincter vaginae
sphincter vesicae
sphingolipid biology in PKD (polycystic kidney disease)
sphingomyelin lipidosis
SPI-Argent II peritoneal dialysis catheter
spiculated breast carcinoma
spider angioma
spidery appearance
Spiegelberg criteria for diagnosis of ovarian pregnancy
Spielmeyer-Sjögren disease
Spielmeyer-Vogt
Spielmeyer-Vogt-Batten
Spielmeyer-Vogt-Sjögren
spike a fever
spike, fever
spike-tooth forceps
spillage from tube
spillage of dye from tube
spill from both tubes
spina bifida
spina bifida occulta
spinal anesthesia
spinal headache
spinal muscular atrophy, type 1 (SMA1)
spinal needle
Spinelli reduction of prolapsed uterus
spinnbarkeit
spinocerebellar ataxia
spinocerebellar ataxia type 3
spinopontive atrophy
spiral arteries
spiral arteriole
spiral-tip catheter
SpiraStent ureteral stent
spirochete
SpiroFlo bioabsorbable prostate stent
spironolactone
Spirtos coaxial catheter
splanchnic blood flow
splanchnic congestion
splanchnic nerves
Splash-shield endoscopic barrier
spleen
  renal surface of
  rupture of
  sago
splenectomy
splenonephric
splenorenal anastomosis
splenorenal arterial bypass graft
splenorenal ligament
splenorenal recess
splenorenal shunt
splice site mutation

splicing
split ejaculate
split-flap technique in vaginal surgery
split-flap vaginal reconstruction
split function
split gene
split-hand deformity
split-hand deformity-mandibulofacial dysostosis
split papules
split renal function decrease
split renal function test
split sperm ejaculate
split-thickness skin graft vaginoplasty
spondyloepiphyseal dysplasia, congenital
spondyloepiphyseal dysplasia tarda
spondylothoracic dysplasia
sponge
  absorbable
  contraceptive
  moist
  Protectaid contraceptive
sponge and needle count
sponge, instrument, and needle count
sponge count
sponge forceps
sponge kidney
sponge-on-a-stick
sponge sticks
spongiositis
spongiosum, corpus
spongiosum penis
spongy body of penis
spongy layer of urethra
spongy layer of vagina
spongy urethra
spongy uterus
spontaneous abortion
  complete
  incomplete
spontaneous bacterial peritonitis
spontaneous cephalic delivery
spontaneous correction of placenta previa
spontaneous cry
spontaneous delivery of placenta
spontaneous fetal movement
spontaneous gangrene of newborn
spontaneous generation
spontaneous labor
spontaneous menses
spontaneous multifetal reductions
spontaneous nipple discharge
spontaneous passage of stone
spontaneous reanastomosis of vas
spontaneous rupture of liver from subcapsular hematoma
spontaneous rupture of membranes (SROM)
spontaneous rupture of symphysis pubis during delivery
spontaneous termination of pregnancy
spontaneous vaginal delivery
spontaneous version
spoon forceps
sporadic
spore
SPOT (salpingitis in previously occluded tubes)
SPOT (sonographic planning of oncology treatment)
spots
  Brushfield
  café au lait
  mongolian
  powder burn
  strawberry
spotting
  contact
  intermenstrual
  postcoital
  vaginal
SprayGel Adhesion Barrier System
spreader
  bladder neck
  Millin bladder neck
  vaginal
Sprengel deformity

spring, intraurethral
spun clean-catch urinalysis
spun urine sediment
spurious pregnancy
squalamine
squamocolumnar junction
squamocolumnar junction of cervix
squamous cell carcinoma
squamous cell carcinoma-in-situ
squamous epithelium
squamous intraepithelial lesion (SIL)
squamous intraepithelial neoplasia (SIN)
squamous metaplasia
square window
squat bar
SRNS (steroid-resistant nephrotic syndrome)
SROM (spontaneous rupture of membranes)
SRT (smoke removal or retrieval tube) vaginal speculum
SRY (sex-specific region of the Y chromosome)
SSCP (single-stranded conformational polymorphism)
SSP (single sequence polymorphism)
SSR (simple sequence repeat)
ST (sacrotransverse) position
stability, detrusor
stab incision
stable CRF (chronic renal failure)
stable diabetes mellitus
stable monogamous relationship
stab wound
stab wound to kidney
Stadol
stage
  breast fibrocystic disease
  Tanner
stage cut
stages of endometriosis (see *American Fertility Society Classification of Endometriosis*)
stages of labor
  first
  second
  third
staghorn calculus
staghorn renal calculus
staghorn stone
staging evaluation
staging, FIGO
staging of cancer, surgical
staging of endometriosis
stagnation mastitis
stain, staining
  acetowhite
  benzidine
  Betke
  cervical Gram
  Giemsa
  Gram
  Hansel
  Kleihauer-Betke
  KOH
  Leder
  meconium
  orthotoluidine
  Papanicolaou (Pap)
  PAS (period acid-Schiff)
  port-wine
  Prescott-Brodie
  Schiller
  Silver
  Silver impregnation
  Sternheimer-Malbin
  Sudan III
  toluidine blue
  toluidine O
  TUNEL (terminal deoxynucleotidyl transferase-mediated deoxyuridine triphosphate)
  Wright
stained urine sediment
staining patterns of ANCA
  cytoplasmic (C-ANCA)
  perinuclear (P-ANCA)

staining the vaginal vault
stale fish syndrome
Stamey bladder neck suspension procedure
Stamey-Malecot catheter
Stamey needle
Stamey percutaneous suprapubic catheter
Stamey suture
Stamey suture carrier
Stamey test for renovascular hypertension
STAMP V (cyclophosphamide, thiotepa, carboplatin [CTCb]) chemotherapy protocol
standard deviations above/below the mean
standard vaginal hysterectomy
Staphylococcus aureus
Staphylococcus epidermidis
Staphylococcus saprophyticus
staple
staple ligated
stapler
  EEA
  Endo-Hernia
  Endo GIA surgical
  Endopath EZ45 No Knife endoscopic linear
  GIA
  Multifire Endo GIA
  Multifire GIA
  Multifire VersaTack
  TA-55
  VersaTack
staples
  metallic
  Proximate
  skin
  surgical
stapling device
STAR (specialized tissue-aspirating resectoscope)
STAR (study of tamoxifen and raloxifene)
StarBAR resection electrode
Stargate falloposcopy catheter
Starion thermal cautery hook
Starling forces
STARRT (selective tubal assessment to refine reproductive therapy) falloposcopy system
START SMART Program for assisted reproductive technology
startle embrace
startle reaction
stasigenesis
stasis
  bladder
  positional
  ureteral
  urinary
  venous
static films
static infantilism
station (-2, -1, 0, +1)
station of fetus within pelvic cavity
statistical genetics
StatLock Dialysis catheter securement device
StatLock Foley catheter securement device
stat urine
status
  endocrine
  nodal
  psychologic
stay suture
STD (sexually transmitted disease) screen, Thayer-Martin
STD treatment, Trovan/Zithromax Compliance Pak
steady-state serum urea nitrogen concentration
steal syndrome
steely hair disease

Steiner-Auvard speculum
Steiner speculum
Steinert disease
Stein-Leventhal syndrome
steinstrasse
stellate lesion on mammogram
Stengel-Batten-Mayou-Spielmeyer-Vogt-Stock disease
Stengel disease
stenosis
  bladder neck
  breast duct
  cervical
  distal urethral
  infrarenal
  interrenal
  meatal
  neovagina
  ostial renal artery
  renal artery
  renal cortical
  suprarenal
  truncal renal artery
  tubal
  ureteral
  urethral
  vaginal
stenosis and induration
stenotic but patent tricuspid valve
stenotic cervix
stenotic lesion
stenotic lesion of renal artery
stenotic ureter
stenotic vagina
Stenotrophomonas
stent
  antegrade ureteral
  balloon uterine
  Beamer
  BioSorb resorbable urologic
  Bridge X3 renal
  Circon
  double-J indwelling catheter
  double-J ureteral

stent *(cont.)*
  Endocare Horizon prostatic
  ENDOcare nitinol urinary
  Fader Tip ureteral
  Greene renal implant
  Horizon nitinol temporary
  Horizon temporary urinary
  hydrophilic-coated urologic
  indwelling ureteral
  IntraStent DoubleStrut renal artery
  IntraStent DoubleStrut XS renal artery
  kidney internal splint/stent (KISS)
  Kwart AQ Retro-Inject
  Kwart Retro-Inject
  LSe Kwart Retro-Inject
  Lubri-Flex urologic
  Multi-Flex urologic
  ostiomeatal
  Percuflex Plus flexible ureteral
  ProstaCoil self-expanding urethral
  Reliance urinary control
  renal
  renovascular
  silicone
  Silitek
  SpiraStent ureteral
  SpiroFlo bioabsorbable prostate
  Surgitek
  Tecoflex
  ureteral
  urethral
  UroCoil self-expanding
  UroLume endoprosthesis wire
  UroLume urethral
  UroLume urinary
  UroLume Wallstent
  Vistaflex biliary
stent placement
step-down unit
step-oblique mammography
step-oblique mammography images
stepping reflex
stereocolposcope

StereoEndoscope
stereotactic (stereotaxic)
stereotactic aspiration biopsy
stereotactic breast biopsy
stereotactic core needle biopsy (SCNB)
stereotactic localization for breast
 biopsy imaging
stereotactic needle biopsy
stereotactic needle breast biopsy
stereotactic vacuum-assisted biopsy
 (SVAB) device
stereotaxic (stereotactic)
stereotaxically guided interstitial laser
 therapy
sterile drapes
sterilely prepared and draped
sterilely prepped and draped
sterile paper drape
sterile vaginal examination
sterility
 aspermatogenic
 dysspermatogenic
 female
 male
 normospermatogenic
sterilization
 elective
 interval
 reverse surgical
 tubal ligation
 voluntary
sterilizing operation
SteriLyte liquid bicarbonate
steri-stripped
Steri-Strips
Sternheimer-Malbin stain
Stern-McCarthy resectoscope
steroid
 circulating gonadal
 corticosteroid
 fluorinated topical
 gonadal
 ovarian
 sex
steroid-binding assay
steroid cell ovarian tumor
steroid-dependent nephrotic syndrome
 (SDNS)
steroid hormone levels
steroid-mediated reabsorption of
 sodium
steroid myopathy
steroid receptors
steroid-resistant nephrotic syndrome
 (SRNS)
stethoscope, DeLee-Hillis
Stevens-Johnson syndrome
Stickler syndrome
stick, sponge
stick-tie
stiff-baby syndrome
stiffening obturator
stiff-man syndrome
stiff ring
stigma (pl. stigmas, stigmata)
 follicular
 malpighian
stigmata of endometriosis
stillbirth
stillborn infant
stimulated cycle
stimulated macrophages
stimulation
 gonadal
 infant
 labor
 ovarian
 pelvic floor electrical stimulation
  (PFS)
 percutaneous Stoller afferent nerve
  stimulation system (PerQ SANS)
 steroid production
 transcutaneous electrical nerve
  (TENS)
 vibroacoustic
stimulator, ureteral
STING (subureteric Teflon injection)
stippled psammomatous calcification

stippling, basophilic
stirrups
  candy-cane
  hanging
  Lloyd-Davis
  Yellofins
stitch (see *suture*)
STMS (sequence tagged microsatellite)
stockinette wrap
Stoller afferent nerve stimulation (SANS) urinary incontinence device
stoma
  cutaneous
  double-loop
  exteriorized
  incontinent external
  nippled
  revision of
stoma site
stoma therapist
stomatitis, gonococcal
stomatocytosis
stone (see also *calculus*)
  bladder
  calcium oxalate
  cystine
  impacted urethral
  "infection"
  intravesical
  kidney
  lower ureteral
  magnesium ammonium phosphate
  noncalcified
  nonopaque
  opaque
  passage of renal
  prostatic
  radiolucent
    matrix
    pure uric acid
    xanthine
  radiopaque
  renal

stone *(cont.)*
  shadowing
  spontaneous passage of
  staghorn
  struvite
  ureteral
  ureteric
  uric acid
  urinary
  urinary tract
  womb
stone analysis
stone basket
  Dormia
  Johnson
  Levant
  Lomac
  Pfister-Schwartz
  SurLok helical
  Surgitek
stone basketing
stone differentiated from tumor
stone disintegration in the ureter
stone extraction
stone formation, vesical
stone former
stone-forming substance in urine
stone fragmentation
stone-grasping forceps
stone-holding basket forceps
stone impaction
stonelike calculus
stonelike mass
stone manipulation, percutaneous
stone migration
stone mole
stone passed spontaneously
stone preserved for analysis
StoneRisk profile
stone snare
stony hard induration of prostate
stony hard prostate
stony mass

stool
  currant jelly
  guaiac-negative
  guaiac-positive
  heme-negative
  rice water
stooling
stopcock, Accel
STOP (selective tubal occlusion procedure) contraceptive device
stopping and starting of stream
stored embryos
Storz cystoscope
Storz cystourethroscope
Storz resectoscope
straight catheterization
straight channel
Straight-In male sling system
straight tubule of testis
straight ureter
straight veins of kidney
strain
strain all urine
strained urine
strain uterography
straining at urine
straining cystogram
straining of urine for residual stones
strand
stranger anxiety
strangulated hemorrhoid
strangulation of inguinal hernia
strangury
Stratasis urethral sling
strawberry cervix
strawberry mark
"strawberry spots"
streaked gonads
streak, gonadal
stream, urinary
strength of urination
streptococcal antigen
streptococcal antigenic products
streptococcal cell-wall antigen
streptococcus A infection
Streptococcus faecalis
Streptococcus pneumoniae
stress cystogram
stress cystography
stress incontinence
stress perfusion scintigraphy
stress test
stress urinary incontinence (SUI)
stretched penile length
stretching of bladder
stretch marks
striae distensae
striae, skin
striation, urothelial
striatonigral disease
stricture
  bulbomembranous urethral
  cervical
  congenital
  male urethral
  postcatheterization urethral
  postobstetric urethral
  postoperative urethral
  prostatic
  rectal
  traumatic urethral
  ureteral
  urethral
  urinary meatal
  vaginal
  vulvar
stricture incision
Stringer laparoscopic suturing technique
string phlebitis
striopallidodentate calcinosis
stripe, endometrial
stroke, thrombotic
stroma
  endometrial
  ovarian
  prostate
  surrounding breast
stromal endometriosis

stromal hyperthecosis
stromal invasion
stromal proliferation
strontium-89 chloride
structural birth defects
structural change
structural gene
structural integrity of vessels
structurally distinct layers
structural properties of membrane
structures
  adnexal
  pelvic
struma ovarii
struma, Hashimoto
struvite stone
StrykeFlow suction irrigator
Stryker endoscopy one-chip camera
Stryker endoscopy three-chip camera
Stryker infant warmer
STS (sequence tagged site)
STS (serologic test for syphilis)
Stuart Prenatal prenatal vitamins
stuck twin syndrome
studding of endometriosis
study
  bladder contractility
  follicular maturation
  immunofluorescence
  immunoperoxidase
  pelvic floor function
  radiopharmaceutical
  renal cyst
  renin
  STAR (study of tamoxifen and raloxifene)
  ureteral reflux
study of tamoxifen and raloxifene (STAR)
stump
  cervical
  distal
  penile
  pregnancy
Stumple familial paraplegia/tremor
stunted fetus
Sturge-Kalischer-Weber syndrome
Sturge-Weber-Dimitri syndrome
Sturge-Weber phakomatosis
Sturge-Weber syndrome
Sturmdorf conical removal of endocervix
stuttering, urinary
Suarez continence ring
subacute cystitis
subacute glomerulonephritis
subacute necrotizing encephalomyelopathy
subacute spongiform encephalopathy
subacute nephritis
subacute thyroiditis
subaortic stenosis
subarachnoid hemorrhage
subareolar abscess
subcapsular hematoma
subclavian catheter
subclavian vein
subcoronal hypospadias
subcortical tumor
subcostal incision
subcostal retractions
subcutaneous arteriovenous (AV) fistula
subcutaneous augmentation material (SAM)
subcutaneous breast implant
subcutaneous catheter tunnel
subcutaneous emphysema
subcutaneous fabric cuff
subcutaneous fat lines
subcutaneous injection artifact on intravenous pyelogram
subcutaneous layer
subcutaneous mastectomy
subcutaneous pocket
subcutaneous tissue flaps
subcutaneous tunnel
subcuticular layer
subcuticular suture

subdermal implantation for contraception
subdural hemorrhage
subepithelial hematoma of renal pelvis
subfascial bleeder
subfascial hematoma
subfascial plane
subfertility
subgaleal hemorrhage
subglandular augmentation mammoplasty
subinvolution of breast
subinvolution of uterus
sublethal gross anatomic defect
subluxation of radial heads at elbows
submammary
submammary abscess
submammary mastitis
submetacentric chromosome
submucosal bleb
submucosal tunneling
submucosal tunnel technique ureterovesiculoplasty
submucous coat of female urethra
submucous cystitis
submucous fibroids
submucous fibromyoma
submuscular breast implant
subpectoral breast implant
subpreputial discharge
subpubic arch
subseptate uterus
subsequent generations
subsequent hernia formation
subserosal fibroid
subserous fibroid
substernal goiter
substitution
substrate
subtelomeric region
subtle distortion of breast architecture on mammogram
subtotal hysterectomy
subtotal thyroidectomy
subumbilical incision
subureteric Teflon injection (STING)
suburethral fascial sling procedure
subvaginal
subvesical duct
subzonal insertion of sperm (SuZI)
Suby G
Suby solution G
succedaneum, caput
succenturiate lobe
succenturiate placenta
succimer
succinylcholine sensitivity
sucrose-iosomaltose malabsorption, congenital
suction
  Berkeley
  bulb
  DeLee
  gentle
  Poole
  Sherwood
suction curet
suction curettage
suction D&C (dilation and curettage)
suctioned
suctioning, bulb
suction/irrigation system, Sherwood intrascopic
suction/irrigation tubing
suction-irrigator
suction lipectomy
sudanophilic leukodystrophy
Sudan III stain
sudden abruption of placenta
sudden infant death syndrome (SIDS)
sufficient cause
suffocative goiter
SUFU (Society for Urodynamics and Female Urology)
sugar in urine
SUI (stress urinary incontinence)
sulbactam
suicide gene

suitable vascular access
sulcus (pl. sulci)
  coronal
  intramammary
sulfamethoxazole/trimethoprim
  (SMX/TMP)
sulfatide lipidosis
sulfatidosis, juvenile, Austin-type
sulodexide
Summer's Eve vaginal douche
Summit acrocephalosyndactyly
Summit syndrome
Sunna circumcision
sunset eyes
SU101 biological agent
superfetation
superficial and deep external pudendal
  arteries
superficial bladder carcinoma
superficial dorsal veins of clitoris
superficial dorsal veins of penis
superficial endometrial implants
superficial endometritis
superficial hematoma of newborn
superficial infection of the breast
superficial inguinal node
superficial inguinal pouch
superficial perineal pouch
superficial tenaculum tear
superficial thrombophlebitis
superficial thrombophlebitis of skin
  of breast
superficial transverse perineal muscles
superficial vulvectomy
superimposed preeclampsia
superimpregnation
superinfection
superior border of suprarenal gland
superior leaf of fascia
superior ligament of epididymis
superior mesenteric plexus
superior pedicle technique reduction
  mammoplasty
superior pole
superior pole of kidney
superior renal segment
superior segmental artery of kidney
superior suprarenal artery
superior vena cava
superior vesical artery
superlactation
supernatant, decanted
supernumerary breast nipple
supernumerary chromosome
supernumerary kidney
supernumerary marker chromosome
supernumerary placenta
superovulation
supersaturation of urine with stone-
  forming salts
supervoltage radiation
superwet reduction mammoplasty
supine position
supplementary menstruation
support
  Gynecare TVT tension-free
  Introl bladder neck
  PelvX pelvic
supportive therapy
suppressed lactation
suppressed menstruation
suppression of lactation
suppression, ovarian
suppressive antibiotic therapy
suppressive anuria
suppressive Gantrisin therapy
suppurative mastitis
suppurative nephritis
suppurative pyelitis
suprapubic arch
suprapubic area
suprapubic catheter
suprapubic catheterization
suprapubic cramping
suprapubic cystoscope
suprapubic cystostomy
  permanent
  punch

suprapubic diversion
suprapubic excision
suprapubic incision
suprapubic introducer
suprapubic lithotomy
suprapubic lithotripsy
suprapubic manipulator
suprapubic midline trocar
suprapubic needle aspiration of bladder
suprapubic palpation
suprapubic region
suprapubic sling
  Goebel-Frangenheim-Stoeckel
  Millin-Read urethrovesical
  Oxford urinary incontinence
suprapubic tenderness
suprapubic tube insertion
suprapubic urodynamic catheter
supracervical hysterectomy
supraclavicular lymph nodes
supraclavicular lymphadenopathy
SupraFoley catheter
Supramid suture
suprarenal aneurysm
suprarenal body
suprarenal cortex
suprarenal extension of aneurysm
suprarenal gland, medulla of
suprarenal impression on liver
suprarenal stenosis
suprascrotal pouch
suprasternal notch
supraumbilical incision
supravaginal hysterectomy
supravaginal part of cervix
supravesical cesarean section
supravesical fossa
supravesical obstruction
supravesical urinary diversion
Supreme II blood glucose monitor
suramin
SureCell Chlamydia test kit
SureCell Herpes (SC-HSV) test kit
SureStep blood glucose monitor
Surete contraceptive gel
surfactant
  homologous
  Human Surf
Surfak (docusate calcium)
Surfaxin (lucinactant)
surf test
surgery (see *operation*)
  cryogenic
  HALS (hand-assisted laparoscopic surgery)
  laparoscopic
  minimally invasive
  pelvic floor
  transsexual
  workbench
surgical abdomen
surgical abortion
surgical aid, CaverMap
surgical capsule of prostate
surgical castration
surgical conversion of genitalia in transsexual patients
surgical excision of fistulous tract
surgical extirpation of gonads
surgical gender reassignment
surgical intervention
surgically implanted hemodialysis catheter (SIHC)
surgically resected
surgical menopause
surgical myomectomy as reproductive therapy (SMART)
surgical repair of atrial septal defect
surgical scar
surgical sealant, Proceed hemostatic
surgical sperm retrieval
surgical staging of cancer
surgical steel skin clips
surgical sterility
Surgicel
Surgiclip
Surgiflex probe
Surgilon suture

Surgiport
SurgiScope robotic surgery device
SurgiSis pubourethral sling
SurgiSis sling/mesh
Surgitek stent
Surgitek OM
Surgiview laparoscope
Surgi-Vision prostate MRI microcoil
Surgi-Vision urethral MRI microcoil
SurLok helical stone basket
surrender of custody
surreptitious vomiting
surrogacy arrangement
Surrogacy Arrangements Act
surrogacy broker
surrogacy contract
surrogacy, gestational
surrogacy termination provisions
surrogate
  gestational
  sex
surrogate contracts
surrogate mother
surrogate parenting
surrogate's right to rescind contract
surrounding breast stroma
Survanta
surveillance, antepartum
survival
  disease-free
  median length of
  overall
susceptibility gene
susceptibility to mutations
Suspend sling implant
suspension
  bladder
  hammock-type pelvic diaphragm
  Infasurf (calfactant) intratracheal
  kidney
  sacrospinous vaginal vault
  uterine
suspensory breast ligament
suspensory ligament of breast
suspensory ligament of clitoris
suspensory ligament of Cooper
suspensory ligament of gonad
suspensory ligament of ovary
suspensory ligament of penis
suspensory ligament of testis
suspensory ligament, scrotal
suspicious calcifications
suspicious mass
sustaining infusion of heparin
Sutralon suture
SutraSilk nonabsorbable silk suture
suture
  Aberdeen knot
  absorbable
  Acier stainless steel
  angle
  atraumatic chromic
  Auto Suture
  Auto Suture ABBI
  baseball
  Biosyn
  Bondek absorbable
  Bralon braided nylon
  catgut
  chromic
  circumferential running stitch
  colposuspension
  Cutalon nylon polyamide surgical
  Dacron
  Dafilon
  Dagrofil
  deep retention
  Dermalon
  Dexon
  double-armed
  Endoknot
  Endo Stitch endoscopic
  Ethibond
  fascial
  fascial absorbable
  figure-of-eight
  Grams nylon nonabsorbable
  Grams polypropylene nonabsorbable

suture *(cont.)*
Grams silk nonabsorbable
helical
imbricating
inverted
Investa
Kelly
Lembert
locking
Lukens PGA synthetic absorbable
mattress
Maxon
Mersilene
Miralene
monofilament nylon
Monocryl
orienting
Panacryl absorbable
PDS
PGA synthetic absorbable
plain
plain gut
polyglactin 910
pop-off
Premilene
Prolene
Pronova nonabsorbable
pursestring
Rapide
retention
Richardson angle
running
running interlocking
running locking
Safil synthetic absorbable surgical
Shirodkar
silk
Surgilon
Sofsilk nonabsorbable silk
Stamey
stay
subcutaneous
subcuticular
Supramid

suture *(cont.)*
Sutralon
SutraSilk nonabsorbable silk
Sutureloop colposuspension
Sutureloop needle/suture
synostotic
Synthofil
Tevdek
Thiersch
through-and-through
Ti-Cron
traction
transfixion
Tycron
undyed Vicryl
Vascufil
Vesica press-in anchor
Vicryl
Vicryl Rapide
whipstitch
Z-stitch

suture carrier
Endoclosure
Sarrett
Stamey
Vesica

suture fastener
ROC
ROC XS

suture grasper, Reddick-Saye
suture granuloma
suture guide, Pilot
suture ligated
suture ligature
suture line
Suture Lok vessel ligator
suture material (see *suture*)
suture needle, Maciol laparoscopic suture needle set

suture passer
Carter-Thomason
MetraPass

suture system, Beacon Technology System (BTS)

suturectomy
Sutured-Clip
Sutureloop colposuspension suture
Sutureloop needle/suture
suturing technique, Stringer laparoscopic
SuZI (subzonal insertion of sperm)
SVAB (stereotactic vacuum-assisted biopsy) device
SVG (seminal vesiculography)
swab and spatula
swabbing, urethral
swab, Calgiswab calcium alginate
swaged needle-suture
swallowed blood syndrome
swallowed maternal blood
Swan-Ganz catheter
sweats, night
Sweetheart clamp
swelling
 breast
 cellular
 genital
 interstitial
 labial
 parenchymatous
 scrotal
 testicular
 vulvar
Swiss cheese cartilage syndrome
Swiss cheese endometrium
Swiss lithoclast lithotriptor
SWL (shock wave lithotripsy)
swollen prostate
Swyer syndrome
Sydney line
Syed obturator
Syed template for placement of perineal interstitial ^{192}Ir implant
Syed-Neblett brachytherapy method
Symmetra ^{125}I prostate brachytherapy seeds
symmetrical breast implant
symmetrical uterus
symmetric fetal growth restriction
sympathomimetic drugs
symphyseal cartilage
symphyseal separation
symphysiotomy for horseshoe kidney
symphysiotomy, obstetrical
symphysis pubis
 diastasis of
 pain at
 separation of
 spontaneous rupture of
 traumatic separation of
Symptom Distress Scale
symptomatic bladder prolapse
symptomatic hyperglycemia
symptomatic neurosyphilis
symptomatic pelvic relaxation
symptomatic rectal prolapse
symptomatic uterine prolapse
symptomatic varicocele
symptoms
 bladder outlet obstructive
 obstructive
 obstructive voiding
 premonitory
symptothermal method
synapsis
synapton
synaptonemal complex
Synarel (nafarelin)
synchronized intermittent mandatory ventilation (SIMV)
synchronized ventilation
synchronizer
syncope, micturition
synctiotrophoblastic elements
syncytial cell
syncytial endometritis
syncytiotrophoblasts in the placenta
syndactylic oxycephaly
syndactyly
syndactyly type 1 with microcephaly and mental retardation
syndesis

syndrome
- Aagenaes
- Aarskog
- Aarskog-Scott
- Aase-Smith
- abdominal muscle deficiency
- ablepharon macrostomia
- Achard
- Achard-Thiers
- "achoo"
- acquired immunodeficiency (AIDS)
- acrocallosal
- acrodermatitis enteropathic
- acute nephritic
- ADAM (androgen decline in the aging male)
- Adams-Oliver
- Adie
- adipogenital-retinitis pigmentosa-polydactyly
- adrenogenital
- adult respiratory distress
- Ahumada-del Castillo
- Aicardi
- Aicardi-Goutieres
- Alagille
- Albers-Schönberg
- Albright
- Aldrich
- Allan-Herndon
- Allan-Herndon-Dudley
- Alport
- Alstrom
- amaurosis congenita of Leber
- amenorrhea-galactorrhea
- AMME (Alport syndrome, mental retardation, midface hypoplasia, and elliptocytosis)
- amnionic fluid
- amniotic band
- Amsterdam dwarf
- Ande
- Anderson-Fabry
- Anderson-Warburg

syndrome *(cont.)*
- androgen decline in the aging male (ADAM)
- androgen insensitivity
- Angelman
- angio-osteohypertrophy
- ankyloblepharon-ectodermal defects-cleft lip/palate
- anterior pituitary hyperhormonotropic
- anticonvulsant hypersensitivity
- Antley-Bixler
- APECED
- Apert
- apple peel
- Aran-Duchenne
- Armenian
- Arnold-Chiari
- Asherman
- Asperger
- asplenia
- auriculo-oculovertebral
- Austin
- autoimmune lymphoproliferative
- autoimmune polyendocrinopathy, candidiasis, ectodermal dysplasia (APECED)
- Baller-Gerold
- Bardet-Biedl
- Barraquer
- Barth
- Bartter
- Bassen-Kornzweig
- Batten-Mayou
- Batten-Vogt
- Beals-Hecht
- Bean
- Beckwith-Wiedemann
- Behçet
- Bernard-Soulier
- bile plug
- Binder
- Bjornstad
- Blackfan-Diamond

syndrome *(cont.)*
- blepharophimosis, ptosis, epicanthus inversus
- blepharospasm-oromandibular-dystonic
- Bloodgood
- Bloom
- blue diaper
- blue dome
- blue rubber bleb nevus
- Bonnevie-Ulrich
- Borjeson
- Borjeson-Forssman-Lehmann
- Bowen Hutterite
- Bowen-Conradi
- Bowen Hutterite
- Brachmann-de Lange
- branchio-oculofacial
- branchio-otorenal (BOR)
- Brandt
- broad ligament laceration
- broad thumb
- broad thumb-hallux
- bronze baby
- Brown
- brown baby
- Brueghel
- Budd-Chiari
- Buerger-Gruetz
- bulldog
- burning vulva
- camptodactyly-cleft palate-clubfoot
- camptodactyly-trismus
- Cantrell
- Cantrell-Haller-Ravich
- carbohydrate deficient glycoprotein
- cardioauditory
- cardiofaciocutaneous
- cardiomyopathy-neutropenia
- cardiorespiratory distress
- Carignan
- carpal tunnel
- Carpenter
- cat's cry

syndrome *(cont.)*
- Catel-Manzke
- cat-eye
- cauda equina
- caudal regression
- Cayler cardiofacial
- central hypoventilation
- cerebellar
- cerebellomedullary malformation
- cerebrocostomandibular
- cerebro-oculofacioskeletal
- cervico-oculoacoustic
- CHARGE
- Charnin-Dorfman
- Cheatle
- Chediak-Higashi
- Chiari-Frommel
- CHILD (congenital hemidysplasia with ichthyosiform erythroderma and limb defects)
- Chotzen
- Christmas tree
- chronic fatigue
- chronic fatigue immune dysfunction
- chronic progressive external ophthalmoplegia
- chronic lead
- chronic nephritic/proteinuric
- Cockayne
- Coffin-Lowry
- Coffin-Siris
- Cohen
- cold injury
- complete androgen insensitivity
- congenital facial dysplasia
- congenital hemidysplasia with ichthyosiform erythroderma and limb defects (CHILD)
- congenital immune deficiency
- congenital nephrotic
- congestion-fibrosis
- conjunctivourethrosynovial
- Conn
- conotruncal anomaly face

syndrome *(cont.)*
- Conradi-Hünermann
- contiguous gene
- Cooper
- Cornelia de Lange
- Costello
- cri du chat
- Crigler-Najjar
- cryptophthalmos-syndactyly
- Cushing
- cyclic vomiting
- Danbolt Cross
- dancing eye
- Dandy-Walker
- deafness, onychodystrophy, osteodystrophy, and mental retardation
- de Morsier
- dead fetus
- defibrination
- de Lange
- delayed pulmonary toxicity
- deletion (see *deletion syndrome*)
- de novo mutation
- Denys-Drash
- DeSanctis-Cacchione
- DeToni-Fanconi
- diabetes mellitus
- diencephalic
- DiGeorge
- digito-otopalatal
- DIMOAD (diabetes insipidus, diabetes mellitus, optic atrophy, and deafness)
- Donahue
- DOOR (congenital deafness, onycho-osteodystrophy, and mental retardation)
- Down
- Drash
- Drummond
- Duane
- Dubin-Johnson
- Dubowitz
- duplication

syndrome *(cont.)*
- Dyggve-Melchior-Clausen
- dysplasia gigantism
- dysplastic nevus
- dystocia-dystrophia
- DYT-1 dystonia
- Eagle Barrett
- ear-patella-short stature
- Eaton-Lambert
- ectrodactyly-electrodermal dysplasia-clefting
- Edwards (trisomy 18)
- Ehlers-Danlos
- 8p deletion
- 8p duplication
- 8p12-p23 duplication
- 8p23.1-8pter deletion
- 18p23.1-8pter
- 18p deletion
- 18q- deletion
- 18q23 deletion
- Eisenmenger
- 11q deletion
- Ellis-van Creveld
- empty sella
- Engelmann
- Escobar
- external chondromatosis
- euthyroid sick (ESS)
- Fabry
- facial-digital genital
- familial nephrotic
- faciocardiocutaneous
- Fanconi
- FAS (fetal alcohol)
- Fechtner
- femoral-facial
- fetal alcohol (FAS)
- fetal aspiration
- fetal face
- fetal hydantoin
- fetal hypokinesis
- fetal trimethadione
- fetal valproate

syndrome *(cont.)*
- fetal varicella (FVS)
- fetal warfarin
- FG
- fibrocystic breast
- fibromyalgia
- Fiessinger-Leroy-Reiter
- fifth digit
- Filippi
- first and second branchial arch
- fish odor
- Fitz-Hugh–Curtis
- 5p deletion
- 5q deletion
- 5q duplication
- 15q11-q13 duplication
- 15q11.2-q14 duplication
- Floating-Harbor
- floppy infant
- FLT3 gene duplication
- Fong
- Fountain
- Forbes-Albright
- 45,X
- 45,XO
- 47,XXY
- 47,XY
- 47,XYY
- 48,XXXX
- 48,XXXY
- 48,XXYY
- 49,XXX
- 49,XXXXX
- 49,XXXYY
- 4p deletion
- 4p15 deletion
- 14q12-q13 duplication
- 4q21-q25 deletion
- 4q21-q28 duplication
- 4q23-q27 duplication
- 4q32-q34 deletion
- 14p16.3 deletion
- 14q31-q32.3 deletion
- 14q32.3 deletion

syndrome *(cont.)*
- fragile X
- Fraley
- Franchetti-Klein
- Francois dyscephalic
- Fraser
- Freeman-Sheldon
- free 21 trisomy
- Fryns
- Fukuhara
- FVS (fetal varicella)
- galactorrhea-amenorrhea
- Gardner
- Genee-Wiedemann
- giant platelet
- Gilbert
- Gilbert-Dreyfus
- Gilford
- Gillespie
- glomerular
- glomerulonephritic
- glycoprotein
- Golabi-Rosen
- Goldberg-Maxwell
- Goldenhar
- Goldenhar-Gorlin
- gonadal dysgenesis
- Goodman
- Goodpasture
- Gordon
- Gorlin-Chaudhry-Moss
- Gottron
- Gougerot-Carteaud
- Gray
- gray baby
- Greig cephalopolysyndactyly
- Greig polysyndactyly craniofacial dysmorphism
- growth hormone insensitivity
- Gruber
- Guerin-Stern
- Guillain-Barre
- Hajdu-Cheney
- Hallerman-Streiff

syndrome *(cont.)*
- Hallerman-Streiff-Francois
- Hallgren
- Hall-Pallister
- hallux duplication, postaxial polydactyly, and absence of corpus callosum
- Hanhart
- happy puppet
- Hartnup
- Hays-Wells
- heart-hand
- Hecht
- HELLP (hemolysis, elevated liver enzymes, and low platelet count)
- hemangiomas-thrombocytopenia
- hemangiomatous branchial clefts-lip pseudocleft
- hemolytic uremic (HUS)
- hepatorenal (HRS)
- heredofamilial nephrotic
- Hermansky-Pudlak
- Holmes-Adie
- Holt-Oram
- HRS (hepatorenal)
- Hunter
- Hurler
- Hurler-Scheie
- HUS (hemolytic-uremic)
- Hutchinson-Gilford progeria
- Hutterite
- hydantoin
- hyper-IgE (hyperimmunoglobulin E)
- hyper-IgM (hyperimmunoglobulin M)
- hyperimmunoglobulin E-recurrent infection
- hyperuricemia-choreoathetosis-self-mutilation
- hyperventilation
- hypomelia-hypotrichosis-facial hemangioma
- hypoplastic left heart
- hypospadias-dysphagia

syndrome *(cont.)*
- hypotonia-hypomentia-hypogonadism-obesity
- IBIDS (icthyosis, brittle hair, impaired intelligence, decreased fertility, and short stature)
- idiopathic primary renal hematuric/proteinuric
- idiopathic respiratory distress
- immotile cilia
- infant of diabetic mother (IDM)
- infant respiratory distress
- infantile nephrotic
- infertile male
- insertion
- inspissated bile
- insulin resistance
- inversion
- iron overload
- irritable bowel
- Ivemark
- Jackson-Weiss
- Jadassohn-Lewandowsky
- Jarcho-Levin
- Jeune
- Job
- Job-Buckley
- Joubert
- Juberg-Marsidi
- jumping gene
- juvenile gout-choreoathetosis-mental retardation
- Kabuki make-up
- Kallmann
- Kanner
- Karsch-Neugelbauer
- Kartagener
- Kasabach-Merritt
- Kast
- Kearns-Sayre
- keratitis-ichthyosis-deafness
- Killian
- Kisbourne
- Klein-Waardenburg

syndrome *(cont.)*
- Klinefelter
- Klipper-Feil
- Klipper-Trenaunay
- Klipper-Trenaunay-Weber
- Kneist
- Laband
- Labhart-Willi
- labyrinthine
- lacrimoauriculodentodigital
- Lambert-Eaton myasthenic
- Landau-Kleffner
- Langer-Giedion
- Lapontre
- Larsen
- Laurence-Moon
- Laurence-Moon-Bardet-Biedl
- Laurence-Moon-Biedl
- LeJeune
- Lennox-Gastaut
- Lenz microophthalmia
- LEOPARD
- Leriche
- Leri-Weill
- Lesch-Nyhan
- Levy-Hollister
- Liddle
- Li-Fraumeni (LFS)
- Lignac-Fanconi
- limb malformations-dentodigital
- lip pseudocleft-hemangiomatous branchial cyst
- lissencephaly
- loin pain hematuria
- Loken-Senior
- Louis-Bar
- Lowe
- Lowe-Bickel
- Lowe-Terrey-MacLachlan
- Lubs
- Lucey-Driscoll
- lupus-like
- lupus obstetric
- luteinized unruptured ovarian follicle

syndrome *(cont.)*
- Lynch
- macrostomia ablepheron
- Maffucci
- malformation
- Mallory-Weiss
- Marden-Walker
- Marfan
- Marinesco-Sjögren
- Marinesco-Sjögren-Gorland
- marker X
- Maroteaux-Lamy
- Marshall-Smith
- Martin-Bell
- MASA
- Masters-Allen
- maternal hypotension
- maternal obesity
- Mayer-Rokitansky
- Mayer-Rokitansky-Küster-Hauser
- MCA (multiple congenital anomaly)
- McCune-Albright
- Meckel
- Meckel-Gruber
- meconium aspiration (MAS)
- meconium blockage
- meconium plug
- megacystic
- megacystic-megaureter
- megacystis-microcolon-intestinal hypoperistalsis
- megalocorneal-mental retardation
- Meige
- Meigs
- MELAS (mitochondrial encephalopathy, lactic acidosis, stroke-like episodes)
- Melkersson
- Melkersson-Rosenthal
- Melnick-Fraser
- Melnick-Needles
- Mendelson
- Menkes kinky hair

syndrome *(cont.)*
- MEN 1 (multiple endocrine neoplasia, type 1)
- menopausal
- mermaid
- MERRF
- microcephaly-hiatal hernia-nephrotic
- microdeletion
- milk-alkali
- Miller
- Miller-Dieker
- minimal change nephrotic
- MLL gene duplication
- Moebius (Möbius)
- Mohr
- monosomy 1p36
- monosomy 2q37.3
- monosomy 10
- monosomy 15q
- monosomy 21q
- monosomy 22
- monosomy 22q11
- monosomy X
- monosomy X with gonadal streak
- Moravcsik-Marinesco-Sjögren
- Morquio
- Morris
- mucosal neuroma
- mulibrey nanism
- multiorgan dysfunction
- multiple congenital anomaly (MCA)
- multiple endocrine deficiency
- multiple endocrine neoplasia (MEN)
- multiple lentigines
- multiple organ dysfunction (MODS)
- multiple pterygium
- Mulvihill-Smith
- myasthenic, of Lambert-Eaton
- Myhre
- myoclonus epilepsy associated with ragged red fibers
- myopathy
- Nager
- nail-patella

syndrome *(cont.)*
- neonatal abstinence
- nephritic
- nephrotic
- Netherton
- Neu-Laxova
- nevoid basal cell carcinoma
- Niikawa-Kuroki
- 9 duplication
- 19 duplication
- Nonne
- Noonan
- Norman-Roberts
- nutcracker
- Obrinsky
- Ochoa
- oculoauriculovertebral
- oculocerebral
- oculocerebrocutaneous
- oculocerebrorenal
- oculogenitolaryngeal
- oculomandibulofacial
- Ohdo
- oligoteratoasthenozoospermia
- 1p21-22 deletion
- 1p22-p36.2 deletion
- 1p36 deletion
- 1p36.3 deletion
- 1q deletion
- 1q41 deletion
- Opitz-Kaveggia
- orocraniodigital
- orofaciodigital
- otopalatodigital
- ovarian hyperstimulation (OHSS)
- ovarian remnant
- ovarian vein
- Paget
- palato-otodigital
- Pallister-Hall
- Pallister-Killian mosaic
- Pallister mosaic
- Pallister W
- Papillon-Léfevre

syndrome *(cont.)*
- Pallister-Killian (PKS)
- Parkes Weber
- Parrot
- Parry-Romberg
- partial androgen insensitivity
- Patau
- P duplication
- pellagra-cerebellar ataxia-renal aminoaciduria
- pelvic congestion
- Pendred
- pentalogy
- pentasomy 8
- pentasomy 8q
- pentasomy sex chromosome
- pentasomy 13q
- pentasomy 21
- pentasomy X
- penta X (also pental)
- Pepper
- Perheentupa
- Perrault
- persistent müllerian duct
- Peutz-Jeghers
- Pfeiffer
- P gene duplication
- Phocas fibrocystic breast
- phocomelia
- Pierre Robin
- Pitt-Rogers-Danks
- PKS (Pallister-Killian)
- placental dysfunction
- placental transfusion
- Poland
- polycystic ovary
- polyglandular deficiency
- Pompe
- postartificial menopausal
- postmastectomy lymphedema
- postpartum hepatorenal
- postpartum pituitary necrosis
- postviral fatigue
- potassium depletion

syndrome *(cont.)*
- Prader-Labhart-Willi
- Prader-Willi
- premature senility
- premenstrual (PMS)
- premenstrual salivary
- premenstrual tension
- primary renal hematuric/proteinuric
- Pringle
- progressive pallid degeneration
- proteus
- prune-belly
- pseudothalidomide
- pterygium
- pterygium colli
- pulmonary hypoperfusion
- quadruplication
- radial aplasia-amegakaryocytic thrombocytopenia
- radial aplasia-thrombocytopenia
- rapidly progressive nephritic
- Rapp-Hodgkin
- rearrangement
- recombinant
- Reifenstein
- Reiger
- Reiter
- renal-retinal
- residual ovary
- resistant ovary
- respiratory distress (RDS)
- restless leg
- retained bladder
- Rett
- Richards-Rundle
- Rieger
- Riley-Day
- ring
- Roberts
- robertsonian translocation
- Robin
- Robinow
- Romberg
- Rosenberg-Chutorian

syndrome *(cont.)*
- Rosewater
- Rothmund-Thomson
- Rotor
- Roussy-Lévy
- Rubenstein
- Rubenstein-Taybi
- Ruhr
- Russell
- Russell-Silver
- Ruvalcaba
- Saethre-Chotzen
- Sakati
- Saldino-Noonan
- salt-losing
- Sanfilippo
- San Luis Valley
- Schimmelbusch
- Schinzel
- Schinzel acrocallosal
- Schinzel-Giedion
- Schmidt
- Schwachman
- Schwachman-Diamond
- Schwartz-Jampel
- Scott craniodigital
- SDNS (steroid-dependent nephrotic)
- Seckel
- Seip
- Setleis
- Sertoli-cell-only
- 7 duplication
- 7p deletion
- 7p11.2-p13 duplication
- 7p15.1-p21.3 duplication
- 7p21.1-p14.2 duplication
- 7q21.3 deletion
- 7q21-q22 deletion
- 7q36 deletion
- 17 duplication
- 17p11.2 duplication
- sex chromosome pentasomy
- shaken baby
- Sheehan

syndrome *(cont.)*
- Shereshevskii-Turner
- SHORT
- short arm
- short stature, telangiectatic erythema of the face
- Shprintzen
- Shy-Drager
- Siemens
- Silver
- Silver-Russell
- Simons
- Simpson dysmorphia
- Simpson-Golabi-Behmel
- Singleton-Marten
- Sipple
- 6p deletion
- 6p duplication
- 6p24 deletion
- 6q23 duplication
- Sjögren
- Sjögren-Larsson
- SLE-like
- sloughed urethra
- Sly
- Smith-Lemli-Opitz
- Smith-Magenis
- Sohval-Soffer
- Sotos
- Souques-Charcot
- spherophakia-brachymorphic
- stale fish
- steal
- Stein-Leventhal
- steroid-dependent nephrotic (SDNS)
- Stevens-Johnson
- Stickler
- Stickler-Marshall
- stiff-baby
- stiff-man
- stuck twin
- Sturge-Kalischer-Weber
- Sturge-Weber
- Sturge-Weber-Dimitri

syndrome *(cont.)*
- sudden infant death (SIDS)
- Sugio-Kajii
- Summit
- Swiss cheese cartilage
- Swyer
- swallowed blood
- systemic capillary leak
- Takahara
- tandem duplication
- TAR (thrombocytopenia-absent radius)
- Tay
- Taybi
- Taylor
- 10p deletion
- 10p11.2-p12.2 duplication
- 10q duplication
- 10qter deletion
- Teschler-Nicola
- Teschler-Nicola-Killian
- testicular feminization
- tethered cord
- tethered spinal cord
- tetrasomy 8
- tetrasomy 9p, partial
- tetrasomy 12p
- tetrasomy 12p-
- tetrasomy 12pter-12p12.3
- tetrasomy 15pter-q13
- tetrasomy 21
- tetrasomy X
- 13p deletion
- 13q deletion
- 13q14 deletion
- 13q23-q25 deletion
- 13q32 deletion
- 13q33-34 deletion
- thoracic endometrial
- thoracoabdominal ectopia cordis
- three M
- 3q duplication
- thrombocytopenia-absent radius (TAR)

syndrome *(cont.)*
- thumbs, hypoplastic-triphalangeal
- thyrohypophysial
- Tillaux-Phocas
- Tillaux-Phocas fibrocystic breast
- tonic pupil
- tooth and nail
- Tourette
- Townes
- Townes-Brocks
- toxic shock
- translocation
- transsexualism
- trapezoidocephaly-multiple synostosis
- Treacher-Collins
- trichodento-osseous
- trichorhinophalangeal
- trigonocephaly C
- trimus pseudocamptodactyly
- triphalangeal thumb
- triple X
- triplication (see *trisomy*)
- triploid
- triploidy
- trisomy C
- trisomy D
- trisomy E
- trisomy mosaicism
- trisomy rescue
- trisomy 1q
- trisomy 4q
- trisomy 6p12-p21.3
- trisomy 7p
- trisomy 7q
- trisomy 8
- trisomy 10p
- trisomy 11
- trisomy 11q
- trisomy 13
- trisomy 13qter
- trisomy 14q
- trisomy 15
- trisomy 15pter-q13

syndrome *(cont.)*
- trisomy 16
- trisomy 16p
- trisomy 16q24.3
- trisomy 17q
- trisomy 18
- trisomy 20
- trisomy 20p
- trisomy 21
- trisomy 22
- trisomy X
- tumor lysis
- Turner
- Turner-Kieser
- Turner-like
- 12 duplication
- 12p11.2-p13.3 duplication
- 2q deletion
- 2q37.1 deletion
- 21 duplication
- 21q deletion
- 22q deletion
- 22q11 deletion
- 22q11.2 deletion
- 22q11-q12 duplication
- 22q13.3 deletion
- twin-twin transfusion
- unusual faces
- upper limb-cardiovascular
- Usher
- uremic
- urethral
- urethro-oculo-articular
- VACTERYL (vertebral anomalies, anal atresia, congenital cardiac disease, tracheoesophageal fistula, renal anomalies, radial dysplasia, and other limb defects)
- van der Hoeve-Habertsma-Waardenburg-Gauldi
- vanished testis
- vanishing twin
- VATER (vertebral, anal, tracheo-esophageal, esophageal, radial)

syndrome *(cont.)*
- velocardiofacial
- venous leak
- Vogt
- Vogt-Koyanagi-Harada
- vomiting
- von Hippel-Lindau
- vulvar vestibulitis
- Waardenburg
- Waardenburg-Klein
- Waelsch
- Walker-Warburg
- wasting
- Watson-Alagille
- Weaver
- Weaver-Smith
- Wegener
- Weill-Marchesani
- Weill-Reyes
- Weismann-Netter-Stuhl
- Weissenbacher-Zweymuller
- Wermer
- West
- wet lung
- whistling face
- whistling face-windmill vane hand
- Whitnall-Norman
- Wieacker
- Wiedemann-Rautenstrauch
- Wildervanck
- Willi-Prader
- Williams
- Williams-Beuren
- Wilms tumor
- Williams-Beuren
- Wilson-Mikity syndrome
- Winchester
- Winchester-Grossman
- Wiskott-Aldrich
- Witkop tooth-nail
- Wittmaack-Eckbom
- Wolf
- Wolf-Hirschhorn
- Wolff-Parkinson-White

syndrome *(cont.)*
  Wolfram
  Wyburn-Mason
  X-linked lymphoproliferative
  XO
  Xp21 deletion
  Xp22.1-Xp22.3 deletion
  Xq22.3 deletion
  Xq23
  Xq23 duplication
  Xq27-28 duplication
  XX male
  XXX female
  XXY
  XY
  XYY
  Young
  Yunis Varon
  Zellweger cerebrohepatorenal
  Zinsser-Cole-Engman
  Zollinger-Ellison
  Zondek
  Zondek-Bromberg-Rozin
synechia (pl. synechiae), intrauterine
synergistic drugs
Synergy ultrasound system
syngeneic transplant
syngeneic transplantation
synorchidism
synorchism
synostotic suture
Synphase oral contraceptive
Synphasic 28 oral contraceptive
Synsorb Pk (8-methoxycarbonyloctyl oligosaccharides)
synteny
synthetic erythropoietin
synthetic high flux material
synthetic membrane
syringomyelia
synthesis, prostaglandin
synthetic conjugated estrogens
synthetic hormonal components of oral contraceptives
synthetic purpurin
synthetic retinoid
synthetic vitamin D prohormone, Hectorol
Synthofil suture
syphilis
  acquired
  benign tertiary
  cardiovascular
  congenital
  early
  early latent
  endemic
  fluorescent treponemal antibody absorption test for (FTA-ABS)
  hemagglutination test for (HATTS)
  hereditary
  late
  late benign
  late latent
  latent
  meningovascular
  microhemagglutination assay for antibodies to *T. pallidum* (MHA-TP)
  nonvenereal
  plasmacrit screening test for
  Porges-Meier flocculation test for
  primary
  rapid plasma reagin (RPR) for
  Reiter complement-fixation test for
  secondary
  standard serologic test for
  tertiary
  Treponema pallidum immobilization test for
syphilis hereditaria tarda
syphilitic aneurysm
syphilitic antibodies
syphilitic aortic regurgitation
syphilitic aortitis
syphilitic cirrhosis
syphilitic gummas
syphilitic meningoencephalitis

syphilitic nephritis
syphilitic node
syphilitic vulvar ulcer
syphiloid
syphilologist
syphilology
syphiloma of Fournier
syringe
  Luer-Lok
  Schimmelbusch bladder
  SofDraw amniocentesis
syringectomy
syringomyelia
syringotome
syringotomy
system
  Aastrom CPS (cell-production system)
  Ablatherm HIFU (high intensity focused ultrasound)
  ACIS (Automated Cellular Imaging System)
  Aksys PHD hemodialysis
  Alexa 1000
  AlloMune
  AMS ProstaJect ethanol injection
  AngioJet rapid thrombectomy
  AngioJet Rheolytic thrombectomy
  argon beam coagulator/bipolar/ unipolar cautery
  Aspen ultrasound
  Aurora MR breast imaging system
  Auto Suture ABBI
  AutoPap 300 QC
  AutoSonix
  Bard flexible endoscopic injection
  BAT (B-mode acquisition and targeting)
  BDProbeTec ET
  Beacon Technology System (BTS)
  Bethesda
  BI-RADS (Breast Imaging Reporting and Data System)
  Bilibed phototherapy

system *(cont.)*
  Biliblanket phototherapy
  Biofield diagnostic
  Brava breast enhancement
  Bridge X3 renal stent
  caliceal (calyceal)
  caliceal drainage
  CathTrack catheter locator
  CEPRATE SC (stem cell) concentration
  Ceprate TCD T-cell depletion
  CFC BioScanner System
  Cheung BPH (benign prostatic hypertrophy) treatment
  ChromaVision digital analyzer
  closed drainage
  Coaguloop
  collecting
  Colormate TLc.BiliTest bilirubinometer
  CRYOcare
  CRYOguide ultrasound
  CS-5 cryosurgical
  CycloTech cyclosporine delivery
  dedicated breast biopsy
  Delta 32 digital stereotactic
  Delta 32 TACT three-dimensional breast imaging
  Derma-Trans roll-on
  Dialock
  Dialock hemodialysis access
  dialog dialysis
  dialysate delivery
  diapact CRRT
  dilated caliceal
  DOBI (Dynamic Optical Breast Imaging System)
  E-Z Tac soft tissue reattachment
  electrical impedance breast scanning
  EnAbl thermal ablation
  EndoLumina II transillumination
  erbium:YAG laser
  ErecAid Classic
  ErecAid system

system *(cont.)*
EVII endoscopic video
female reproductive
Fletcher-Suit-Delclos (FSD) mini-colpostat tandem and ovoids
Flo-Stat fluid management
FSD (Fletcher-Suit-Delclos)
GE Senographe 2000D digital mammography
genital
genitourinary
GVHD (graft versus host disease) grading
Gynecare Verascope hysteroscopy
Gyrus endourology
hemodialysis
HercepTest HER2 protein expression
HLA
Home Choice automated PD (peritoneal dialysis)
HTA (Hydro ThermAblator)
HydroThermAblator
Illumina PROSeries laparoscopy
implantable vascular valve
Indigo LaserOptic
Indigo LaserOptic Treatment
KOH colpotomizer
KTP/532 laser
Laparolift gasless laparoscopy
LCx probe
LifeSite hemodialysis
LifeSite hemodialysis access
LigaSure vessel sealing
lithotriptor gantry
LORAD full field digital mammography
LuMax cystometry
Maestro fluid-management
male reproductive
Mammex TR computer-aided mammography diagnosis
MammoReader

system *(cont.)*
MammoSite RTS (radiation therapy)
Mammotest breast biopsy
Mammotest Plus breast biopsy
Mammotome ultrasound
MCAS (modular clip application)
MediClenze perineal lavage
Medstone STS-T transportable lithotripsy
MIBB breast biopsy
MicroSpan microhysteroscopy
MicroSpan minihysteroscopy
Microsulis microwave endometrial ablation
modular clip application (MCAS)
MultAvalue laparoscopic
NeoControl pelvic floor therapy
Neonatal Facial Coding System
Neotrend
normal collecting
NovaSure endometrial ablation
OnCyte newborn sepsis detection
OPERA STAR
OptiVu HDVD (high definition video display)
Ovation falloposcopy
Oxifirst fetal oxygen monitoring
PadKit sample collection
pelvicaliceal
pelvicaliceal collecting
PenRad mammography clinical reporting
Persist incontinence treatment
phagocytic
PHD (personal hemodialysis)
Precision Office TUNA
Precision Tack transvaginal anchor
Precision Twist transvaginal anchor
PREP System for Pap smear
Prisma CRRT
Profile Mammography
ProstaJect ethanol injection
ProstaScint

system *(cont.)*
  Quantum PD night exchange
  radiofrequency interstitial tissue ablation (RITA)
  RenaClear dialyzer cleaning
  renal collecting
  RITA (radiofrequency interstitial tissue ablation)
  Sadowsky breast marking
  SalEst salivary estriol measurement
  Salute tissue fixation
  selective tubal assessment to refine reproductive therapy (STARRT) falloposcopy system
  Senographe 2000D digital mammography imaging
  SenoScan mammography
  SiteSelect breast biopsy
  SJM Rosenkranz pediatric retractor
  SoftScan laser mammography
  Soprano cryoablation
  STARRT falloposcopy
  Straight-In surgical
  takedown of urethral sling
  Tesla imaging
  ThermaChoice uterine balloon therapy (UBT) system
  ThermoChem-HT
  Thermoflex
  Thermoflex WIT (water-induced thermotherapy)
  THL (Transvaginal Hydro Laparoscopy)
  Thrombex PMT (percutaneous mechanical thrombectomy)
  Transvaginal Hydro Laparoscopy (THL)

system *(cont.)*
  transvaginal suturing (TVS)
  T-TAC (transcervical tubal access catheter)
  T3 targeted transurethral thermo-ablation
  Tylok cerclage cabling
  Ultraseed brachytherapy
  ultraviolet light irradiation
  upper collecting
  urinary
  urinary collecting
  urogenital
  UROS bladder infusion
  VidaMed TUNA
  Visica fibroadenoma cryoablation
  Vocare bladder
  VTU-1 vacuum erection
  Wallaby phototherapy
  water purification
  XenoMune
  Xplorer 1000 digital x-ray imaging
systematic dilation
systemic anticoagulation
systemic capillary leak syndrome
systemic infection
systemic inflammatory disease
systemic iodine allergy
systemic lupus erythematosus (SLE)
  diffuse
  focal
systemic necrotizing arteritis
systemic sclerosis
systemic therapy
systolic mammary souffle

T, t

T_4 (L-thyroxine)
T (serum testosterone)
T (thymine)
TAB (tumescent absorbent bandage)
tabes dorsalis
tabetic neurosyphilis
table, cystoscopy
tachycardia
  fetal
  maternal
tachypnea
  idiopathic
  transitory
tack, Origin Tacker laparoscopic
tacrolimus
TAE (total abdominal evisceration)
TA-55 autostapler
TA-55 staper
tag of Spence in mammography
tag, tagged
TAG 72.3 ovarian cancer test
TAH (total abdominal hysterectomy)
TAH/BSO (total abdominal hysterectomy and bilateral salpingo-oophorectomy)
tail, axillary
tail of breast in mammography
tail of breast tissue
tail of Spence
Takahara syndrome
Takayasu arteritis
Take-apart scissors and forceps
takedown of adhesions
takedown of urethral sling
talipes equinovarus
talipes equinus
talipes valgus
talipes varus
Talon balloon dilation catheter
Talon curved needle driver
Tamm-Horsfall mucoprotein
Tamm-Horsfall proteinuria
tamoxifen
tamoxifen citrate
tamponade
  antepartum
  obstetric
tampon, vaginal
tamsulosin
tamsulosin
Tanafem douche
Tanagho anterior bladder flap
tandem and ovoids
tandem duplication (see *duplication syndrome*)
tandem repeat sequence

tangential breast fields
Tangier disease
Tanner Developmental Scale (list)
Tanner staging of genital development
tape
  Mersilene
  Prolene mesh
  tension free vaginal (TVT)
  umbilical
tapered reimplantation
tapiroid cervix
TAR (thrombocytopenia-absent radius) syndrome
targeted ablation therapy
targeted cryosurgery
target organ deterioration of diabetes
Targis catheter
Targis microwave system
Targis transurethral thermoablation system
Targretin
tarsoepiphyseal aclasis
tarsomegaly
TATA box
Tauri disease
taxane therapy
taxanes
  docetaxel
  modified
  paclitaxel
  synthetic
  Taxotere (docetaxel)
Taxol (paclitaxel)
Taxotere (docetaxel)
Taybi syndrome
Taylor syndrome
Tay-Sachs disease (TSD)
Tay syndrome
TB (tuberculosis)
TBM (tubular basement membrane)
TBS ICSI ("to be sure" intracytoplasmic sperm injection)
TBT (transcervical balloon tuboplasty)
Tc (technetium)
TCCB (transitional cell carcinoma of bladder)
TCD (tapetochoroidal dystrophy)
TDOS (trichodento-osseous syndrome)
^{99m}Tc-DMSA
^{99m}Tc-DTPA
T cells
  cytotoxic T lymphocyte (CTL)
  helper (Th)
  suppressive (TS)
TCIC (transabdominal cervicoisthmic cerclage)
TCI-31 Lifelong Ovulation Tester
^{99m}Tc-labeled HAG3
^{99m}Tc-labeled MAG3
TCu380A IUD (intrauterine device)
TD Glucose monitor
Td (tetanus-diphtheria toxoids)
TDD (thoracic duct drainage)
TDMS (Trex digital mammography system)
tear
  anal mucosa
  bladder
  capsular
  cervical
  hymenal
  labial
  perineal
  periurethral
  rectal mucosa
  rectovaginal septum
  secondary perineal
  tentorial
  urethral
  uterine
  vaginal
  vaginal muscle
  vulvar
teardrop breast implant
tear of fourchette
teceleukin (recombinant interleukin-2)
teceleukin and alfa-2a
TechneScan DMSA

TechneScan DTPA
TechneScan MAG3 (^{99m}Tc mertiatide) renal diagnostic imaging
technetium (Tc)
technetium-labeled sulfur colloid scan
technetium mercaptoacetyltriglycine
technetium pentetic acid
technetium pertechnetate (^{99m}Tc)
technique (see also *approach; maneuver; operation*)
  abdominal pedicled inverted penile skin
  Ayre spatula-Zelsmyr Cytobrush
  bipolar surgical
  bladder washout
  buttonhole
  buttonhole puncture
  clamp, cut and tie
  digital subtraction
  fetoscopic
  full-bladder
  full-bladder ultrasound
  Hibbard
  low dose film mammographic
  microsurgical
  molecular
  perineal surgical apron
  polymerase
  renal imaging
  Seldinger
  sequential clamp and suture
  Tzanck
  ultrasound dilution
  ureteral compression
  videofetoscopic
  videolaparoscopic
  whiplash
technology
  assisted reproductive
  XenoMouse
technology transfer
Technos ultrasound system
Tecoflex stent
TEF (tracheoesophageal fistula)
Tefcat intrauterine catheter
Teflon-coated guidewire
Teflon paste
  Ethicon
  Polytef
Teflon paste injection for incontinence
Tegretol (carbamazepine)
telecanthus with associated abnormalities
TeleMed reusable biopsy forceps
telescope, M3G
telescopic urine
television monitor
Telfa dressing
Telfa pad
TeLinde modified radical hysterectomy
telocentric chromosome
telomerase
telomere length
telomeric (T) chromosome staining method
telomeric detection
telophase
temafloxacin
TEMP (tamoxifen, etoposide, mitoxantrone, Platinol) chemotherapy protocol
temperature
  axillary
  basal body
  core body
  intrascrotal
  oral
  rectal
temperature probe
template, Syed
temporal pole
temporary access to circulation
temporary atony of ureter
temporary hypoestrogenism
10p deletion syndrome
10p11.2-p12.2 duplication syndrome
10q duplication syndrome
10qter deletion syndrome

Tenacath HSG (hysterosalpingography) catheter
tenaculum
  double-tooth
  double-toothed
  Gynex Emmet
  Hulka
  Hulka uterine
  Lahey
  Pozzi
  Schroeder
  single-tooth
  single-toothed
  triple-tooth
tenaculum site
Tenckhoff catheter
Tenckhoff peritoneal dialysis catheter
Tenckhoff silicone catheter
tender, exquisitely
tenderness
  abdominal
  breast
  cervical motion
  costovertebral angle (CVA)
  focal
  kidney
  left costovertebral angle
  left lower quadrant
  motion
  prostate
  rebound
  right lower quadrant
  slight costovertebral angle
  suprapubic
  ureteral
  uterine
tenderness of vulvar vestibule
tenderness over kidney and ureter
tender to motion
Tender Touch Ultra cup
tender uterus
tendon, conjoint
tenesmus, urinary
tennis racquet-type closure
TENS (transcutaneous electrical nerve stimulation)
tension-free anastomosis in the perineum
tension-free vaginal tape (TVT) procedure
tension hydrocephalus
tension, premenstrual
tent
  intracervical
  laminaria
tentorial tear
Tenzel forceps
TEP (totally extraperitoneal) hernia repair
Tequin (gatifloxacin)
terahertz waves
teratocarcinoma
teratogenesis
teratogenic effect
teratogens
teratology, drug-induced
teratoma
  cystic
  fetal sacral
  malignant
  malignant ovarian
  ovarian
  testis
teratophobia
Terazol 3 (terconazole)
Terazol 7 (terconazole)
terazosin
terbutaline
terconazole
teres major muscle
term birth, living infant
term by dates
term infant
term intrauterine pregnancy
term pregnancy
terminal deletion
terminal dribbling
terminal hematuria

terminal renal failure
terminate a pregnancy
termination codon
termination of parental rights
termination of surrogate's parental relationship
terminator
termination of pregnancy
- elective
- induced
- spontaneous
- selective

term
- estimated at
- high head at
- pregnancy estimated at

terodiline
Terry-Mayo needle
tertiary syphilis
tertipara
Terumo Clirans dialyzer
TES (thoracic endometrial syndrome)
Teschler-Nicola-Killian syndrome
Teschler-Nicola syndrome
TESE (testicular sperm extraction)
TESE-ICSI (testicular sperm extraction-intracytoplasmic sperm injection)
Tesio hemodialysis access catheter
Tesla imaging system
test (also *assay*)
- Access Ostase
- Accu-Dx bladder cancer
- Accupoint hCG Pregnancy Test Disc
- acetowhite
- acid load
- ACS:180 BR breast cancer screening
- ACTH stimulation
- adhesive cellulose tape
- Affirm one-step pregnancy
- Affirm pregnancy
- AFP (alpha-fetoprotein)
- age-specific PSA
- aggregated human IgG

test *(cont.)*
- AHuG (aggregated human IgG)
- alanine aminotransferase (ALT)
- AlaSTAT latex allergy
- Alatest latex-specific IgE
- aldosterone
- Alexagram breast lesion diagnostic
- Allen-Doisy hormone evaluation
- alpha-fetoprotein (AFP)
- ALT (alanine aminotransferase)
- AMAS (antimalignan antibody in serum)
- AmnioStat-FLM
- Amplicor Chlamydia Assay
- Amplicor CT/NG
- ANA (antinuclear antibody)
- ANCA (antineutrophil cytoplasmic antibodies)
- AneuVysion assay
- Answer pregnancy
- antimalignan antibody in serum (AMAS)
- antineutrophil cytoplasmic antibodies (ANCA)
- antinuclear antibody (ANA)
- Apt
- Aschheim-Zondek pregnancy reaction
- AuraTek rapid cancer
- Auto-Lyte cotinine EIA (enzyme immunoassay)
- BabyStart ovulation prediction
- bacterial inhibition assay (BIA)
- BAER (brain stem auditory-evoked response)
- basal body temperature
- Bard BTA recurrent bladder cancer
- Bayer HER-2/neu serum
- B-D Basal Thermometry
- BDProbeTec ET system
- Bence-Jones protein
- Be Sure One Step pregnancy
- Betke-Kleihauer
- BIA (bacterial inhibition assay)

test *(cont.)*
bicarbonate titration
Biocept-5 pregnancy
Biocept-G pregnancy
Biofield
bladder tumor assay (BTA)
Bonney stress incontinence
BRACAnalysis genetic susceptibility
BRACAnalysis test for detection of hereditary breast and ovarian cancer
brain stem auditory-evoked response (BAER)
Brite-Life One Step pregnancy
BTA stat test of urine for cancer
BTA TRAK bladder tumor assay
CA 15-3 RIA radioimmunoassay for monitoring breast cancer
CA 19-9 ovarian cancer
Candida
Capture-S syphilis
carcinoembryonic antigen (CEA)
CARDS Q.S. hCG serum/urine
CBC (complete blood count)
CEA (carcinoembryonic antigen)
cervical mucus penetration
chemiluminescent
Chiron Diagnostics ELISA assay
Chlamydia enzyme
Chlamydia slide
Chlamydia trachomatis (CT) assay
chromohydrotubation
chromopertubation
chromosomal analysis
ClearBlue Easy One-Step pregnancy
ClearBlue Easy pregnancy
ClearPlan Easy pregnancy
Colaris molecular diagnostic
colony count
Colorgene DNA Hybridization
complete blood count (CBC)
Conceive Ovulation Predictor
Concise Performance Plus hCG-Combo pregnancy

test *(cont.)*
Concise Performance Plus pregnancy
Confirm 1-Step pregnancy
contraction stress
Coombs
CPK (creatine phosphokinase)
creatine phosphokinase (CPK)
creatinine clearance, 24-hour
cryptorchid
CT (*Chlamydia trachomatis*) assay
CVS pregnancy
Cycle Check ovulation prediction
cystometry
DA (direct agglutination) latex pregnancy
DBest pregnancy
Delta OD450
DHEA (dehydroepiandrosterone)
DHEA-S (dehydroepiandrosterone sulfate)
Diacyte DNA ploidy analysis
DiaScreen urine chemistry
differential renal function
differential ureteral catheterization
dinitrophenylhydrazine screening for maple sugar urine disease
dipslide
direct Coombs
direct IBT (immunobead)
Directigen latex agglutination
DNA ploidy analysis
DPPC (dipalmitoyl phosphatidylcholine)
E-cadherin expression breast carcinoma
ectopic
EGFR (epidermal growth factor receptor)
Elecsys total PSA immunoassay
EMIT (enzyme-multiplication immunoassay technique)
Emit 2000 cyclosporine specific assay

test *(cont.)*
- epidermal growth factor receptor (EGFR)
- e.p.t. pregnancy
- ESR (erythrocyte sedimentation rate)
- estradiol
- EZ-Screen Profile (urine drug screen)
- Fact Plus pregnancy
- Fact Plus Pro pregnancy
- FastPack PSA
- fecal occult blood
- fern
- fern-negative Nitrazine
- fern-positive Nitrazine
- Fertil MARQ male infertility
- fetal fibronectin (tFN)
- First Response ovulation prediction kit
- First Warning breast cancer screening device
- flow cytometry
- fluorescent treponemal antibody absorption (FTA-ABS)
- foam stability test for fetal pulmonary maturity
- follicle-stimulating hormone (FSH)
- follicular maturation
- Fortel ovulation prediction
- free PSA
- free thyroxine (T_4) index
- free/total PSA (prostate-specific antigen) index
- Friberg
- fructosamine
- FSH (follicle-stimulating hormone)
- FTA-ABS (fluorescent treponal antibody absorption)
- FTI (free thyroxine index)
- *Gardnerella*
- GAT (gelatin agglutination)
- gelatin agglutination (GAT)
- Gen-Probe amplified CT assay

test *(cont.)*
- germ (germination) tube
- Glofil-125 renal function
- Gluco-Protein
- glucose tolerance (GTT)
- Glycosal diabetes
- GnRH (gonadotropin-releasing hormone)
- Gono Kwik
- Gravindex
- HealthCheck One-Step One Minute pregnancy
- hemizona assay
- hemoagglutination inhibition (HI) titer
- HercepTest
- Heritage Panel genetic screening
- High Risk Hybrid Capture HPV
- HOS (hypo-osmotic swelling)
- Hubner postcoital
- Hybrid Capture CMV DNA
- Hybrid Capture HPV DNA
- Hybrid Capture II human papillomavirus
- Hybritech free PSA
- Hybritech Tandem PSA ratio
- hypo-osmolar swelling
- hypo-osmotic swelling (HOS)
- HZA (hermizona) assay
- IMMULITE 2000 PSA
- Immulite third-generation PSA assay
- Immuno 1 complex PSA (cPSA)
- immunobead
- immunobead antisperm antibody
- ImmunoCyt bladder cancer
- immunologic pregnancy
- indirect IBT (immunobead)
- Inform HER-2/neu for breast cancer recurrence
- InPath cervical cancer screening
- insulin tolerance
- intracavernous injection
- in vitro sensitivity assay
- INVOS 2100 (for breast cancer)

test *(cont.)*
Isletest and Isletest-ICA islet cell autoantibodies
Isojima antisperm antibody
KetoSite
Kibrick antisperm antibody
kidney function
KidneyScreen At Home
Kleihauer
Kleihauer-Betke
Kurzrok postcoital fertility
Lady-Q saliva ovulation prediction
LAL (*Limulus amoebocyte* lysate)
LASA-P (lipid associated sialic acid in plasma)
leukocyte esterase dipstick
LH (luteinizing hormone)
LifeSign1 midstream pregnancy
Limulus amoebocyte lystate
lipid-associated sialic acid (LSA)
LSA (lipid-associated sialic)
L/S ratio
lupus anticoagulant
luteinizing hormone (LH)
mammary aspiration specimen cytology (MASCT)
Mammotest Plus breast biopsy system
Marshall
Marshall-Marchetti
MAS (mammary aspiration specimen) cytology
MASCT/MAS (mammary aspiration specimen cytology)
maternal serum alpha-fetoprotein (MSAFP) screening
Matritech NMP22
metyrapone
MHA-TP (microhemagglutination assay for antibodies to *T. pallidum*)
Micral urine dipstick
microimmunofluorescence (micro-F)
Miraluma breast imaging

test *(cont.)*
Miyazaki-Bonney stress urinary incontinence
MSAFP (maternal serum alpha-fetoprotein) screening
MSAP (maternal screening alpha-fetoprotein)
MultiVysion PB assay
NB/70K ovarian cancer
neuron-specific aldolase
nipple stimulation
Nitrazine
NMP22 transitional cell CA of bladder
nonstress
NTx Assay
O&P (ova and parasites)
Oncotech Extreme Drug Resistance Assay
one-hour glucose tolerance
Osteomark
Ovulplan ovulation prediction
OvuQuick ovulation prediction
OvuSign midstream ovulation prediction
OvuStick
oxytocin challenge
pad (for urinary incontinence)
PAH (para-aminohippuric) acid
PAP (prostatic acid phosphatase)
Pap (Papanicolaou)
Pap Plus HPV Screen
Papanicolaou (Pap)
PapNet
PAPP A (pregnancy-associated plasma protein A)
Pathfinder DFA (direct fluorescent antigen)
peritoneal equilibration (PET)
PET (peritoneal equilibration)
pHEM-ALERT vaginosis
placental alkaline phosphatase
plasma renin
plasmacrit screening

test *(cont.)*
- Porges-Meier flocculation
- positive Marshall
- postcoital cervical mucus at ovulation
- postejaculatory urinalysis
- Premier Type-Specific HSV-1 IgG ELISA
- Premier Type-Specific HSV-2 IgG ELISA
- PrePaQ pregnancy
- progesterone challenge
- prolactin level
- ProstAsure
- protein truncation (PTT)
- PSA (prostate-specific antigen)
- PSA-ACT (prostate-specific antigen bound to alpha$_1$-antichymo-trypsin)
- PSA4 home prostate cancer
- PSA velocity
- PSMA (prostate-specific membrane antigen)
- Pyrilinks-D
- Q tip urethral mobility
- QuickVue one-step hCG-Combo pregnancy
- QuickVue UrinChek 10+ urine
- radioisotope renal excretion
- rapid plasma reagin circle-card (RPR-CT) for syphilis
- Rapoport differential ureteral catheterization
- Reiter complement-fixation
- renal function
- RPR (rapid plasma reagin)
- RPR-CT (rapid plasma reagin circle-card)
- Rubin
- SalEst system
- Schiller test for cervical carcinoma
- SelfCare pregnancy
- serum creatinine
- semen fructose

test *(cont.)*
- serum hCG (human chorionic gonadotropin)
- serum pregnancy
- shake
- Sims-Huhner sperm-mucus interaction
- SPA (sperm penetration assay)
- SpermCheck
- sperm-mucus interaction
- sperm-oocyte interaction
- sperm penetration assay (SPA)
- split renal function
- spun urine sediment
- Stamey
- standard serologic syphilis
- StoneRisk
- SureCell Chlamydia
- SureCell Herpes (SC-HSV)
- surf
- TAG12
- TAG 72.3 ovarian cancer
- TAT (tray agglutination)
- TestPackChlamydia
- Thayer-Martin
- thin-layer chromatography
- ThinPrep and ThinPrep 2000
- ThinPrep Pap
- Thorn
- thrombus precursor protein (TpPTM)
- thyroid function
- thyroid-stimulating hormone (TSH)
- thyrotropin-releasing hormone (TRH)
- tissue polypeptide-specific (TPS) antigen
- TN-alpha
- toluidine blue dye
- TORCH screening titer
- total (free) PSA (prostate-specific antigen) test
- total serum T_3 (total serum triiodothyronine)

test *(cont.)*
total serum T_4 (total serum thyroxine)
TPA (tumor peptide antigen)
TpPTM (thrombus precursor protein)
Treponema pallidum immobilization
TRH
Trichomonas
Truquant BR in vitro
Truquant BR RIA (radioimmunoassay)
TSH (thyroid-stimulating hormone)
tumor peptide antigen (TPA)
24-hour creatinine clearance
24-hour urine collection
U-Titer
uPM3 urine
urecholine supersensitivity bladder
Uri-Test
Uricult dipslide
urinary concentration
urinary creatinine
urinary electrolytes
URiprobe
Uriscreen
Uriscreen urine specimen
UriSite microalbumin/creatinine urine
vaginal cornification
vaginal mucification
Vas MARQ male fertility
vasopressin
VDRL (Venereal Disease Research Laboratory)
ViraPap
Virgo ANCA (antineutrophil cytoplasmic antibodies) screen
Virgo cANCA assay
Virgo pANCA assay
VLDL
Wallace pipette
washout
water deprivation

test *(cont.)*
WEST (Weinstein Enhanced Sensory Test) for diabetic neuropathy
Westergren sedimentation rate
wet mount for *Candida*, *Gardnerella*, and *Trichomonas*
whiff
Whitaker pressure-perfusion test for impediment of urinary flow
X-chromosome determination test
Yellow IRIS urinalysis
zona-free hamster egg
zona hamster egg

testalgia
Tes-Tape reagent strip
test-cross
testectomy
testes (see *testis*)
testes gland
testicle (pl. testicles)
atrophic
atrophy of
bilaterally descended
descended
pain in the
ptosis of
swelling in the
torsion of
undescended

testicle-sparing surgery
testicular abnormality
testicular adrenal rest tissue
testicular appendage
testicular appendix
testicular artery
testicular atrophy
testicular biopsy
testicular blood flow, occlusion of
testicular cancer
testicular cord
testicular core biopsy
testicular cyst
testicular degeneration

testicular duct
testicular dysgenesis
testicular feminization
testicular feminization syndrome
testicular hematoma
testicular histopathology
testicular implant
testicular infarction
testicular injury
testicular interstitial fluid (TIF)
testicular mapping by multiple biopsy
testicular mass
testicular microlithiasis
testicular nodule
testicular pain
testicular prosthesis
testicular shrinkage
testicular sperm extraction (TESE)
testicular torsion
testicular tumor
  choriocarcinoma
  embryonal cell
  functional interstitial cell
  nonseminomatous-type
  seminoma
  teratocarcinoma
  teratoma
testicular vein
testing, genetic
testis (pl. testes)
  abdominal
  absence of the
  anterior border of
  appendix
  appendix of
  bilateral descended
  cryptorchid
  descended
  detorsion of
  ectopic
  efferent ductule of
  free-floating
  hydrocele of

testis *(cont.)*
  infarcted
  lobule of
  movable
  parenchyma of
  peeping
  posterior border of
  retained
  rete
  retractile
  scrotal
  septula of
  straight tubule of
  suspension ligament of
  torsion of
  undescended
  vascular layer of
testis cord
testis-determining factor (TDF)
testis ectopia
testis sparing
testis teratoma
testitis
Testoderm patch
Testoderm TTS (testosterone transdermal system) patch
testolactone
testosterone
testosterone effect
testosterone-estrogen-binding globulin
testosterone flare
testosterone gel, Androgel
testosterone precursor
testosterone stimulation of malignant disease
testosterone transdermal patch
testosterone transdermal system (TTS), Testoderm
TestPackChlamydia
test strip, Excel GE
test-tube baby
TET (tubal embryo transfer)
tetanic contraction

tetanus
  neonatal
  postpartum
  puerperal
  uterine
tetanus-diphtheria toxoids (Td)
tetanus neonatorum
tetanus omphalitis
tetany
  alkalosis-induced
  hypocalcemic
  latent
  neonatal
  neonatal hypocalcemic
  uterine
tethered cord syndrome
tethered spinal cord syndrome
tethering of bladder
tetracycline
tetrad
tetrahydrobiopterin deficiency
tetralogy of Fallot
tetraploidy
tetrasomy (see also *syndrome*)
  age-dependent
  isolated
  mosaic
  mosaic 5p
  partial
tetrasomy 8 syndrome
tetrasomy 9p, partial syndrome
tetrasomy 12p syndrome
tetrasomy 12p- syndrome
tetrasomy 12pter-12p12.3 syndrome
tetrasomy 15pter-q13 syndrome
tetrasomy 21 syndrome
tetrasomy X syndrome
Tevdek
TFD (tight fingertip dilated)
TFE uterine sound
tFN (fetal fibronectin)
TGEF (transabdominal thin-gauge embryofetoscopy)
TGGE (thermal gel gradient electrophoresis)
thalassemia (pl. thalassemias)
  alpha-thalassemia
  beta-thalassemia
  sickle cell
thalassemia major
thalassemia minor
thalidomide
thalidomide embryopathy
thalidomide-related birth defects
thanatophoric dwarfism
thawed cycle
Thayer-Martin cell culture
Thayer-Martin culture medium
Thayer-Martin test
THBR (thyroid hormone-binding ratio)
The Bandeau postaugmentation bra
theca cell
theca-lutein cyst of ovary
theca lutein ovarian cyst
thecal hyperplasia
The Female Condom
thelarche
theophylline
TheraCys (BCG live intravesical)
TheraCys (BCG vaccine, live)
Theradigm-HPV
therapeutic abortion
therapeutic cancer vaccine
therapeutic douche
therapeutic infarction
therapeutic insemination
therapeutic option
therapeutic therapy
therapist, stoma
therapy (pl. therapies)
  adjunctive suppressive medical
  adjuvant
  adjuvant systemic
  androgen ablation
  androgen deprivation
  antegrade scrotal sclerotherapy

therapy *(cont.)*
- anthracycline
- anticoagulant
- antimicrobial
- bacille Calmette-Guérin instillation
- biphosphonate
- breast-conserving (BCT)
- calcium-vitamin D
- chronic dialysis
- chronic suppressive
- continuous renal replacement (CRRT)
- cytolytic
- dialytic
- diuretic
- "dose-dense"
- electrocautery
- electroporation
- endocrine
- estrogen replacement (ERT)
- ESWT (extracorporeal shock wave)
- extracorporeal
- extracorporeal shock wave (ESWT)
- fibrinolytic
- Foscan (temoporfin, mTHPC) mediated photodynamic
- helmet-molding
- herbal
- high dose oral estrogen
- hormonal
- hormone replacement (HRT)
- HRT (hormone replacement)
- immunosuppressive
- instillation
- InterStim implantable continence-control
- intrauterine thermal balloon ablation
- laser
- maternal blood clot patch
- mineralocorticoid replacement
- monotherapy
- multiagent
- natural hormone replacement

therapy *(cont.)*
- neoadjuvant hormonal (NHT)
- palliative
- palliative radiation
- parenteral antibiotic
- photodynamic
- Pitocin
- postmastectomy radiation
- pulse
- pulse steroid
- radiation
- retrograde sclerotherapy
- "shotgun" vitamin
- STARRT (selective tubal assessment to refine reproductive therapy)
- suppressive Gantrisin
- systemic
- tamoxifen
- targeted ablation
- taxane
- therapeutic
- ThermaChoice uterine balloon
- 30-minute TUMT (transurethral microwave thermotherapy)
- thrombolytic
- TMx-2000 BPH thermotherapy
- Ultraseed brachytherapy system
- UroVive intrinsic sphincter deficiency
- uterine balloon
- Vocare Bladder System
- WIT (water-induced thermotherapy)

TheraDerm-MTX

TheraSeed implant

Therex (huHMFG1) humanized monoclonal antibody

ThermaChoice uterine balloon therapy (UBT) system

Therma Jaw hot urologic forceps

thermal ablation system
- EnAbl
- Targis transurethral
- Urologic Targis transurethral

thermal annealing
thermal gel gradient electrophoresis (TGGE)
thermally induced phase-separation membrane formation
ThermoChem-HT system
Thermoflex system for urinary obstruction
Thermoflex WIT (water-induced thermotherapy) system
thermoregulation
thermotherapy
  microwave
  transurethral microwave (TUMT)
  Urowave
  water-induced (WIT)
  WIT (water-induced)
The Whittlestone Physiological Breastmilker
THI (transient hypogammaglobulinemia of infancy)
thiazolidinediones (TZDs)
thick discharge
thickened bladder
thickening in area of wide excision
thickening in breast
thickening, skin
thick meconium in labor
thickness, epithelial
thickness of bladder wall
thickness of parenchyma
Thiersch-Duplay urethroplasty
Thiersch suture
thin discharge
thin-layer chromatography
thinning
ThinPrep and ThinPrep 2000 screening test for cervical cancer
ThinPrep Pap test
thin-walled vagina
Thioplex (thiotepa)
third and fourth pharyngeal pouch syndrome
third degree perineal laceration
third degree prolapse of uterus
third degree uterine prolapse
third-party donor
third-party reproduction
three-quarter strength formula
third spacing of fluids
third stage hemorrhage
third stage of labor
third trimester
third trimester abortion
third trimester bleeding
third trimester placenta
30-minute TUMT (transurethral microwave thermotherapy)
THL (Transvaginal Hydro Laparoscopy) system
Thomas-Allis vulsellum forceps
Thomas-Gaylor biopsy punch
Thomas-Gaylor uterine biopsy forceps
Thomas uterine curette
Thomas vascular access shunt for dialysis
Thompson retractor
Thomsen disease
thoracic duct drainage (TDD)
thoracic endometrial syndrome (TES)
thoracic kidney
thoracic-pelvic-phalangeal dystrophy
thoracoabdominal ectopia cordis syndrome
thoracoabdominal incision
thoracoabdominal radical nephrectomy
thoracodorsal nerve
thoracomelus
thoracopagus
thoracoparacephalus
Thorn test of uric acid excretion
threatened abortion
threatened labor
threatened loss of pregnancy
threatened premature labor
3-androstanediol glucuronide
3-beta-hydroxysteroid dehydrogenase deficiency

3-D gadolinium-enhanced MR angiography
3Dscope laparoscope
3-hydroxy fatty acids
three-chip camera
three-dimensional reconstruction of tissue
3M breast implant
3M Clean Seals waterproof bandage
three M syndrome
three-vessel cord
three-way catheter
three-way stop suprapubic drainage tube
thrice-weekly hemodialysis
thrill in vessel
thrive, failure to
thrombasthenia of Glanzmann and Naegeli
thrombectomy, Thrombex PMT (percutaneous mechanical thrombectomy)
Thrombex PMT (percutaneous mechanical thrombectomy) system
thrombocytopenia
  essential
  idiopathic maternal
  intrauterine
  neonatal
  transient neonatal
thrombocytopenia absent radii (TAR) syndrome
thrombocytopenic purpura, adult immune
thrombocythemia, essential
thromboembolic disease in pregnancy
thromboembolism
thromboendarterectomy
thrombolytic therapy
thrombophlebitis
  breast
  deep vein
  pelvic
  postpartum pelvic
  superficial
thrombophlebitis migrans
thrombophlebitis of superficial breast vein
thrombosed cord
thrombosed hemorrhoid
thrombosis
  cerebral venous
  deep vein
  intracranial venous sinus
  pelvic vascular
  placental
  renal artery
  renal vein
  vascular access
thrombosis of cord
thrombosis of cord vessels
thrombosis of corpus cavernosum
thrombosis of penis
thrombotic stroke
thrombotic thrombocytopenic purpura
thrombus precursor protein (TpPTM)
through-and-through incision
through-and-through suture
Thrumond-Rösch hysterocath
thrush in newborn
thumbs, hypoplastic-triphalangeal
thymidine phosphorylase
thymine (T)
thymoglobulin (antithymocyte globulin, rabbit)
thymoglobulin polyclonal antibody therapy
thymus, enlarged
Thyrogyn (thyrotropin alfa)
thyrohypophysial syndrome
thyroid "C" cells
thyroid deficiency
thyroid gland
thyroid hormone binding ratio (THBR)
thyroid microsomal autoantibodies (MSA)
thyroid scan
thyroid storm

thyroidectomy, subtotal
thyroiditis
  autoimmune
  chronic lymphocytic
  de Quervain
  giant cell
  granulomatous
  Hashimoto
  painless
  silent
  subacute
thyrotoxicosis factitia
thyrotoxicosis, neonatal
thyrotropin-releasing hormone (TRH) test
thyroxin-binding globulin capacity
thyroxine-binding globulin
thyroxine-binding protein
Ti-Cron suture (also Tycron)
ticarcillin
Tice BCG
tidal drainage of urinary bladder
tidal fashion
tidal volume
tie-over dressing
TIF (testicular interstitial fluid)
Tigan suppositories
tight fingertip dilated (TFD)
tight foreskin
tight hymenal ring
tight introitus
tight metabolic control
tight prepuce
Tillaux-Phocas fibrocystic breast syndrome
tilted
tilt of uterus
tilted uterus
Timberlake obturator
time
  dwell
  pyelographic appearance
  transit
times three (x 3)
timing contractions
tin mesoporphyrin (SnMP)
tin protoporphyrin (SnPP)
tip (see *catheter tip*)
tip of penis
tipped uterus
Tischler biopsy punch
Tischler cervical biopsy punch forceps
Tis disease
Tisseel "surgical glue"
tissue
  apical
  areolar
  breast
  dense breast
  desiccating
  endometrial
  fatty
  fibrofatty
  fibroglandular
  glandular
  hypertrophied
  mesenchymal
  nodal
  passage of
  perinephric
  periprostatic
  perivesical
  polypoid
  tail of breast
  testicular adrenal rest
  trophoblastic
tissue anoxia
tissue approximation
tissue engineering
tissue expander
  AccuSpan
  Becker
  Cox-Uphoff International (CUI)
  Heyer-Schulte toxic diffuse goiter
tissue glue for tissue welding
tissue-grasping forceps
tissue ingrowth at skin and/or preperitoneal fascia

tissue invasion
tissue irrigation
tissue mass
tissue morcellator
  Cook
  Elmore radiofrequency
tissue of fetus
tissue penetration
tissue polypeptide-specific (TPS) antigen
tissue-selective estrogens
tissue solder for tissue welding
tissue-sparing technique
tissue specific
tissue stabilization
tissue type
tissue typing
tissue vascularity
Tis-U-Trap endometrial suction catheter
titer
  HI (hemoagglutination inhibition)
  rubella
  TORCH screening
TLI (total lymphoid irradiation)
TM (transport maximum)
TMNS (total motile normal sperm)
TMP/SMX (trimethoprim/sulfamethoxazole)
TMx-2000 BPH thermotherapy
tocolytic medication
tocophobia
Tofranil (imipramine)
toilet retraining
tokos *or* tocos (slang for tokodynamometer)
Toldt
  line of
  white line of
tolerance, high renal
tolrestat
tolterodine
tolterodine tartrate
toluidine blue
toluidine O stain
tomography
  computed (CT)
  kidney
  positron emission (PET)
  single photon emission computed (SPECT)
  PET (positron emission)
tones, fetal heart
tonic neck reflex
tonic pupil syndrome
tongue, fissured
tonsillar clamp
Toomey evacuator
Toomey irrigating syringe
tooth and nail syndrome
Topel cyst aspirator
Topel disposable endoscopic cyst aspirator
Topel endoscopic cyst aspirator
Topel knot
topical radioprotectant
Topiglan (SEPA/alprostadil) gel
Toradol (ketorolac tromethamine)
Toray Filtryzer dialyzer
TORCH (toxoplasmosis, other infections, rubella, cytomegalovirus infection, and herpes simplex) screening titer
Torek two-stage operation for undescended testicle
toremifene citrate
torque
torque control of catheter
torque wire
torsed ovary
torsed testicular appendage
torsemide
torsion
  adnexal
  appendage
  dystonia
  epididymis
  extravaginal
  fallopian tube

torsion *(cont.)*
  intravaginal
  ovarian cyst
  ovarian pedicle
  perinatal
  renal pedicle
  spermatic cord
  testicular
  umbilical cord
torsion dystonia
torsion of appendage
torsion of epididymis
torsion of fallopian tube
torsion of ovarian cyst
torsion of ovarian pedicle
torsion of ovary
torsion of renal pedicle
torsion of spermatic cord
torsion of testicle
torsion of testis
torsion of umbilical cord
tortuosity of ureter
tortuous ureter
torus (pl. tori)
torus uretericus
torus uterinus
Tostrex (transdermal testosterone gel)
total abdominal evisceration (TAE) organ harvesting technique
total abdominal hysterectomy (TAH)
total abdominal hysterectomy with anterior vaginal colporrhaphy
total abdominal hysterectomy with bilateral salpingo-oophorectomy (TAH/BSO)
total amniotic T_3 and T_4
total anomalous pulmonary venus (PV) connection
total blood loss
total cystectomy with urethrectomy
total estrogen blockade
total filtration surface
total/free PSA (prostate-specific antigen) test
total hematuria
total incontinence
total lymphoid irradiation (TLI)
total mastectomy
total motile normal sperm (TMNS)
total parenteral nutrition (TPN)
total pelvic exenteration
total placenta previa
total serum T_3 (total serum triiodothyronine) test
total serum T_4 (total serum thyroxine) test
total vulvectomy
Touhy needle
Tourette syndrome
towel clamp
Townsend mini-bite cervical biopsy punch forceps
Townes-Brocks syndrome
Townes syndrome
toxemia of pregnancy
toxemia, severe
toxemic retinopathy of pregnancy
toxic drug concentration in blood/tissues
toxic end products
toxic goiter
toxicity
  drug
  GI
  hepatic
  renal
toxic nephritis
toxic nephropathy
toxic nephrosis
toxic nodular goiter
toxic shock syndrome
toxic shock syndrome toxin-1 (TSST-1)
toxins
toxoplasmosis, congenital
TPA (tumor peptide antigen)
TPAL terminology (A, abortions; L, living children; P, premature infants; T, term infants)

TP-40 chemotherapy drug
TPH (*Treponema pallidum* hemagglutination) test for syphilis
TPN (total parenteral nutrition)
TpP, TpPTM (thrombus precursor protein) test
TPS (tissue polypeptide-specific) antigen
TQa (transcutaneous access flow) device
trabeculated bladder
trabeculation, bladder
trace edema
trace pedal edema
Tracer blood glucose monitor
trachelorrhaphy
trachelotomy
tracheoesophageal fistula (TEF)
tracheoesophageal fistula with (or without) esophageal atresia
track-etch membrane formation
tract
  fistulous
  genital
  genitourinary
  lower
  mammilopeduncular
  mammilotegmental
  mammilothalamic
  outflow
  reproductive
  upper
  urinary
traction balloon
traction suture
traction, urinary
tractor, Lowsley prostatic
traditional birth attendant
traditional surrogacy arrangement
training, incontinence
trait
transabdominal amniocentesis
transabdominal approach
transabdominal aspiration of fluid from amniotic sac
transabdominal cervicoisthmic cerclage (TCIC)
transabdominal chorionic villus sampling
transabdominal hysterectomy
transabdominal ovum retrieval
transabdominal radical nephrectomy
transabdominal retroperitoneal lymph node dissection
transabdominal sampling of the chorionic villi for genetic analysis
transabdominal thin-gauge embryofetoscopy (TGEF)
transaxillary subpectoral mammoplasty
transcatheter embolization
transcellular transport
transcervical balloon tuboplasty (TBT)
transcervical catheter
transcervical catheterization of fallopian tube
transcervical chorionic villus sampling
transcervical introducer
transcervical sampling of chorionic villi for genetic analysis
transcervical tubal access catheter (T-TAC)
trans configuration, cis-
transcript
transcription control mechanism
transcription factor
transcription start site
transcutaneous electrical nerve stimulation (TENS)
transdermal (dihydrotestosterone) DHT
transdermal system
  Climara (estradiol)
  CombiPatch (estradiol/norethindone)
  Esclim (estradiol)
  Estalis (estrogen/progesterone)
transducer
  abdominal
  piezoelectric

tranducer *(cont.)*
  pressure
  rectal
  rectal multiplane
  vaginal
transduction
transect
transected vaginal cuff
transection of ureter
transection of uterosacral ligaments
transfection
transfer
  EIFT (embryo intrafallopian)
  embryo intrafallopian (EIFT)
  gamete intrafallopian (GIFT)
transfer gene
transfer of frozen embryo to surrogate mother
transference of muscle and blood supply
transferrin
transfer RNA (tRNA)
transfixion suture
transformation, malignant
transformation zone of cervix
transforming gene
transfundal insertion of catheter
transfusion
  donor twin
  donor-specific (DST)
  exchange
  fetofetal
  fetomaternal
  fetoplacental
  intrauterine
  intrauterine fetal
  maternal-fetal
  twin-to-twin transplacental
  twin-twin
transfusion hepatitis
transfusion nephritis
transfusion of packed cells
transfusion reaction
transgender identity
transgender person
transgenic
transient bacteremia
transient hypertension of pregnancy
transient hyperthyroidism
transient hypogammaglobulinemia of infancy (THI)
transient neonatal pustular melanosis
transient neonatal neutropenia
transient neonatal thrombocytopenia
transient septicemia
transient tachypnea of newborn (TTN, TTNB)
transilluminate
transilluminated
transillumination
transillumination and drainage
transillumination of scrotum
transillumination of ureter
transition
transitional cell carcinoma
  nonpapillary
  papillary
transitional cell carcinoma of bladder (TCCB)
transitional cell carcinoma of prostate
transitional cell carcinoma of renal pelvis
transitory fever of newborn
transitory ileus of newborn
transitory tachypnea
translation
translocation (pl. translocations)
  balanced
  de novo
  reciprocal
  robertsonian
translocation chromosome
translucency, nuchal
translumbar introduction of contrast agent
transluminal angioplasty needle
transmembrane driving force
transmission, sexual

- transparent polyurethane dressing
  - Op-Site
  - Tegaderm
- transpectral impedance scanner, T-Scan 2000
- transpelvic urethral sling
- transperineal approach
- transperineal needle biopsy of prostate
- transperineal prostate implantation of radioactive seeds
- transperineal prostatic cryoablation
- transperineal template placement
- transperineal ultrasonography
- transperitoneal approach to uterus
- transperitoneal cesarean section
- transperitoneal classical cesarean section
- transplacental access
- transplacental carcinogenesis
- transplacental transmission of maternal antibody
- transplant, transplantation
  - allogenic renal
  - bone marrow (BMT)
  - cadaveric
  - combined kidney and pancreatic (CKPT)
  - gracilis muscle
  - human islet
  - islet-cell
  - isolated pancreas
  - kidney
  - kidney-pancreas
  - Lich-Gregoire kidney
  - liver
  - living-donor
  - living-related
  - pancreas
  - renal
  - solid organ
  - syngeneic
  - xenogeneic
- transplantation genetics
- transplantation of ureter into ileum with external diversion
- transplant coordinator
- transplanted kidney
- transplant kidney
- transplant operation
- transplant team
- transplant waiting list
- transport
  - renal epithelial
  - transcellular
  - tubular sodium
- transport maximum (TM) for glucose
- transport properties of a membrane
- transport of solute
  - convective
  - diffusive
- transposable element
- transposase
- transposition
- transposition of the great arteries
- transposon
- transrectal needle biopsy of prostate
- transrectal prostatic ultrasonographic biopsy
- transrectal sonography
- transrectal ultrasonography
- transrectal ultrasound (TRUS)
- TransScan TS2000 electrical impedance breast scanning system
- transseptal orchiopexy
- transsexualism syndrome
- transsexual surgery
- transsphenoidal exploration of pituitary
- transudate
- transudation of vaginal fluid
- transumbilical augmentation mammoplasty
- transumbilical breast augmentation (TUBA)
- transureteroureteral anastomosis
- transureteroureterostomy (TUU)
- transureteroureterostomy anastomosis
- transurethral balloon Laserthermia prostatectomy
- transurethral biopsy
- transurethral collagen injection

transurethral cystoscope
transurethral cystoscopy
transurethral enucleation
transurethral fistulectomy
transurethral Foley catheter to stent urethral injury
transurethral incision of prostate (TUIP)
transurethral lysis of adhesions
transurethral microwave thermotherapy (TUMT)
transurethral microwave (TURM) treatment for benign prostatic hyperplasia/hypertrophy
transurethral needle ablation (TUNA) of prostate
transurethral occlusive device (TUOD)
transurethral prostatectomy
transurethral resection of bladder neck
transurethral resection of bladder tumor (TURBT)
transurethral resection of prostate (TURP)
transurethral resection (TUR)
transurethral thermoablation system, Urologic Targis
transurethral ultrasound-guided laser-induced prostatectomy (TULIP)
transurethral ureteroscopic lithotomy
transurethral ureteroscopic lithotripsy
transurethrally
transvaginal approach
transvaginal echography
transvaginal enterocele repair
Transvaginal Hydro Laparoscopy (THL) system
transvaginal hysterectomy
transvaginal oocyte retrieval
transvaginal ovum retrieval
transvaginal sacrospinous colpopexy
transvaginal sonography
transvaginal suturing (TVS) system
transvaginal ultrasound (TVS)
transvaginal ultrasound-guided drainage with trocar method
transvaginal ultrasound, Sassone score of appearance in
transvaginal uterine cervical dilation with fluoroscopic guidance
transversalis fascia
transverse abdominal incision
transverse arrest of fetal head
transverse cervical cesarean section
transverse hermaphroditism
transverse incision
transverse lie (presentation)
transverse Pfannenstiel incision
transverse plane
transverse presentation
transverse rectus abdominis myocutaneous (TRAM) flap
transverse septum
transverse vesical fold
transversion
transversus abdominis
transvesical prostatectomy
transvesicle approach
transvesicle ovum retrieval
transvestism
transvestite
transvestitism
TRAP (twin reversed arterial perfusion) sequence
trapezoidocephaly-multiple synostosis syndrome
trapped oocyte
trapped placenta
trastuzumab (anti-HER2 humanized monoclonal antibody)
trauma
  anal
  birth
  bladder
  blunt
  breast
  homosexual rectal
  kidney
  obstetrical
  penile

trauma *(cont.)*
  rectal
  renal
  scrotal-testicular
  urethral
traumatic amenorrhea
traumatic anemia
traumatic avulsion of penis
traumatic dissection of renal artery aneurysm
traumatic glaucoma
traumatic hematuria
traumatic orchitis
traumatic rupture of bladder
traumatic scar
traumatic separation of symphysis pubis
traumatic urethral stricture
tray agglutination test (TAT)
Treacher-Collins syndrome
treated premalignant lesion
treatment modalities
Treitz, ligament of
Trelex mesh
Trelstar Depot (injectable triptorelin pamoate)
Trelstar depot (triptorelin pamoate)
Trelstar LA (triptorelin pamoate)
tremor
Trendelenburg position
treponal tests
Treponema genitalis
Treponema pallidum
Treponema pallidum hema-agglutination (TPH) test
Treponema pallidum immobilization test
Trevor disease
Trex digital mammography system (TDMS)
TRH (thyrotropin-releasing hormone)
trial
  Canadian Urology Oncology Group (CUOG)
  Radiation Therapy Oncology Group (RTOG)
trial forceps
trial of labor after cesarean section
triamcinolone acetonide cream
triamterene
triangle
  anal
  iliofemoral
  Langenbeck
  Pawlik
  urogenital
  vesical
Triangle gelatin-sealed sling material
triangle of doom
triangle of pain
TriAngle sling
triangular excision of redundant vaginal mucosa
triangular fontanelle
triangular uterus
triangular vaginal patch sling
tribrachia
tribrachius
Tribulus Terrestris extract
trichloroacetic acid
trichoepithelioma
trichomonads
trichomonal cystitis
trichomonal prostatitis
trichomonal vaginitis
trichomonal vulvovaginitis
Trichomonas test
Trichomonas vaginalis
trichomoniasis
trichomoniasis vaginitis
trichodento-osseous syndrome (TDOS)
trichopoliodystrophy
trichorhinophalangeal syndrome
tricuspid atresia
Triella oral contraceptive
trifurcation of renal vessels
trigeminal embryonic groove
trigonectomy
Trigonella foenum-graecum (fenugreek)
trigone of bladder

trigone of urinary bladder
trigone, vesical
trigonitis
  acute
  chronic
trigonocephaly
trigonocephaly C syndrome
Tri-Levlen oral contraceptive
trilobar enlargement of prostate
trilobar hyperplasia of prostate
trilobar hypertrophy of prostate
Trilucent breast implant
trimester
  first
  second
  third
trimethoprim/sulfamethoxazole (TMP/SMX)
trimethylaminuria
trimus pseudocamptodactyly syndrome
Tri-Norinyl (norethindrone/ethinyl estradiol) oral contraceptive
Trinovin dietary supplement
Trinovum 21 oral contraceptive
trinucleotide repeat
trinucleotide repeat analysis
trinucleotide repeat expansions
trinucleotide repeat mutation
triopathy
triphalangeal thumb syndrome
Triphasil (levonorgestrel/ethinyl estradiol)
triple-lumen catheter
triple-lumen umbilical catheter
triple screen test (AFP, uEST, hCG)
triple-tooth tenaculum
triplet codons
triplet gestation
triplet pregnancy
triple voiding cystography
triple X syndrome
triplication syndrome
triploid triploidy
triptolide
triptorelin pamoate
trisomy (pl. trisomies) (see also *syndrome*)
  age-dependent
  free 21
  isolated
  mosaic
  mosaic 5p
  partial
  sex chromosome
trisomy C syndrome
trisomy D syndrome
trisomy E syndrome
trisomy mosaicism
trisomy rescue
trisomy 1q syndrome
trisomy 4q syndrome
trisomy 6p12-p21.3 syndrome
trisomy 7p syndrome
trisomy 7q syndrome
trisomy 8 syndrome
trisomy 10p syndrome
trisomy 11 syndrome
trisomy 11q syndrome
trisomy 13 syndrome
trisomy 13qter syndrome
trisomy 14q syndrome
trisomy 15 syndrome
trisomy 15pter-q13 syndrome
trisomy 16 syndrome
trisomy 16p syndrome
trisomy 16q24.3 syndrome
trisomy 17q syndrome
trisomy 18 syndrome
trisomy 20 syndrome
trisomy 20p syndrome
trisomy 21 syndrome
trisomy 22 syndrome
trisomy X syndrome
tritanopia
Trivagizole 3 (clotrimazole vaginal cream, 2%)
Trivora (levonorgestrel/ethinyl estradiol) oral contraceptive

Trivora-21 (ethinyl estradiol/levonorgestrel)
Trivora-28 (ethinyl estradiol/levonorgestrel)
tRNA (transfer RNA)
trocar
  Add-A-Cath
  Bluntport disposable
  Core
  DeRoyal surgical cannula/
  Endopath laparoscopic
  Hasson
  hysteroscopic
  infraumbilical
  Iotec
  laparoscopic
  Lawrence Add-A-Cath
  Origin Medsystems
  PediPort disposable
  Reuter
  Reuter suprapubic
  Saber BT blunt-tip surgical
  sharp
  suprapubic midline
  Surgiport
trocar guides
trocar puncture into bladder
trocar sheath
trocar tent
trocar with built-in reduction sleeves
Troisier node
trophic hormones manufactured by placenta
trophoblast cell
trophoblastic disease
trospium
trovafloxacin
Trovan (trovafloxacin)
Trovan/Zithromax Compliance Pak
Trovert
true breeding
true hermaphrodite
true hermaphroditism
true pelvis
true precocious puberty
true uterine inertia
TruJect auto-injector drug delivery system
Trulife silicone breast implant
Trumpet Valve hydrodissector
truncal renal artery stenosis
truncated protein product
truncus arteriosis, persistent
Truquant BR in vitro test
Truquant BR RIA
TRUS (transrectal ultrasound)
Tru-Scint AD imaging agent
tryptophan malabsorption
Trysul vaginal cream
T-Scan 2000 transpectral impedance scanner
TS2000 (TransScan 2000)
TSH immunoassay test
TSH-01 transdermal tape with natural estrogen and 17-beta-estradiol
TSST-1 (toxic shock syndrome toxin-1)
T3 (liothyrine sodium)
T3 resin uptake
T3 targeted transurethral thermo-ablation system for BPH
T-TAC (transcervical tubal access catheter) system
TTN (transient tachypnea of newborn)
TTNB (transient tachypnea of newborn)
Tuason laparoscopic knot pusher
TUBA (transumbilical breast augmentation)
tubae, hydrops
tubal abortion
tubal anastomosis
tubal blockage
tubal dye perfusion
tubal dysmenorrhea
tubal embryo transfer (TET)
tubal extremity of ovary
tubal factor
tubal fimbriectomy
tubal gestation

tubal infantilism
tubal insufflation
tubal ligation
  bilateral
  Falope-Ring
  Irving
  laparoscopic
  Pomeroy
  reproductive sterilization
  occlusion of
tubal lumen
tubal lumen support
tubal nephritis
tubal obstruction
tubal occlusion
tubal occlusion device
  Falope-Ring
  Silastic band
  spring-loaded clip
tubal occlusive disease
tubal ostia
tubal ostium
tubal patency
tubal perfusion pressure
tubal phimosis
tubal pregnancy
tubal reanastomosis
tubal reconstructive surgery
tubal reticular inclusion
tubal ring
tubal rugae
tubal spasm
tubal spillage, postprocedural
tubal stenosis
tubal sterilization by electrocoagulation
tube
  abscess of fallopian
  accessory fallopian
  ampullary folds of uterine
  Baggish
  collecting
  Cope nephrostomy
  cutaneous nephrostomy
  cystostomy

tube *(cont.)*
  damaged fallopian
  edematous fallopian
  endotracheal
  Falcon
  fallopian
  feeding
  fimbriae of uterine
  fold of uterine
  hollow musculomembranous
  infundibulum of uterine
  lumen of
  mucosa of uterine
  nasogastric
  nephrostomy
  nonfunctioning fallopian
  serosa of uterine
  Silastic
  urostomy
  uterine
  uterine part of uterine
tube cast
tubectomy
tube graft urethral reconstruction
tubeless lithotripsy
tubeless percutaneous renal surgery
tubercle
  genital
  pubic
tuberculosis (TB)
  congenital
  genitourinary
  renal
tuberculosis of kidney
tuberculosis of ureter
tuberculous cystitis
tuberculous endometritis
tuberculous epididymitis
tuberculous nephritis
tuberculous orchitis
tuberculous salpingitis
tuberous sclerosis
tuberous sclerosis complex

tube transfer (ZIFT), zygote intrafallopian
tubing, suction/irrigation
tuboabdominal pregnancy
tubointerstitial nephropathy
tuboligamentary pregnancy
tubo-ovarian abscess
tubo-ovarian adhesions
tubo-ovarian inflammatory disease
tubo-ovarian pregnancy
tubo-ovarian varicocele
tubo-ovariectomy
tubo-ovaritis
tuboperitoneal
tuboplasty
 balloon
 transcervical balloon (TBT)
 transcervical balloon tuboplasty
 ultrasound transcervical
tubotorsion
tubouterine pregnancy
tubovaginal
tubular basement membrane (TBM)
tubular breast deformity
tubular cell
tubular cell casts
tubular cell secretion
tubular defect
tubular dilation
tubular dysfunction
tubular dysplasia
tubular ectasia
tubular epithelium
tubular fullness
tubular lumina
tubular necrosis
tubular nephritis
tubular obstruction
tubular protein droplets
tubular secretion
tubular sodium retention
tubular sodium transport
tubular transport
 distal
 proximal
tubule
 collecting
 convoluted
 distal convoluted
 kidney
 metanephric
 proximal
 paragenital
 proximal convoluted
 renal
 seminiferous
 uriniferous
tubuloglomerular feedback
tubulointerstitial disease
tubulointerstitial inflammation
tubulointerstitial lesion
tubulointerstitial nephritis, allergic
tubulointerstitium
tubuloreticular inclusions
tubulorrhexis
Tucker-McLane forceps
Tudor "rabbit ear" urethropexy
tuft, glomerular
TUIP (transurethral incision of prostate)
TULIP (transurethral ultrasound-guided
 laser-induced prostatectomy)
tumefaction
tumescence, compromised
tumescent absorbent bandage (TAB)
tummy tuck flap
tumor
 adenomatoid
 adenomatoid oviduct
 aggressive angiomyxoma
 AML (angiomyolipoma) solid renal
 androgen-secreting
 aneuploid
 angiomyxoma
 benign
 bladder
 borderline ovarian
 Brenner
 bulky
 cystic
 dysgerminoma

tumor *(cont.)*
- endometriod
- estrogen-producing ovarian
- estrogen-receptor positive (ER+)
- estrogen-receptor-negative (ER-)
- estrogen-secreting testicular
- fatty
- fetal
- fibrous
- genital tract
- granulosa-theca cell
- invasive ductal
- invasive lobular
- kidney
- Krukenberg
- malignant
- malignant teratoma
- medullary
- mixed mesodermal
- necrotic
- nonseminomatous germ cell
- ovarian
- ovarian granulosa cell
- papillary
- pedunculated
- pedunculated vesical tumor
- placental site trophoblastic
- poorly differentiated
- pregnancy
- progesterone-receptor-positive
- renal cell
- seeding of
- Sertoli-Leydig cell ovarian
- Sertoli stromal cell ovarian
- steroid cell ovarian
- stone differentiated from
- subcortical
- tubular
- urinary
- urothelial
- uterine
- virilizing
- vulvar
- well-differentiated

tumor *(cont.)*
- Wharton
- Wilms

tumor ablation, focused-heat
tumor base
tumor blush
tumor cell deposit, occult
tumor cell homogenate
tumor debulking
tumor dissemination
tumor embolization
tumor encroachment
tumor-free margin of normal tissue
tumor invasion
tumor invasion of bladder wall
tumor involvement
tumor lysis syndrome
tumor marker
- antimalignan antibody
- CA 15-3
- CA 19-9
- CA27.29 antigen
- CEA
- CYFRA 21-1
- CYFRA 21-1 tumor necrosis factor
- HER-2-neu oncogene breast cancer
- neuron-specific aldolase
- p21 (Kip1) protein prostate cancer
- sigmaS serum
- TAG12
- TAG72.3
- TN-alpha
- TPA (tumor peptide antigen)
- TPS (tumor polypeptide-specific) antigen

tumor necrosis factor
tumor progesterone receptor
tumor-reductive surgery
tumor seeding
tumor suppressor
tumor suppressor gene, APC
tumor thrombus
TUMT (transurethral microwave thermotherapy)

TUNA (transurethral needle ablation)
TUNEL (terminal deoxynucleotidyl transferase-mediated deoxyuridine triphosphate) stain
tunica mucosa uteri
tunica vaginalis
  chylocele
  congenital hydrocele of
  hydrocele of
tunica vaginalis testis
tunnel
  subcutaneous
  subcutaneous catheter
tunnel infection
TUOD (transurethral occlusive device)
Tuohy-Borst valve
TUR (transurethral resection)
turbid urine
TURBT (transurethral resection of bladder tumor)
turgor
  poor tissue
  skin
TURM (transurethral microwave) treatment for BPH
Turner biopsy needle
Turner-Kieser syndrome
Turner-like syndrome
Turner syndrome
Turner-Warwick self-retaining retractor
Turner-Warwick urethroplasty
TURP (transurethral resection of prostate)
turricephaly
Tuttle forceps
TUU (transureteroureterostomy)
TVH (total vaginal hysterectomy)
TVS (transvaginal suturing system)
TVS (transvaginal ultrasound)
TVT (tension-free vaginal tape) procedure
12 mm port site
12p tetrasomy
12p- tetrasomy
12pter-12p12.3 tetrasomy
22q11 deletion syndrome
22q11.2 deletion syndrome
22q deletion syndrome
24-hour creatinine clearance
24-hour urine collection
21-hydroxylase deficiency
twin
  binovular
  bipartite diamnionic
  conjoined
  conjoined asymmetric
  conjoined equal
  conjoined symmetric
  conjoined unequal
  diamnionic
  diamniotic
  dichorionic
  di-di (dichorionic-diamniotic)
  diovular
  dizygotic
  enzygotic
  fraternal
  heterologous
  identical
  incomplete conjoined
  locked
  monoamniotic
  monochorial
  monochorionic
  mono-ovular
  monozygotic
  polyzygotic
  Siamese
  stuck
twin-coil dialyzer
twin gestation
twinning
twin placenta
twin pregnancy
  dichorionic
  monochorionic
twin reversed arterial perfusion (TRAP) sequence

twins (see *twin*)
twin-to-twin transplacental transfusion
twin-twin transfusion syndrome
twisted ovarian cyst
twisting of pedicle
2q deletion syndrome
2q37.1 deletion syndrome
two-layer closure
two-stage technique of mastectomy
two-vessel cord
Tycron suture (also Ti-Cron)
Tylenol (acetaminophen)
Tylenol No. 3 (acetaminophen, codeine)
Tylok cerclage cabling system
tympany
type 1 plasminogen activator inhibitor (PAI-1)
type 3 LAVH (laparoscopic-assisted vaginal hysterectomy) procedure
type 5 hyperlipidemia
tyrosinuria
tyrosinemia, hereditary, hepatorenal-type
tyrosinemia type 1
tyrosyluria
Tzanck preparation
Tzanck smear
TZDs (thiazolidinediones)

U, u

U (uracil)
UA (urinalysis)
UAC (umbilical artery catheter)
UAE (uterine artery embolization)
UBE3A gene
UBT (Uterine Balloon Therapy)
UCAC (uterine cornual access catheter)
UCLA pouch
UD-BMT (unrelated donor, bone
  marrow transplantation)
uEST (unconjugated estrogen)
UHMM (ultra-high magnification
  mammography)
UKM (urea kinetic modeling)
ulcer
  cluster of
  decubitus
  diabetic
  endophytic
  genital
  gonococcal vulvar
  Hunner
  labial
  mucosal
  nipple
  penile
  perforating
  plantar

ulcer *(cont.)*
  pressure
  pudendal
  rodent
  scrotal
  shallow discrete
  skin
  stasis
  stercoraceous
  stercoral
  syphilitic vulvar
  urethral meatus
  urinary
  vaginal
  venereal
  vulvar
ulceration
  gummatous
  mucosal
  vulvar
ulcerative colitis
ulcer scrapings
Uldall (*not* Udall) subclavian
  hemodialysis catheter
UltraCision ultrasonic knife
ultrafast CT electron beam tomography
ultrafilter
ultrafiltrate

ultrafiltration (UF)
  hydraulic
  osmotic
  rapid
ultrafiltration of excess fluid across the membrane
ultrafiltration procedures
ultra-high magnification mammography (UHMM)
Ultramark 4 ultrasound
Ultraseed brachytherapy system for prostate cancer
UltraSling
ultrasonic dissector
ultrasonic guidance for amniocentesis
ultrasonic guidance for intrauterine fetal transfusion
ultrasonic lithotripsy
ultrasonic lithotripsy probe
ultrasonographer
ultrasonography (see *ultrasound*)
ultrasound, ultrasonography (US)
  Aloka
  BABE
  BabyFace 3-D surface rendering
  BladderScan
  breast
  CRYOguide
  endoanal
  endovaginal (EVUS)
  fetal
  focused extracorporeal
  HDI 3000
  high intensity focused
  high resolution
  intracavitary prostate
  laparoscopic
  laparoscopic intracorporeal
  Mammotome
  neonatal adrenal
  obstetric
  pelvic
  real-time
  renal
ultrasound *(cont.)*
  Sonablate 200
  sonohysterography
  Sonopsy 3-D
  Synergy
  Technos
  transabdominal
  transperineal ultrasonography
  transrectal (TRUS)
  transvaginal (TVS)
  vaginal
ultrasound analysis of prostate
ultrasound augmented mammography
ultrasound biopsy needle
ultrasound devices (see also *imaging*)
  Aspen system
  NeuroSector
  Philips ultrasound machines
  PocketDop
  Sonablate 200
  Ultramark 4 ultrasound
ultrasound dilution technique
ultrasound disruption of stones
ultrasound examinations, serial
ultrasound guidance
ultrasound-guided transcervical tuboplasty
ultrasound-guided transvaginal aspiration of eggs
ultrasound-guided TULIP (transurethral laser-induced prostatectomy)
ultrasound monitoring of ovarian follicle diameter
ultrasound needle guidance for amniocentesis
ultrasound needle guidance for fetal transfusion
ultrasound transcervical tuboplasty
ultrasound velocity dilution
UltraStat 10 laser system
ultraviolet light irradiation system
ultraviolet phototherapy
UMB-E umbilical catheter anchor
umbilical artery catheter (UAC)

umbilical artery in fetus
umbilical artery velocimetry
umbilical blood
umbilical coiling index
umbilical cord
umbilical cord around neck x 2
umbilical cord blood sampling, percutaneous (PUBS)
umbilical cord compression
umbilical cord compromise
umbilical cord entanglement
umbilical cord knot
umbilical cord prolapse
umbilical cord torsion
umbilical cord varices
umbilical duct
umbilical endometriosis
umbilical eversion
umbilical fistula
umbilical fungus
umbilical granuloma
umbilical hemorrhage
umbilical hernia
umbilical ligament
umbilical ring
umbilical scissors
umbilical souffle
umbilical stump infection
umbilical tape
umbilical vein
umbilical vein catheter (UVC)
umbilical venous catheter (UVC)
umbilicalis, funiculus
Umbili-Cath Tecoflex umbilical catheter
umbilicus (pl. umbilici)
  amniotic
  bluish discoloration around
  decidual
  endometriosis of
  everted
  infection of
umbrella cell
UMCD (uremic medullary cystic disease) complex
Unasyn (ampicillin; sulbactam)
unbalanced chromosome complement
uncentrifuged fresh urine sample
uncircumcised male
uncircumcised male phallus
uncircumcised penis
unclassified carcinoma
uncoiling of stent
unconscious homosexuality
unconjugated estrogen (uEST)
uncontrolled maternal diabetes
underdeveloped jaw
underlying etiology
underlying structures
undermethylation
undermine
undermined
undermining of muscle
undermining of skin edges
undermining of tissue
undermining of wound edges
underperfusion, renal
undescended testicle
undescended testes
undesired fertility
undesired postpartum fertility
undyed Vicryl sutures
unenhanced scan
unequal crossing over
unesterified fatty acids
uneventful prenatal course
unexplained cause of infertility
unexplained infertility
unfavorable cervix
unicellular organism
unicorn uterus
unicornuate uterus
Uniform Parentage Act (UPA)
Uniform Status of Children of Assisted Conception Act
unilateral groin dissection
unilateral hemidysplasia
unilateral hermaphroditism
unilateral orchiectomy

unilateral renal agenesis
unilateral renal bleeding
unilateral small kidney
unilateral vulvectomy
unilocular cyst
Unimar J-Needle
uninhibited bladder
uninhibited neurogenic bladder dysfunction
union of the labia majora
uniparental disomy (UPD) analysis
unit
- Belzer organ preservation
- beta subunit of hCG
- Bovie cautery
- Bovie electrosurgical
- CNS-hypothalamic-pituitary
- colony-forming (CFU)
- crossed ectopic renal unit
- cryosurgical unit
- Crystal Vision smoke evacuation
- dialysis
- electrosurgical (ESU)
- family-centered obstetric
- free alpha subunit of hCG
- hypothalmic-pituitary
- intensive care (ICU)
- membrane
- Montevideo
- nicked-free beta subunit of hCG marker
- neonatal intensive care unit (NICU)
- perinatal evaluation and treatment (PETU)
- pilosebaceous
- renal
- satellite hemodialysis
- step-down

United Network for Organ Sharing (UNOS)
United States Public Health Service (USPHS)
universal donor cells
universal infantilism
universal vacuum release (UVR)
unmethylated (active) X-chromosome
unobstructed neourethra
unopposed estrogen
UNOS (United Network for Organ Sharing)
unpaired chromosome
unregulated cell growth
unripe cervix
unsafe sex
unsensitized Rh negative
unsex
unstable ARF (acute renal failure)
unstable bladder
unstable lie
unstable lie of fetus
unstimulated cycle
UOAC (uterine ostial access catheter)
UP (ureteropelvic) junction
UPD (uniparental disomy) analysis
uphill transport
UPJ (ureteropelvic junction) obstruction
UPLIFT (uterine positioning via ligament investment fixation and truncation) procedure
uPM3 urine test
upper collecting system
upper genital tract
upper GI (gastrointestinal) atresia
upper inner quadrant of breast
upper lateral quadrant of breast
upper limb-cardiovascular syndrome
upper medial quadrant of breast
upper outer quadrant of breast
upper pole
upper pole calix (calyx)
upper pole collecting system
upper pole moiety
upper pole of kidney
upper pole of renal pelvis
upper pole of testis
upper pole ureter
upper tract diversion
upper tract obstruction

upper tracts
upper urinary tract infection
upper uterine segment
Uprima (apomorphine)
upstream
upstream face of asymmetric membrane
upstream side of the membrane
uptake, focal areas
urachal carcinoma
urachal cyst
urachal sinus
urachus, patent
urachus remnant
uracil (U)
uracil mustard
urate crystals
urate nephrolithiasis
urates
Urban extended radical mastectomy
urea
urea clearance
urea clearance values
urea cycle defects or disorders
urea generation
urea kinetic modeling (UKM)
urea reduction ratio (URR)
urea-splitting organism
Ureaplasma urealyticum
ureaplasmal infection
ureasepsis
Urecholine (bethanechol)
urecholine supersensitivity bladder test
Ureflex ureteral catheter
uremia
  chronic
  extrarenal
  prerenal
uremic acidosis
uremic colitis
uremic coma
uremic encephalopathy, acute
uremic frost
uremic medullary cystic disease
  (UMCD) complex
uremic myopathy
uremic neuropathy
uremic neuropathy/myopathy
uremic pericarditis
uremic poisoning
uremic solutes
uremic syndrome, hemolytic
uresiesthesia
uresis
ureter
  abdominal part of
  angulation of
  atonic
  bifid
  circumcaval
  construction of intestinal
  crushing of
  curlicue
  dilation of
  dilated
  distal right
  ectatic
  ectopic
  extraperitoneal excision of lower
    one-third of
  fishhook appearance of
  hook-shaped
  ileal
  intramural portion of distal ureter
  intravesical
  J-hook deformity of distal
  kinked
  kinking of
  left
  looped
  lower pole
  moderately dilated
  mucosa of
  muscular layer of
  native dilated
  occlusion of
  orthotopic
  partial obstruction of
  polyp of

ureter *(cont.)*
- postcaval
- retrocaval
- retroiliac
- right
- rigid
- scar tissue in
- stenotic
- stone disintegration in
- straight
- stricture of
- tenderness over
- tortuosity of
- tortuous
- tuberculosis of
- upper pole

ureter adhesions
ureter and kidney tenderness
ureter calculus
ureter constriction
ureter kinking
ureter location
ureter placement
ureteral achalasia
ureteral advancement
ureteral bougie
ureteral branch
ureteral bud, accessory
ureteral bud bifurcation
ureteral calculi in pregnancy
ureteral calculus
ureteral catheter
ureteral catheter with an olive-shaped tip
ureteral catheterization
ureteral colic
ureteral compression, extrinsic
ureteral compression technique
ureteral continuity
ureteral dilation
- segmental
- total

ureteral dissection
ureteral distention
ureteral division
ureteral duplication, bilaterality of
ureteral ectasia
ureteral ectopia
ureteral electromyogram (EMG)
ureteral endometriosis
ureteral endoscopy
ureteral filling
ureteral filling defect
ureteral fistula
ureteralgia
ureteral hypoperistalsis during pregnancy
ureteral illuminating catheter
ureteral insertion
ureteral lithiasis
ureteral meatotomy
ureteral notching
ureteral obstruction
- bilateral (BUO)
- functional

ureteral obstruction by calculi
ureteral occlusion
ureteral opening
ureteral orifice
ureteral pelvis
ureteral peristalsis
ureteral reflux
ureteral reflux imaging
ureteral reflux study
ureteral segment, aperistaltic distal
ureteral smooth muscle
ureteral stasis
ureteral stenosis
ureteral stent (see *stent*)
ureteral stent placement
ureteral stimulator
ureteral stone
ureteral stone extraction
ureteral stone lithotripsy
ureteral stricture
ureteral vascular compromise
ureteral-vesical reflux
ureteral wall

ureterectasia
ureterectasis
ureterectomy
ureteric branch
ureteric branches of the inferior
  suprarenal artery
ureteric branches of the ovarian artery
ureteric branches of the patent part
  of umbilical artery
ureteric branches of the renal artery
ureteric branches of the testicular artery
ureteric dilation
ureteric dysmenorrhea
ureteric fold
ureteric obstruction
ureteric orifice
ureteric pelvis
ureteric peristalsis
ureteric polyp
ureteric stone
ureteris, mons
ureteritis
ureteritis cystica
ureterocaliceal anastomosis
ureterocalicostomy
ureterocele
  ectopic
  orthotopic
ureterocelorraphy
ureterocervical fistula
ureterocervical fistulectomy
ureterocolic
ureterocolostomy
ureterocutaneous fistula
ureterocystoplasty
ureterocystoscope
ureterocystostomy
ureteroenteric
ureteroenterostomy
ureterogram, retrograde
ureterography, retrograde
ureterohydronephrosis
ureteroileal anastomosis
ureteroileal conduit
ureteroileal loop, Cordonnier
ureteroileocutaneous anastomosis
ureteroileoneocystostomy
ureteroileostomy
  Bricker
  cutaneous
ureterointestinal anastomosis
  Coffey
  Higgins technique for
ureterolithiasis, left
ureterolithotomy
ureterolysis
ureteroneocystostomy
ureteronephrectomy
ureteropathy
ureteropelvic (UP) junction
ureteropelvic junction (UPJ) obstruction
ureteropelvic obstruction, congenital
ureteropexy
ureteroplasty
ureteroplication
ureteroproctostomy
ureteropyelitis
ureteropyelogram, retrograde
ureteropyelography, retrograde
ureteropyeloscope (see also *endoscope*)
  AUR
  DUR
  flexible
  Karl Storz flexible
  Gautier
ureteropyelostomy
ureteropyosis
ureterorectostomy
ureterorenal reflux
ureterorenoscopy
  flexible retrograde
  rigid
ureterorrhagia
ureterorrhaphy
ureteroscope (see also *endoscope*)
  AUR-7 flexible
  flexible
  Gautier

ureteroscope *(cont.)*
  Karl Storz flexible
  MRD-6 micro
  rigid
  semirigid
  Wolf
ureteroscopic stone removal
ureteroscopy
ureterosigmoid
ureterosigmoid anastomosis
ureterosigmoidostomy
ureterostenosis
ureterostomy
  cutaneous
  cutaneous intubated
  cutaneous loop
  loop cutaneous
  tube
ureterotomy
ureterotrigonoenterostomy
ureteroureteral anastomosis
ureteroureterostomy
ureterovaginal fistula
ureterovesical junction (UVJ),
  competence of
ureterovesical obstruction
ureterovesical orifice
ureterovesical prosthesis
ureterovesical reflux
ureterovesicostomy
ureterovesiculoplasty
urethra
  angle of inclination of
  anterior
  blocked
  bulbous
  distal
  distal part of prostatic
  female
  hypermobile
  intermediate part of
  male
  membranous
  mucosa of

urethra *(cont.)*
  muscular layer of
  muscular layer of spongy
  navicular fossa of
  nontraumatic rupture of
  patent
  pendulous
  penile
  polyp of
  posterior
  prostatic
  prostatomembranous
  proximal
  proximal part of prostatic
  ruptured
  shortening of
  spongy
urethrae, sphincter
urethral abscess
urethral and vesical neck damage
urethral artery
urethral atresia
urethral bulking agent
urethral burning
urethral calculus
urethral calibration
urethral carcinoma
urethral caruncle
urethral catheter
urethral cause of urinary incontinence
urethral compression and stability
  of bladder base
urethral crest
urethral cyst
urethral damage
urethral dilation
urethral dilation
urethral discharge
urethral diverticulectomy
urethral diverticulum
urethral drainage
urethral false passage
urethral fever
urethral fistula

urethral flora
urethral fluid
urethral gland
urethral gland abscess
urethral glands of female
urethral glands of male
urethral gonorrhea
urethral granuloma
urethral groove
urethral hair
urethral hematuria
urethral hypermobility
urethral induration
urethral injury
urethral instrumentation
urethral lacuna
urethral marking ring
urethral meatoplasty
urethral meatotomy
urethral meatus
urethral meatus ulcer
urethral obstruction
  congenital valve
  meatal stenosis
  stricture
urethral opening
urethral orifice of bladder
urethral papilla
urethral perforation
urethral plate
urethral plication
urethral plug, Avina female
urethral pressure profile study
urethral prolapse
urethral septum
urethral sling (see also *sling*)
  Aldridge-Studdiford
  autologous
  bioabsorbable
  BioSling
  Bio-Vascular remodelable tissue
  bulbar
  bulbourethral
  Cook Stratasis

urethral sling *(cont.)*
  implantable
  in situ
  in vivo
  laparoscopic
  modified bulbar
  REMEEX
  SIS (small intestine submucosal)
    technology
  SPARC
  Stratasis
  suburethral
  takedown of
  transpelvic
  TVT (tension-free vaginal tape)
    modified
  Veritas
  Vesica
urethral sound
urethral sounding
urethral sphincter deficiency
urethral sphincter electromyogram
urethral stenosis
urethral stent
urethral stricture
  acquired
  bulbar
  bulbomembranous
  bulbous
  congenital
  pendulous
  postcatheterization
  postobstetric
  postoperative
  traumatic
urethral stricture disease
urethral surgical reconstruction
urethral suspension (see *urethral sling*)
urethral swabbing
urethral syndrome
urethral tear
urethral trauma
urethral tube graft
urethral valve

urethral wall, saclike outpouching of
urethralgia
urethralis, anulus
urethrectomy
urethremorrhagia
urethrism
urethrismus
urethritis
  anterior
  bacterial
  follicular
  gonococcal
  gonorrheal
  granular
  nongonococcal
  nonspecific (NSU)
  nonsymptomatic
  posterior
  proximal
  simple
urethro-oculoarticular syndrome
urethrobulbar
urethrocele
urethrocutaneous fistula
urethrocystocele
urethrocystogram
urethrocystography
  retrograde
  voiding (VCU)
urethrocystometrography
urethrocystopexy
urethrocystoscopy
urethrodynia
urethrogram, retrograde
urethrography, retrograde
urethroileal anastomosis
urethrolysis
urethrometer
urethro-ocular articular syndrome
urethropenile
urethroperineal fistula
urethroperineoscrotal
urethroperineovesical fistula
urethropexy
  Burch retropubic
  retropubic
  Schwartz-Pregenzer
  Tudor "rabbit ear"
urethroplasty
  Cecil
  dorsal onlay graft
  Polytef augmentation
  Thiersch-Duplay
  Turner-Warwick
urethroprostatic
urethrorectal
urethrorectal fistula
urethrorrhagia
urethrorrhea
urethroscope
urethroscopic
urethroscopy, perineal
urethroscrotal fistula
urethrospasm
urethrostaxis
urethrostenosis
urethrostomy through the perineum
urethrostomy, perineal
urethrotome, Otis
urethrotomy
  direct-vision internal (DVIU)
  external
  internal
  perineal
urethrotrigonitis
urethrovaginal fistula
urethrovaginal sphincter
urethrovesical angle (UVA)
urethrovesical fistula
urethrovesical junction
urethrovesicopexy
urethrovesicovaginal fistula
urge incontinence
urgent dialysis
urge urinary incontinence
urgency incontinence

urgency, severe
uric acid
uric acid level
uric acid lithiasis
uric acid nephrolithiasis
uric acid nephropathy
uricosuria
uricosuric drugs
Uricult dipslides
uridine diphosphate glucuronosyltransferase deficiency
urinalysis (UA)
  automated manual dipstick
  chromatographic
  clean-catch
  cytometric
  first-voided
  immunoassay
  midstream
  routine
  spun clean-catch
  24-hour
  Yellow IRIS
urinary 5-HIAA
urinary 17-hydroxycorticosteroid
urinary 3-methylhistidine
urinary aldosterone
urinary aldosterone level
urinary amino acids
urinary amylase
urinary antiseptic medication
urinary apparatus
urinary bladder
  anterior wall of
  apex of
  dome of
  epithelium of
  fundus of
  lateral wall of
  peak flow of
  posterior wall of
  removal of
  trigone of
urinary blood
urinary burning
urinary calcium excretion
urinary calculus
urinary carcinogen
urinary cast
urinary catecholamines
urinary citrate
urinary clot
urinary clot retention
urinary collecting system
urinary concentrating capacity
urinary concentration test
urinary conduit
urinary creatinine
urinary cyst
urinary diversion
  internal
  permanent
  supravesical
urinary diversion procedure for intestinal urinary conduit
urinary drainage bag
urinary electrolytes
urinary eosinophils
urinary erythrocyte volume
urinary exertional incontinence
urinary extravasation
urinary fever
urinary fistula
urinary flow rate
urinary formed elements
urinary free cortisol
urinary frequency
urinary glucose
urinary hesitancy
urinary incontinence (see *incontinence*)
urinary incontinence device (see also *incontinence device*)
  Aldridge-Studdiford urethral sling
  AlloSling
  Autocath 100 bladder-control
  autologous urethral sling
  Avina female urethral plug
  barrier

urinary incontinence device *(cont.)*
bioabsorbable urethral
BioSling urethral sling
BioVascular remodelable tissue urethral sling
bulbar urethral sling
bulbourethral sling
CapSure shield
collagen injection
continence ring
Cook incontinence ring
Cook Stratasis urethral sling
Dumontpallier pessary
Duth pessary
Emmet-Gelhorn pessary
fascial sling
fascia lata suburethral sling
fat injection
female incontinence ring
FemSoft insert
Findley folding pessary
FortaPerm surgical sling
Gariel pessary
Gelhorn pessary
Guhrung pessary
Gynecare TVT (tension-free vaginal tape)
Hodge pessary
implantable urethral sling
Impress Softpatch foam pad
incontinence ring
InnoSense sling
in situ urethral sling
InterStim implantable continence-control therapy
Introl bladder neck support prosthesis
in vivo urethral sling
laparoscopic urethral sling
levator muscle sling
Macroplastique implantable
Mayer pessary
Medworks
Menge pessary

urinary *(cont.)*
Miniguard
modified bulbar urethral sling
musculofascial sling
NeoControl
pessary
Prentif pessary
Prochownik pessary
ProteGen vaginal sling
PTFE (polytetrafluoroethylene) suburethral sling
pubococcygeal sling
pubovaginal sling
Raz sling
Reliance Urinary Control Insert
REMEEX urethral sling
ring pessary
SANS (Stoller afferent nerve stimulation)
SPARC urethral sling
stiff ring
Stoller afferent nerve stimulation (SANS)
Straight-In male sling
Stratasis urethral sling
Suarez continence ring
suburethral fascial sling
SurgiSis pubourethral sling
SurgiSis sling-mesh
Suspend sling
TriAngle sling
triangular vaginal patch
TVT (tension-free vaginal tape) modified urethral sling
transpelvic urethral sling
UltraSling
urethral sling
UroMed incontinence patch
Veritas urethral sling
Vesica urethral sling
woven sling
Zwanck pessary
Z-stitch bladder neck stabilization

urinary incontinence treatment (see also *incontinence treatment*)
- Acutrainer
- Antibacterial Personal Catheter
- appendicovesicotomy
- AS-800 artificial sphincter
- bladder neck support prosthesis
- Camey reservoir
- Camey supravesical bowel urinary diversion
- Contigen glutaraldehyde cross-linked collagen injection
- Cunningham clamp for male urinary incontinence
- Ditropan XL (oxybutynin chloride)
- Duke continent urinary diversion
- Durasphere injectable bulking agent
- estrogen replacement therapy (ERT)
- fascia lata suburethral sling
- FemSoft insert
- Florida pouch
- fria
- glutaraldehyde cross-linked collagen injections
- ileal conduit
- ileal neobladder
- Indiana pouch
- Innova home therapy system
- intrinsic sphincter deficiency
- Introl bladder neck support prosthesis
- InVance male sling procedure
- laparoscopic urinary diversion procedure
- LeBag reservoir
- LeDuc anastomosis
- Macroplastique implant
- Mainz pouch urinary reservoir
- Mitrofanoff appendicovesicotomy
- Neocontrol
- Nichol vaginal suspension procedure
- On-Command catheters
- pelvic floor electrical stimulation (PFS)

urinary *(cont.)*
- Penn pouch
- percutaneous bladder neck stabilization (PBNS)
- periurethral collagen injection
- promontofixation
- Protect-a-Pass suture passer
- PTFE (polytetrafluoroethylene) suburethral sling material
- Raz sling operation
- Reliance urinary control insert
- Repliform
- ROC and ROC XS suture fasteners
- Straight-In surgical system
- Stratasis urethral sling
- suburethral sling procedure
- SurgiSis sling/mesh
- Suspend sling implant
- Teflon paste injection for incontinence
- transurethral collagen injection
- transvaginal suturing (TVS) system
- Triangle gelatin-sealed sling material
- triangular vaginal patch sling
- TVT (tension-free vaginal tape) procedure
- UCLA pouch
- urethral surgical reconstruction
- urinary diversion procedure
- UroVive balloon system
- vaginal wall sling procedure
- Vesica percutaneous bladder neck stabilization kit
- W-stapled urinary reservoir
- Z-stitch

urinary ketones

urinary leakage

urinary leakage with stress

urinary lithiasis

urinary meatus stricture

urinary metanephrine

urinary mucosa

urinary obstruction

urinary organs

urinary osmolality
urinary output
urinary pathogen
urinary pH
urinary potassium
urinary precipitancy
urinary prosthesis (see *urinary incontinence devices*)
urinary protein loss
urinary reservoir, W-stapled
urinary retention
urinary sediment
urinary sediment cytology
urinary sediment examination
urinary smear
urinary sodium excretion
urinary sodium wastage
urinary solute excretion
urinary sphincter, artificial
urinary sphincter mechanism
urinary sphincter muscle
urinary sphincter resistance
urinary stasis
urinary stone
urinary stream, intermittent
urinary stress incontinence
urinary stuttering
urinary system
urinary tenesmus
urinary tract
urinary tract anatomy
urinary tract anomaly
urinary tract calculus
urinary tract epithelial neoplasia
urinary tract fistula
urinary tract infection (UTI)
  bacterial
  lower
  recurrent
  relapsing
  superimposed
  upper
urinary tract inflammation
urinary tract neoplasia
urinary tract obstruction
urinary tract stone
urinary tract symptoms
urinary traction
urinary tract, irrigation of
urinary tumor
urinary ulcer
urinary VMA (vanillylmandelic acid)
urinary volume, reduction of
urination
  burning on
  copious
  force of
  frequency of
  frequent
  involuntary
  painful
  precipitant
  strength of
  stuttering
urination journal
urine
  acid
  alkaline
  a.m.
  ammoniacal
  appearance of
  bacilli in
  black
  blood in
  blood-tinged
  bloody
  brick dust
  casts in
  chylous
  clean-catch
  clean-voided
  clean-voided midstream
  cloudy
  Coca-Cola
  concentrated
  crude
  dark
  diabetic

urine *(cont.)*
- double-voided
- double-voided a.m.
- dyspeptic
- excretion of
- excretion of acid in
- febrile
- fetal
- feverish
- first a.m.
- first morning
- freshly voided
- frothy
- glucose in
- gouty
- hypotonic
- incontinence of
- involuntary discharge of
- ketones in
- large residual of
- leakage of
- maple syrup
- milky
- morning
- nebulous
- occult blood in
- postvoid residual
- production of
- protein in
- radiopaque
- red blood cells in
- residual
- retained
- seepage of
- smoky
- stat
- strain all
- strained
- straining at
- sugar in
- telescopic
- turbid
- 24-hour

urine *(cont.)*
- voided
- white blood cells in

urine bilirubin
urine cortisol
urine creatinine
urine creatinine/serum creatinine ratio
urine culture, quantitative
urine cytology
urine dipstick
urine discharge during sleep, involuntary
urine effluent
urine flow
urine formation, absence
urine-free cortisol
urine incubation
urine leakage with coughing, sneezing, or laughter
urine loss
urine osmolality
urine output
urine output variations
urine pH
urine potassium
urine production in excess of 30 mL/h
urine protein electrophoresis
urine reflux
urine sediment
- abnormal
- stained

urine smear
urine solute concentration
urine stream
urine urobilinogen
urine vanillylmandelic acid (VMA) and catecholamine excretion
urine volume
uriniferous
uriniferous tubule
urinific
uriniparous
urinogenital

urinogenous
urinoma
urinometer
urinometry
urinoscopy
urinosexual
urinous
uriposia
URiprobe test
Uriscreen urine specimen test
Urised (methenamine; phenyl salicylate; atropine sulfate; methylene blue; hyoscyamine; benzoic acid)
UriSite microalbumin/creatinine urine test
Uristat Urinary Pain Relief
Uri-Test
uroammoniac
urobilin
urobilinogen
urobilinuria
urocanic aciduria
urocele
urochesia
UroCoil self-expanding urethral stent
UroCoS (uroporphyrinogen cosynthase)
urocyanin
urocyanosis
urocyst
urocystic
urocystis
Urocyte diagnostic cytometry system
urocytogram
urodynamic assessment
urodynamic loop catheter
urodynamic pressure/flow studies
urodynamics
urodynia
uroflowmeter
uroflowmetry
urofollitropin
urofuscohematin
urogenital aging
urogenital apparatus
urogenital cleft
urogenital diaphragm
urogenital duct
urogenital fistula
urogenital membrane
urogenital peritoneum
urogenital region
urogenital ridge
urogenital septum
urogenital sinus
urogenital sinus anomaly
urogenital system
urogenital triangle
urogenous pyelitis
urogonadotropin
Urografin-76
Urografin 290 imaging agent
urogram
  excretory
  intravenous (IVU)
urography
  antegrade
  cystoscopic
  excretory
  intravenous
  magnetic resonance (MRU)
  retrograde
urogravimeter
urogynecologist
urohematoporphyrin
uroheparin
urohypertensin
urolagnia
Urolase fiber visual laser ablation of prostate
urolith
urolithiasis, calcium oxalate
urolithic
urolithology
urological
urologic evaluation
urologic history
urologic imaging
urologic investigation

Urologic Targis transurethral thermo-ablation system
urologist
urology
Uroloop electrosurgical device
UroLume endoprosthesis
UroLume endoprosthesis wire stent
UroLume flow-directed microcatheter
UroLume stent
UroLume Wallstent
UroMax II catheter
UroMax II urethral balloon catheter
UroMed incontinence patch
uromelanin
uroncus
uropathy, obstructive
urophanic
urophein
uropoiesis
uropoietic
uroporphyria, erythropoietic
uroporphyrinogen cosynthase (UroCoS)
UroQuest On-Command catheter
uroradiology
urorectal
urorubrohematin
UROS bladder infusion system
uroschesis
uroscopic
uroscopy
urosemiology
urosepsis
urothelial cancer
urothelial carcinoma
urothelial carcinoma in situ
urothelial cell sediment
urothelial neoplasia, preinvasive
urothelial striations
urothelial tumor
urothelium
urothorax
Urovist Cysto imaging agent
Urovist Meglumine imaging agent
Urovist Sodium imaging agent
UroVive balloon treatment for urinary stress incontinence
UroVive intrinsic sphincter deficiency therapy
Urowave microwave thermotherapy device
UroXatral (alfuzosin)
URR (urea reduction ratio)
urticaria neonatorum
US (ultrasound)
USA series hysteroscope
U.S. Food and Drug Administration (FDA)
U-shaped incision
usher syndrome
USPHS (United States Public Health Service)
uteri
  cervix
  descensus
  leiomyomata
  myomatous
  os
uterine adenomyosis
uterine adnexa
uterine anomaly
uterine appendage
uterine arteries were skeletonized
uterine artery
uterine artery embolization (UAE) procedure
uterine atony
uterine balloon therapy (UBT)
uterine band
uterine bleeding
  abnormal (AUB)
  diminished
  dysfunctional
  irregular
uterine calculus
uterine cancer
uterine cavity
uterine cervix
uterine cervix carcinoma

uterine chondrosarcoma
uterine cirsoid aneurysm
uterine clots
uterine colic
uterine contraction
  frequent
  hypertonic
  incoordinate
  intense
  irregular
  light
  painless
  prolonged
  regular
uterine cornual access catheter (UCAC)
uterine corpus
uterine corpus carcinoma
uterine cramps
uterine cry
uterine cul-de-sac
uterine curette
uterine curettings
uterine descensus
uterine didelphia
uterine didelphys
uterine dilation, progressive
uterine distention
uterine distention medium
uterine dressing forceps
uterine dysmenorrhea
uterine dyssynergia
uterine dystocia
uterine elevation
uterine elevator
uterine endometriosis
uterine endometrium
uterine enlargement from fibroids
uterine evacuation
uterine factor
uterine fibroid, pedunculated
uterine fistula
uterine fundus
uterine gland
uterine hemorrhage
uterine horn
uterine hypertrophy
uterine hypoplasia
uterine hypotonia
uterine impression on bladder
uterine inertia
uterine inhibitor
uterine insufficiency
uterine inversion
uterine involution
uterine irregularity
uterine laceration
uterine leiomyoma
uterine leiomyosarcoma, right atrial extension of
uterine ligament
uterine lining, scarring of
uterine manipulator/injector
  acorn
  Harris-Kronner uterine manipulator injector (HUMI)
  Kronner Manipujector
  Majoli
  RUMI
  Valtchev
  Zinnanti uterine manipulator injector (ZUMI)
uterine massage
uterine mobilization
uterine mobilizer
  Hulka
  Valtchev
uterine morcellation
uterine mucous membrane
uterine muscular wall pregnancy
uterine myoma (pl. myomata)
uterine neck
uterine opening of uterine tubes
uterine ostial access catheter (UOAC)
uterine part of uterine tube
uterine pedicle
uterine perforation
uterine peritoneal covering
uterine peritoneum

uterine polyp
uterine positioning via ligament investment fixation and truncation (UPLIFT) procedure
uterine pregnancy
uterine preservation
uterine prolapse
  complete
  first degree
  second degree
  severe
  third degree
uterine resectoscope
uterine retroflexion
uterine rupture
uterine scar
uterine septectomy
uterine septum
uterine softening
uterine souffle
uterine sound
uterine stent (see *stent*)
uterine subinvolution
uterine surface of discoidal placenta
uterine suspension
uterine tear
uterine tenderness
uterine tetanus
uterine tetany
uterine tilt
uterine tone
uterine-tubal junction
uterine tube
  ampulla of
  ampullary folds of
  infundibulum of
  muscular layer of
  uterine part of
  vesicular appendices of
uterine tumor
uterine veins
uteroabdominal pregnancy
uterocervical
uterocystostomy
uterogram
uterography
uterolith
uterometer
utero-ovarian ligament
utero-ovarian varicocele
uteroparietal
uteropelvic
uteroperitoneal fistula
uteropexy
uteroplacental apoplexy
uteroplacental circulation
uteroplacental insufficiency
uteroplacental perfusion
uteroplacental vasoconstriction
uteroplasty
uterorectal fistula
uterosacral ligament
uterosalpingography
uteroscope
uteroscopy
uterotonic
uterotropic
uterotubal insufflation
uterotubal pregnancy
uterotubography
uteroureteric fistula
uterovaginal fistula
uterovaginal plexus
uterovaginal prolapse, incomplete
uteroventral
uterovesical fistula
uterovesical fold
uterovesical ligament
uterovesical pouch
uterus (pl. uteri)
  anomalous
  anteflexed
  anterior lip of
  anteversion of
  anteverted
  aplastic
  arcuate
  atonic

uterus *(cont.)*
- atony of
- band of
- bicameral
- bicornate
- bicornis
- bicornuate
- bifid
- biforate
- bilocular
- bimanual abdominorectal palpation of
- bimanual abdominovaginal palpation of
- bipartite
- body of
- boggy
- border of
- cervical glands of
- cervix of
- cochleate
- consistency of
- cordiform
- cornu of
- Couvelaire
- didelphic
- double
- double-mouthed
- duplex
- empty
- endometriosis of
- external os of
- fetal
- fibroid
- firm
- fluid-filled mass in
- fundus of
- Gilliam suspension of
- gravid
- heart-shaped
- helicine artery of
- hemi-
- horn of
- hourglass

uterus *(cont.)*
- hourglass contraction of
- incarcerated gravid
- incudiform
- infantile
- inversion of
- inverted
- inverted pear-shaped
- involuted
- isthmus of
- large for dates
- lateral angle of
- malposition of
- masculine
- midposition
- mobile
- mobility of
- multiparous
- myomatous
- neck of
- normal-size
- one-horned
- opening of
- orifice of
- outline of
- pear-shaped
- position of
- posterior lip of
- postpartum subinvoluted
- pregnant
- prolapse of
- prolapse of gravid
- prostatic
- pubescent
- retroflexed
- retroflexion of
- retroversion of
- retroverted
- retroverted gravid
- ribbon
- round ligament of
- rupture of
- saddle-shaped
- septate

uterus *(cont.)*
serosa of
size of
slightly retroflexed
soft
spongy
subseptate
symmetrical
tender
tipped
triangular
unicorn
unicornuate
uterus acollis
uterus amputated at the lower uterine segment
uterus anteverted, anteflexed
uterus bicornis
uterus didelphys
uterus exteriorized
uterus freely mobile
uterus normal in size, shape, and consistency
uterus normal in size, shape, and contour
uterus-to-abdominal wall fistula
UTI (urinary tract infection)
U-Titer
utricle, prostatic
utricular cyst
utricular opening
UV (ureterovesical) junction
UVA (urethrovesical angle)
UVC (umbilical vein catheter)
UVJ (ureterovesical junction)
UVR (universal vacuum release)
UVS (umbilical venous catheter)
uvula of bladder

V, v

Vabra aspiration
Vabra aspirator
Vabra cannula
Vabra curet or curette
VAB-6 chemotherapy protocol for testicular cancer
VAC (vinblastine, actinomycin D, Cytoxan) chemotherapy protocol
VACA (vinblastine, actinomycin D, Cytoxan, Adriamycin) chemotherapy protocol
VACAD (vincristine, Adriamycin, Cytoxan, actinomycin D, dacarbizine) chemotherapy protocol
vaccine
  AIDSvax
  Avicine therapeutic cancer
  chickenpox
  DT (diphtheria-tetanus)
  DTaP or DTP (diphtheria, tetanus, and pertussis)
  DTP (diphtheria-tetanus-pertussis)
  hepatitis B (HBV)
  Hib (*Haemophilus influenzae*)
  IPV (inactivated polio vaccine)
  JT1001 prostate cancer
  measles-mumps-rubella (MMR)
  O-Vax therapeutic

vaccine *(cont.)*
  pneumococcal
  polio
  Provenge vaccine
  Ovarex vaccine
  TheraCys (BCG live)
  therapeutic cancer
  varicella (chickenpox)
VACP (VePesid, Adriamycin, Cytoxan, Platinol) chemotherapy protocol
VACTERL (vertebral anomalies, anal atresia, congenital cardiac disease, tracheoesophageal fistula, renal anomalies, radial dysplasia, and other limb defects) syndrome
VacuLink vascular access graft
vacuolar nephrosis
vacuolization of renal tubules
Vacurette suction curet
vacuum aspiration abortion
vacuum aspirator-cannula
vacuum-assisted delivery
vacuum-assisted vaginal delivery
vacuum delivery
vacuum delivery system, Mityvac
vacuum erection device (VED)
Vacuum Erection Technology (V.E.T.)
vacuum extraction delivery

vacuum extractor
  Bird
  CMI
  Malmstrom
  Mityvac
  Murless
  O'Neil
vacuum forceps
vacuum marks
vacuum pump, CMI
vacuum-type breast pump
VAD (vincristine, Adriamycin, dexamethasone) chemotherapy protocol
VAD/V (vincristine, Adriamycin, dexamethasone, verapamil) chemotherapy protocol
VAG (vascular access graft)
Vagifem vaginal tablets (estradiol hemihydrate)
Vagi-Guard douche
vagina (pl. vaginae)
  anterior fornix of
  anterior part of
  anterior wall of
  apex of
  azygos artery of
  bipartite
  clear cell adenocarcinoma of
  congenital absence of
  distended
  double
  elastic
  expulsion of gas from
  fornices of
  fornix of
  highly vascular
  mucosa of
  muscular layer of
  narrowness of
  parous
  posterior wall
  septate
  spongy layer of
  stenotic

vagina *(cont.)*
  stenosis of
  stricture of
  surgical creation of functional
  thin-walled
  vestibule of
  well-epithelialized
vagina dentata
vaginal aplasia
vaginal-abdominal approach in surgery
vaginal adenosis
vaginal agenesis
vaginal apex
vaginal approach in gynecologic surgery
vaginal approach in surgery
vaginal artery
vaginal atresia
vaginal atrophy
vaginal birth
vaginal birth after cesarean (VBAC)
vaginal bleeding
vaginal breech delivery, failed
vaginal burning
vaginal candidiasis
vaginal candle
vaginal carcinoma
vaginal celiotomy
vaginal cellulitis
vaginal-cervical Ahluwalia retractor-elevator (VCARE)
vaginal cesarean section
vaginal column
vaginal conduit
vaginal condyloma
vaginal cone irradiation
vaginal constriction ring
vaginal construction technique
  Abbe-McIndoe
  colocolponeopoiesis
  Davydov
  Frank and McIndoe
  Frank nonsurgical perineal autodilation

vaginal construction *(cont.)*
McCraw gracilis myocutaneous flap
McIndoe
split-flap
Williams vulvovaginoplasty
Yang-Monti
vaginal contraceptive film (VCF)
vaginal cornification test
vaginal cuff
vaginal cuff cellulitis
vaginal cuff smear
vaginal culture
vaginal delivery (see *delivery*)
vaginal dilation
vaginal discharge
vaginal dome
vaginal douche (see *douche*)
vaginal dysmenorrhea
vaginal endometriosis
vaginal enterocele
vaginal eversion, massive
vaginal eversion repair
vaginal examination
vaginal fistula
vaginal flap
vaginal flap reconstruction of urethra and vesical neck
anterior bladder flap approach
posterior bladder flap approach
vaginal flap approach
vaginal flora
vaginal fornix (pl. fornices)
anterior
lateral part of
posterior part of
vaginal fundus
vaginal gland
vaginal hematoma
vaginal hysterectomy
vaginal hysterectomy and anterior repair
vaginal infection
vaginal intercourse
vaginal interruption of pregnancy, with dilation and curettage (VIP-DAC)
vaginal intraepithelial neoplasia
vaginal introitus
vaginal itching
vaginal laceration
vaginal lengthening
vaginal lithotomy
vaginal lubricant
vaginal lubrication
vaginal maturation index
vaginal microflora
vaginal mucification test
vaginal mucosa, triangular excision of redundant
vaginal muscle tear
vaginal myomectomy
vaginal nerves
vaginal orifice
vaginal outlet, relaxation of
vaginal pack
vaginal packing
vaginal pad
vaginal pain
vaginal part of cervix
vaginal pessary, elastic
vaginal plexus
vaginal pool
vaginal portion of procedure
vaginal prolapse
vaginal protrusion
vaginal reconstruction (see *vaginal construction)*
vaginal relaxation
vaginal replacement
vaginal ring, Estring (estradiol-loaded silicone vaginal ring)
vaginal secretions
vaginal septum
vaginal shortening
vaginal sling, FortaPerm
vaginal smear
vaginal speculum
vaginal sphincter
vaginal spotting
vaginal stenosis

vaginal stricture
vaginal suspension
vaginal tampon
vaginal tear
vaginal transducer
vaginal transudate
vaginal ultrasound
vaginal vault
vaginal vault prolapse
vaginal vestibule
vaginal wall
vaginal wall collapse
vaginal wall graft
vaginal wall hammock
vaginal wall plication
vaginal wall prolapse
vaginal wall scrapings
vaginal wall sling procedure
vaginal was well epithialized
vaginal yeast infection
vaginalis, tunica
vaginapexy
vagina rugous
vaginate
vagina was entered anteriorly
vagina well epithelialized
vaginectomy
  complete
  partial
  partial upper
vaginism
vaginismus
  acquired-type
  functional
  generalized-type
  lifelong-type
  posterior
  psychogenic
  situational-type
vaginismus due to combined factors
vaginismus due to psychological factors
vaginitis (pl. vaginitides)
  adhesive
  atrophic
vaginitis *(cont.)*
  bacterial
  Candida
  candidal
  desquamative inflammatory
  emphysematous
  foreign body
  Gardnerella
  granular
  nonspecific
  pinworm
  postirradiation
  postmenopausal atrophic
  radiation
  senile
  trichomonal
  trichomoniasis
vaginoabdominal
vaginocele
vaginodynia
vaginofixation
vaginogram
vaginohysterectomy
vaginolabial
vaginomycosis
vaginopathy
vaginoperineal fistula
vaginoperineoplasty
vaginoperineorrhaphy
vaginoperineotomy
vaginoperitoneal
vaginopexy
vaginoplasty
vaginoscopy
vaginosis, bacterial (BV)
vaginotomy
vaginovesical
vaginovesical fistula
vaginovulvar
Vagisec Plus vaginal suppositories
Vagistat (tioconazole)
vagitus uterinus
VAI (vincristine, actinomycin D, ifosfamide) chemotherapy protocol

valacyclovir
valdecoxib
Valentine position for urethral irrigation
Valergen (estradiol)
Valergen 20 (estradiol)
Valergen 40 (estradiol)
valgus calcaneus (clubfoot)
valinemia
valine transaminase deficiency
Valle hysteroscope
ValleyLab laparoscopic and electrosurgical instruments
VALOP-B (etoposide, doxorubicin, cyclophosphamide, vincristine, prednisone, bleomycin)
valrubicin
Valertest No. 1
valproate fetal
Valsalva maneuver
valsartan and hydrochlorothiazide
Valstar (valrubicin)
Valtchev uterine manipulator
Valtchev uterine mobilizer
Valtrex (valacyclovir)
valve
  anterior urethral
  failed nipple
  posterior urethral
  stenotic but patent tricuspid
  Tuohy-Borst
  urethral
valve infusion port
VAM (VP-16, Adriamycin, methotrexate) chemotherapy protocol
van Andel catheter
Van Buren sound
Van Buren urethral bougie
vancomycin-resistant enterococcus
van der Hoeve-Habertsma-Waardenburg-Gauldi syndrome
van Heuven anatomic classification of diabetic retinopathy
Vaniqa
vanished testis syndrome
vanishing twin phenomenon
vanishing twin syndrome
Vantage Graves vaginal speculum
Vantin (cefpodoxime proxetil)
VaporTrode roller electrode
vardenafil
variable expression
variable expression of X-linked recessive disorders
variable number of tandem repeats (VNTR)
variability
  baseline
  beat-to-beat
  deceleration
variable decelerations
variable fetal heart rate deceleration
variable penetrance
variation
varicella
varicella vaccine
varices (sing. varix)
  pelvic
  perineal
  prostatic
  umbilical cord
  vulvar
varicocele
  ovarian
  symptomatic
  tubo-ovarian
  utero-ovarian
varicocele ligation
varicocelectomy
varicomphalus
varicophlebitis
varicose veins
  perineal
  vulvar
varicosity (pl. varicosities)
  lower extremity
  pelvic
  vulvar
varicotomy

variety
VariSeed software for prostate brachytherapy
varix (pl. varices)
vas (pl. vasa)
vasa deferentia (plural of vas deferens)
vasa previa
Vas-Cath catheter
Vas-Cath Flexxicon II catheter
Vas-Cath Opti-Flow catheter
Vas-Cath Opti-Flow hemodialysis catheter
Vas-Cath Opti-Flow long-term dual-lumen hemodialysis catheter
Vas-Cath Soft-Cell catheter
Vas-Cath Soft-Cell permanent dual-lumen hemodialysis catheter
Vascufil suture
vascular access
vascular access graft (VAG)
vascular access thrombosis
vascular anastomosis
vascular anatomy
vascular anomaly
vascular birthmarks
vascular bundle
vascular clamp
vascular congestion
vascular endothelial cells
vascular endothelial growth factor (VEGF)
vascular layer of testis
vascular lesion
vascular lesion of cord
vascular malformations of brain
vascular nephritis
vascular nephropathy
vascular occlusion
vascular pedicle
vascular permeability
vascular proliferation
vascularity
  cervical
  tissue
vascularized omental and myocutaneous flaps
vasculitis
  renal
  small-vessel
vasculitis disease
vasculogenic loss of erectile functioning
Vascu-Sheath introducer
vas deferens (pl. vasa deferentia), artery to
vasectomy
  bilateral
  cross-over
  elective
  elective bilateral
  prophylactic
  recanalization
vasectomy reversal
Vaseline gauze dressing
vasitis
Vas MARQ male fertility test
vasoactive amines
vasoactive substances
vasocongestion of pelvis
Vasodilan (isoxsuprine)
vasodilation from sepsis
vasodilator drugs
vasoepididymal obstruction
  acquired
  congenital
vasoepididymostomy
Vasofem vaginal suppository
vasogram, contrast
vasography
vasoligation (see *vasectomy*)
Vasomax (phentolamine mesylate)
vasomotor instability in menopause
vasomotor symptoms related to menopause
vaso-orchidostomy
vasopermeability factor
vasopressin
vasopressin-resistant renal concentrating defect

vasopressin-sensitive diabetes insipidus
vasopressin stimulation
vasopressin tannate in oil
vasopressin test
vasopressor drip
vasospasm
vasospastic ischemia
vasotomy
vasovagal response
vasovasostomy
vasovasotomy
vasovesiculectomy
vastomy
VATER (vertebral defects, imperforate anus, tracheoesophageal fistula, renal defects) syndrome
vault, vaginal
VBAC (vaginal birth after cesarean [section])
VBMCP (vincristine, BCNU, melphalan, Cytoxan, prednisone) chemotherapy protocol
VBMF (vincristine, bleomycin, methotrexate, fluorouracil) chemotherapy protocol
VBP (vinblastine, bleomycin, cisplatin) chemotherapy protocol
VCARE (vaginal-cervical Ahluwalia retractor-elevator)
VCE (vagina, cervix, endocervix) smear
VCF (vaginal contraceptive film)
VCFS (velocardiofacial syndrome)
VCU (voiding urethrocystography)
VCUG (vesicoureterogram)
VCUG (voiding cystourethrogram)
VD (venereal disease)
VDRL (Venereal Disease Research Laboratory) diagnostic test for syphilis
vectis
vector
Vector, Vector X large-lumen guiding catheters
Vectra VAG (vascular access graft)
VED (vacuum erection device)
VEGF (vascular endothelial growth factor)
vein
  adrenal
  arterialization of
  axillary
  cephalic
  dilation of forearm
  femoral
  great suprarenal
  internal jugular
  internal pudendal
  internal spermatic
  left ovarian
  left testicular
  left umbilical
  lumbar
  posterior labial
  posterior scrotal
  renal
  right ovarian
  right testicular
  scrotal
  spermatic
  subclavian
  testicular
  umbilical
  uterine
  vesical
VeIP (vinblastine, ifosfamide, Platinol) chemotherapy protocol
Veit maneuver
velamentous insertion of umbilical cord
velamentous placenta
VELBNS (video-assisted extraperitoneal laparoscopic bladder neck suspension)
velocardiofacial syndrome (VCFS)
velocity, PSA
Velosulin BR insulin
vena (pl. venae)
vena cava, inferior

venacavography, inferior
Venaflo vascular graft
venereal arthritis
venereal condyloma
venereal disease (see *sexually transmitted disease*)
venereal disease phobia
Venereal Disease Research Laboratory (VDRL)
venereal lymphogranuloma
venereal proctocolitis
venereal sore
venereal ulcer
venereal warts
venereology
venereophobia
veneris, mons
venipuncture
Venofer (iron sucrose)
venogram
venography
veno-occlusive mechanism of corpora cavernosa
venous access device
venous circle of mammary gland
venous compression
venous drainage
venous flow controller, Actis
venous hum
venous leak dysfunction
venous leak syndrome
venous oozing
venous port
venous segments of the kidney
venous sinus
venovenous bridging via a filter
venovenous bypass
venovenous hemodialysis
ventilation
  bag and mask
  high frequency (HFV)
  positive-pressure (PPV)
  synchronized intermittent mandatory (SIMV)
ventilator
  BABYbird II
  Babyflex
  Bear Cub infant
  high frequency oscillating (HFOV)
  Infant Star
  Siemens Servo 300
  Siemens Servo 900C
ventilatory support, compromised
ventouse, delivery by
ventral apron prepuce
ventral chordee
ventral hernia
ventral hood, persistent
ventral penile foreskin
ventral strip anastomosis
ventral wall
ventricular dilation
ventricular septal defect (VSD)
ventriculoperitoneal (VP) shunt
Veress needle (*not* Verres)
Veridien umbilical clamp
Veritas urethral sling
vermis cerebellar agenesis
vernix, fetal
VerreScope microlaparoscope
Versadopp 10 Doppler ultrasound probe
VersaPoint coagulator
VersaPoint hysteroscopic fibroid removal device
Versaport trocar system
VersaPulse Select holmium laser
VersaTack stapler
version
  abdominal
  bimanual
  bipolar
  Braxton Hicks
  cephalic
  combined
  external
  external cephalic
  Hicks
  internal

version *(cont.)*
  internal cephalic
  internal podalic
  pelvic
  podalic
  postural
  Potter
  spontaneous
  Wigand
  Wright
vertex, ballotable
vertex delivery
vertex presentation
vertex was manually rotated
vertical bipedicle flap technique reduction mammoplasty
vertical fundal incision
vertical incision
vertical mastopexy
vertical midline Pfannenstiel incision
vertical reduction mammoplasty
veru (verumontanum)
verumontanitis
verumontanum
very low birth weight (VLBW) infant
very low density lipoprotein (VLDL)
Vesica percutaneous bladder neck stabilization kit
Vesica press-in anchor
Vesica sling kit
vesica urinaria
vesical artery
vesical calculus
vesical distention
vesical diverticulum
vesical dysfunction
vesical fistula
vesical gland
vesical hematuria
vesical lithotomy
vesical neck damage
vesical neck, elevation of
vesical outlet obstruction
vesical plexus
vesical stone formation
vesical triangle
vesical trigone
vesical veins
vesical venous plexus
vesicalis anus
vesicle hernia
vesicles, seminal
vesicoabdominal
vesicobullous eruptions
vesicocele
vesicocervical
vesicocervicovaginal fistula
vesicoclysis
vesicocolic fistula
vesicocutaneous fistula
vesicoenteric fistula
vesicointestinal fistula
vesicolithiasis
vesicolithotomy
vesicoperineal fistula
vesicoprostatic
vesicopsoas hitch procedure
vesicopubic
vesicopustular
vesicopustule
vesicorectal fistula
vesicorectostomy
vesicosigmoid
vesicosigmoidostomy
vesicosigmoidovaginal fistula
vesicospinal
vesicostomy, cutaneous
vesicotomy
vesicoumbilical ligament
vesicoureteral reflux (VUR)
  familial
  acquired
  congenital
vesicoureteral scintigraphy
vesicoureteric reflux (VUR)
vesicoureterine pouch
vesicoureterogram (VCUG)
vesicoureterovaginal fistula

vesicourethral anastomosis
vesicourethral angle
vesicourethral canal
vesicourethral orifice
vesicourethral suspension, Marshall-Marchetti-Krantz
vesicouterine fistula
vesicouterine ligament
vesicouterine peritoneal reflection
vesicouterine peritoneum
vesicouterine pouch
vesicouterovaginal
vesicovaginal fistula
vesicovaginal fistula repair
vesicovaginal lithotomy
vesicovaginal space
vesicovaginorectal fistula
vesicovisceral
vesicula (pl. vesiculae)
vesicular appendices of uterine tube
vesicular cystitis
vesicular mole
vesicular ovarian follicle
vesiculectomy, prostatoseminal
vesiculitis, seminal
vesiculopathy, seminal
vesiculoprostatitis
vesiculotomy
vessel
  aberrant
  atypical
  communicating
  inadvertent perforation of
  inferior epigastric
  thrombosis of cord
vessel loop
vessels were clamped, divided, and ligated
vessels were skeletonized
vestibular adenitis
vestibule
  vaginal
  vulvar
vestibulitis, focal vulvar
vestibulodynia
vestibulourethral
vestige of ductus deferens
vestige of processus vaginalis
vestige of vaginal process
vestigial
V.E.T. (Vacuum Erection Technology)
V gene
VHL tumor suppressor gene
viability, fetal
viable female infant
viable fetus
viable infant
viable male infant
viable pregnancy
viable sperm
Viadur (leuprolide implant)
Viagra (sildenafil citrate)
ViaSpan organ preservation solution
vibroacoustic stimulation
VIC (vinblastine, ifosfamide, CCNU) chemotherapy protocol
vicarious menstruation
vicious hyperemesis
Vicryl Rapide synthetic absorbable suture
VID (vitellointestinal duct)
VidaMed TUNA system
vidarabine
video-assisted extraperitoneal laparoscopic bladder neck suspension
video colposcope
videoendoscopic augmentation mammoplasty
videofetoscope
videofetoscopic technique
VideoHydro laparoscope
videolaparoscopic technique
videoresectoscope, Wolf
VIE (vincristine, ifosfamide, etoposide) chemotherapy protocol
view
  craniocaudal (of breast)
  mammographic
  retromammary space

villi, hydropic
villose
villous edema
villous placenta
villus (pl. villi)
VIN (vulvar intraepithelial neovaginal construction technique)
vinblastine
vinegar douche
Vioxx (rofecoxib)
VIP-B (VP-16, ifosfamide, Platinol, bleomycin) chemotherapy protocol
VIP-DAC (vaginal interruption of pregnancy, with dilation and curettage)
viral culture
viral cystitis
viral DNA polymerase
viral hepatitis
viral infection
viral replication
viral shedding
ViraPap human papillomavirus detection test
Virchow hydatid
virga
virgin
virgin generation
virginal introitus
virginity
Virgo ANCA (antineutrophil cytoplasmic antibodies) screen
Virgo cANCA assay
Virgo pANCA assay
virilism, adrenal
virilization
  drug-induced
  isosexual
virilizing tumor of adrenal origin
virilizing tumor of ovarian origin
virtual azoospermia
virtual labor monitor (VLM)
virus
  herpes simplex
  HIV-1E

virus *(cont.)*
  HMTV (human mammary tumor)
  HPV (human papillomavirus)
  human herpesvirus 6 (HHV-6)
  human mammary tumor (HMTV)
  lymphocytic choriomeningitis
  oncogenic
virus-host interaction
viscera
  abdominal
  adherence of
  pelvic
visceral peritoneum
visceral xanthogranulomatosis
viscous (adj.); viscus (noun)
viscus, hollow
viscus puncture
Visi-Black surgical needle
Visica fibroadenoma cryoablation system
Visicath cystoscope
Visidex, Visidex II blood glucose testing strips
Visilex mesh
Visipaque intravascular injection
Visipaque (iodixanol) nonionic contrast medium
Vistaflex biliary stent
visual amnesia
visualization
  direct
  excellent
  good
  inadequate
  poor
visual laser ablation of prostate (VLAP)
visual laser ablation of the trigone (VLAT)
visual response to light
vital signs monitor
vitamin
  Cenogen-OB prenatal formula
  Chromagen OB
  Pramet FA

vitamin *(cont.)*
  Pramilet FA
  prenatal
  Prenavite
  Stuart Prenatal
  water soluble
vitamin C
vitamin D intoxication
vitamin K deficiency of newborn
vitelline cord
vitelline duct
vitelline fistula
vitellointestinal duct (VID)
vitiligo
Vivelle (estradiol transdermal system)
Vivelle-Dot transdermal estrogen patch
Vivonex infant formula
VLAP (visual laser ablation of prostate)
VLAT (visual laser ablation of the trigone)
VLBW (very low birth weight) infant
VLDL (very low density lipoprotein)
V+Loop cutting electrode
VLM (virtual labor monitor)
VMA (vanillylmandelic acid), urine
VNTR (variable-number tandem-repeat)
VNTRs (single-stranded conformational polymorphism)
vocal cords, meconium aspiration below
Vocare bladder system
Vogt cephalosyndactyly
Vogt Kayanagi Harada syndrome
Vogt syndrome
void
voiding
  burning on
  difficulty
  pain on
voiding cystography
voiding cystourethrogram (VCUG)
voiding cystourethrography
voiding dysfunction
voiding flow rate
voiding internal urethral orifice
voiding painlessly
voiding pressure
voiding urethrocystography (VCU)
voiding without difficulty
Voltaren (diclofenac)
volume
  dwell
  extracellular
  extracellular fluid
  increase in urine
  postvoid residual urine
  reduction of urinary
  residual (RV)
volume acquisition
volume analysis
volume depletion
volume element
volume overload
volume overloaded patient
volume rendering of helical CT data
volumetric segmentation
voluming artifact
voluntary guarding
voluntary relinquishment of surrogate's parental rights
voluntary sterilization
volvulus, midgut
vomiting
  excessive
  morning
  pernicious
  surreptitious
vomiting of pregnancy
vomiting syndrome
von Gierke disease
von Hansemann cells
von Hippel-Lindau syndrome
von Recklinghausen disease
von Willebrand disease
Voorhees needle (do not confuse with *Veress needle*)
voxel (volume element)
voyeurism

V-pad
VPCA (vincristine, prednisone, Cytoxan, ara-C) chemotherapy protocol
VP (ventriculoperitoneal) shunt
VRE (vancomycin-resistant enterococcus)
Vrolik disease type 2
VSD (ventriculoseptal defect)
VTE (pregnancy-related venous thromboembolism)
VTU-E vacuum erection system
VTU-1 vacuum erection system
vulgaris, acne
vulva (pl. vulvae)
  abscess of
  carbuncle of
  cyst of
  dystrophy of
  edema of
  endometriosis of
  furuncle of
  hyperesthesia of
  hypertrophy of
  kraurosis of
  leukoplakia of
  oral stimulation of
  preinvasive lesion of
  senile atrophy of
  stricture of
  tumor of
  ulceration of
  varicose veins of
vulval
vulvar abscess
vulvar atrophy
vulvar carcinoma in situ
vulvar cellulitis
vulvar commissure
vulvar cyst
vulvar deformity, reconstruction of
vulvar dystrophy
  atrophic
  atypical
  hyperplastic
vulvar edema
vulvar endometriosis
vulvar epithelium, hyperkeratotic white patches of the
vulvar erythema
vulvar fistulectomy
vulvar hematoma
vulvar hypertrophy
vulvar intraepithelial neoplasia (VIN)
vulvar itching
vulvar kraurosis
vulvar lymphatics
vulvar melanoma
vulvar pain
vulvar pain of vestibular origin
vulvar tear
vulvar tumor
vulvar varices
vulvar varicose veins
vulvar varicosities
vulvar vestibule
vulvar vestibule tenderness
vulvar vestibulitis
vulvar vestibulitis syndrome
vulvectomy
  Basset en-bloc radical
  bilateral
  modified
  radical
  skinning
  superficial
  total
  unilateral
vulvectomy without node dissection
vulvismus
vulvitis
  atrophic
  candidal
  chronic
  chronic atrophic
  chronic hypertrophic
  creamy
  diabetic
  eczematiform
  erosive

vulvitis *(cont.)*
- focal
- follicular
- infectious pustular
- leukoplakic
- monilial
- phlegmonous
- plasma cell
- pseudovulvitis
- senile
- ulcerative

vulvocrural
vulvodynia
vulvovaginal candidiasis
vulvovaginal cystectomy
vulvovaginal gland
vulvovaginitis
- candidal
- monilial
- trichomonal

vulvovaginoplasty, Williams
VUR (vesicoureteral reflux)
VUR (vesicoureteric reflux)
V-Y plasty of bladder neck

W, w

Waardenburg-Klein syndrome
Waardenburg syndrome
Waelsch syndrome
WAGR syndrome
Waldmann disease
Waldman episiotomy scissors
Walker-Warburg syndrome
wall
  bladder
  cystic
  lateral pelvic
  vaginal
  ventral
Wallaby phototherapy system
Wallaby pouch
Wallace pipette
Wallach ColpoStar colposcope
Wallach Endocell endometrial cell sampler
Wallach PentaScope colposcope
Wallach TriScope colposcope
Wallach Tristar colposcope
Wallach ZoomScope Quantum colposcope
Wallstent, Urolume
Walsh radical retropubic prostatectomy
Walther dilator
WAMBA (Wise areola mastopexy breast augmentation)
wandering goiter
wandering kidney
wandering spleen
wand, laser
Wappler cystoscope
Wappler cystourethroscope
warmed resuscitation bassinet
warmer
  Bair Hugger
  Isolette infant
  Kreiselman infant
  Ohio infant
  open radiant infant
  overhead
  radiant
  Stryker infant
Warren shunt
Warren splenorenal shunt
wart
  genital
  intra-anal
  perianal
  venereal
wash back
washed semen sample

washed sperm
washed spermatozoa
washings
  peritoneal
  preputial
washout curve
washout phase
washout test for estimating renal obstruction
waste, nitrogenous
wasting syndrome
waterbath lithotripsy
water birth
water breaking
water, degassed, demineralized
water deprivation
water deprivation test
water diuresis
water drinking
  compulsive
  psychogenic
water-induced thermotherapy (WIT) system
watering-can perineum
watering-can scrotum
water-jet dissector
water purification system
  deionization
  reverse osmosis
water resorption
Waters extraperitoneal cesarean section with supravesical approach
water soluble contrast medium
water soluble radiopaque contrast medium
water soluble vitamins
water tablets
water-tight closure
watery discharge
Watkins uterine interposition operation
Watson-Alagille syndrome
watts of suprapulse power
waveform, segmental renal artery
waves, terahertz
waxy cast
waxy kidney
WBC (white blood cell)
W chromosome
weak bonds
weak urinary stream
weakness and lethargy
Weaver-Smith syndrome
Weaver syndrome
webbed penis
Weck clip
Weck laparotomy pads
Wedge electrosurgical prostate resection device
wedge of perineal skin
wedge resection
wedge resection of bladder
wedge resection of kidney
wedge resection of ovary
weekly taxane therapy
Wegener granulomatosis
Wegener syndrome
weight
  average for gestational age (AGA)
  estimated fetal (EFW)
  extremely low birth (ELBW)
  high birth
  large for gestational age (LGA)
  low birth (LBW)
  micropreemie
  small for gestational age (SGA)
  very low birth (VLBW)
weighted cone for incontinence
weighted posterior retractor
weighted Sims speculum
weighted speculum
Weill-Marchesani syndrome
Weill-Reyes syndrome
Weisman Graves vaginal speculum
Weismann-Netter-Stuhl syndrome
Weissenbacher-Zweymuller syndrome
Welch Allyn colposcope
Welch Allyn vaginal speculum
Welch Allyn Video Path colposcope

well-baby care
well-being, fetal
well-circumscribed neoplasm
well-epithelialized cervix
well-epithelialized vagina
Wenckebach heart block
Werdnig-Hoffman disease
Werlin-Ischida coaxial catheter
Wermer syndrome (polyendocrinopathy)
Werner syndrome (WS)
Wertheim-Cullen forceps
Wertheim excision of vagina and wide lymph node excision
Wertheim radical hysterectomy with pelvic lymph node dissection
Wertheim radical operation for carcinoma of uterus
Wertheim-Schauta procedure
Wertheim vaginal forceps
Westergren sedimentation rate
WEST (Weinstein Enhanced Sensory Test) for diabetic neuropathy
West syndrome
wet-field cautery
wet lap sponge
wet lung syndrome
wet mount
wet mount for *Candida, Gardnerella,* and *Trichomonas*
wet-phase separation membrane formation
wet prep
wet-technique reduction mammoplasty
Wharton jelly
Wharton tumor
wheezing
whiff test
whiplash technique
whipstitch
whistle-tip ureteral catheter
whistling face syndrome
whistling face-windmill vane hand syndrome
Whitaker pressure-perfusion test for impediment of urinary flow
white and cheesy discharge
white blood cell (WBC)
white blood cells in urine
White classification for diabetes mellitus
white discharge
white line of Toldt
whitlow
Whitnall-Norman syndrome
Whittlestone Physiological Breastmilker, The
WHO (World Health Organization)
whole blood clotting time
whole pelvis irradiation
whole pelvis radiation
whole sperm ejaculate
whooping cough
WIC (Women, Infants, Children) program
wide conization
wide excision
wide glucose excursions
wide-mouthed mucosal diverticulum
width of myometrium
width of tumor invasion
Wieacker syndrome
Wiedemann-Rautenstrauch syndrome
Wildervanck syndrome
wild-type allele
Willett forceps
Williams-Beuren syndrome
Williams syndrome
Williams vulvovaginoplasty
Willi-Prader syndrome
Willy Meyer incision for mastectomy
Wilms tumor
Wilson disease
Wilson-Mikity syndrome
Winchester-Grossman syndrome
Winchester syndrome
window in broad ligament
window, square

wind-up phenomenon
Winter procedure
Winter shunt
wire
  Hawkins localization
  Sadowsky hook
  torque
wire guide canalization
Wise areola mastopexy breast
  augmentation (WAMBA)
Wise mastopexy
Wise pattern reduction mammoplasty
Wiskott-Aldrich syndrome
WIT (water-induced thermotherapy)
withdrawal bleed
withdrawal bleeding
within normal limits (WNL)
Witkop tooth-nail syndrome
Wittmaack-Eckbom syndrome
Wittner uterine biopsy punch
WNL (within normal limits)
Wohlfart-Kugelberg-Welander disease
Wolf cystoscope
Wolfe breast carcinoma classification
Wolfe mammographic parenchymal
  patterns
wolffian duct
wolffian ridge
Wolff-Parkinson-White (WPW)
  syndrome
Wolf-Hirschhorn syndrome
Wolfram syndrome
Wolf syndrome
Wolf ureteroscope
Wolf videoresectoscope
Wolman disease
womb (see *uterus*)
  falling of
  neck of
womb stone
Women's Health Initiative
Woods corkscrew maneuver
Woods screw maneuver
Woody Guthrie disease
workbench surgery
working in a clockwise direction
World Health Organization (WHO)
wound
  dehiscence of uterine
  disruption of perineal
  scalpel
  stab
wound approximation
wound care, Composite Cultured Skin
wound cleanser, DiabKlenz
wound dehiscence
wound was steri-stripped
woven sling in continence device
wrap
  Ace
  bias stockinette
  Snugs mastectomy bandage
  stockinette
wrap-around ghosting artifact
wrapping, omental
Wright stain
Wright version
wrist drop
W-stapled ileal neobladder
W-stapled urinary reservoir
W syndrome
WT1 (Wilms tumor 1)
  gene
Wyburn-Mason syndrome

X, x

Xanar 20 Ambulase CO_2 laser
xanthine oxidase deficiency
xanthinuria deficiency, hereditary
xanthogranulomatosis, generalized
xanthogranulomatous pyelonephritis
Xatral OD (alfuzosin)
Xatral SR (alfuzosin)
X-chromosome determination test
X-chromosome inactivation
Xeloda (capecitabine)
xenogamy
xenogeneic transplantation
XenoMouse technology
XenoMune system
xenotransplant
xenotransplantation
xeroderma pigmentosum
Xeroform ("zero-form") gauze dressing
xeromammogram
xeromammography
X-linked copper deficiency
X-linked copper malabsorption
X-linked disorders
X-linked dominant
X-linked ichthyosis, recessive
X-linked inheritance
X-linked juvenile retinoschisis
X-linked locus
X-linked lymphoproliferative (XLP) syndrome
X-linked mental retardation with macro-orchidism
X-linked recessive disorder
X-linked recessive mutation
X-linked spondyloepiphyseal dysplasia
XMG (x-ray mammogram)
XO genetic female
XO gonadal dysgenesis
XO syndrome
Xpeedior catheter
XPlan radiation treatment software
Xplorer 1000 digital x-ray imaging
Xp deletion syndrome
Xp21 deletion syndrome
Xp22.1-Xp22.3 deletion syndrome
Xq22.3 deletion syndrome
Xq23 syndrome
Xq27-28 syndrome
x-ray mammogram (XMG)
x-ray mammography (XMG)
x-ray, pouchogram
XX gonadal dysgenesis
XX male syndrome
XXX female
XXY male
XXY syndrome

XY gonadal dysgenesis
Xylocaine
Xylocaine jelly
XY syndrome
XYY syndrome
XYY male

Y, y

YAC (yeast artificial chromosome)
Yachia incisionless bladder suspension
YAG (yttrium-aluminum-garnet) laser
Yang-Monti concept of intestinal reconfiguration for neovagina
Yankauer scissors
Yasmin 28 (dospirenone/ethinyl estradiol) oral contraceptive
yeast artificial chromosome (YAC)
yeast infection
yeast, selenium
Yellofins stirrups
yellow atrophy
yellow discharge
Yellow IRIS urinalysis
yellow leukorrhea
Yeoman uterine biopsy forceps
Y-linked inheritance
Y-linked locus
Yocon (yohimbine)
yogurt douche
yohimbine
Yohimex (yohimbine)
yolk sac
Yoon fallopian tube ligation ring
Young-Dees-Leadbetter bladder-neck reconstruction
Young syndrome
Yours Truly breast implant
YSI neonatal temperature probe
yttrium-aluminum-garnet (YAG) laser
Y-type infusion and drainage set
Yunis Varon syndrome
Yutopar (ritodrine)
Yuzpe protocol of oral contraception
Yuzpe regimen
Y-V-plasty

Z, z

Z allele
Zavanelli maneuver
Z chromosome
Z-Clamp hysterectomy forceps
Zeiss colposcope
Zellweger cerebrohepatorenal syndrome
Zelsmyr Cytobrush
Zemplar (paricalcitol)
Zenapax (daclizumab)
"zero-form" (see *Xeroform gauze dressing*)
Z gene
zidovudine
Ziehen-Oppenheim disease
ZIFT (zygote intrafallopian transfer)
Zimmer automatic pump
zinc finger protein
zinc ion binding site
zinc mesoporphyrin
zinc oxide
Zinnanti uterine manipulator/injector (ZUMI)
Zinsser-Cole-Engman syndrome
zipper sphincterotomy
Zoladex (goserelin implant)
zoledronic acid for injection
Zollinger-Ellison syndrome
Zometa (zoledronic acid for injection)
zona drilling
zona-free hamster egg test
zona-free hamster oocyte test
zona hamster egg test
zona pellucida
zona pellucida binding test
zonary placenta
Zondek-Bromberg-Rozin syndrome
Zondek syndrome
zone
  electric
  erogenous
  transformation
  triangle of doom
  triangle of pain
zonula occludens
Zoomscope colposcope
Zovia (ethynodiol diacetate/ethinyl estradiol) oral contraceptive
Z-Scissors hysterectomy scissors
Z-stitch
ZUMI uterine manipulator
Zwanck pessary
zygosity
  heterozygous
  homozygous

zygosity testing
zygote
zygote intrafallopian tube transfer (ZIFT)
zygotene
Zyloprim (allopurinol)